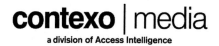

ICD-9-CM
Volumes 1 & 2, Expert for Physicians

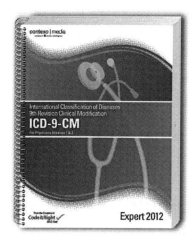

$107.95

Item ID: MICD9-12
ISBN: 978-1-58383-732-0
Spiralbound
Available September 2011

Promo Code: FOBA12

Choosing the right diagnosis and procedure codes is the key to reducing denials. Physician coding and billing staff can rely on this resource to help find the right code quickly, comply with HIPAA and reduce claims denials.

- Detailed, full-page anatomy illustrations plus over 350 code-specific illustrations that have been integrated into the book—allows better interpretation of clinical notes to help you code with more specificity

- Definitions of Diagnoses, Conditions and Injuries—medical terms defined in plain English to help identify specific diagnoses quickly and efficiently

- ICD-9-CM Official Coding Guidelines integrated into tabular listing with the affected code(s)—one-stop code and guideline look-up

- All 2012 new and revised codes with a summary of all code changes plus official ICD-9-CM Appendixes—using official and updated information is essential to complying with HIPAA and getting paid

- Intuitive icons for age and sex edits, new or revised text and 4th and 5th digit requirements—helps ensure specificity and validity

- *AHA Coding Clinic® for ICD-9-CM* references noted with applicable codes—lets you know exactly where to look for more guidance

- Valid three-digit list—identify a condition or disease when an additional digit is not available

ICD-9-CM ASCII File

- Two sets of descriptions: short (28 characters) and full (unabbreviated)
- New and revised code status indicator
- Fourth or fifth digit status field
- Fixed-width and tab-delimited file formats available
- Keep computer systems current and up-to-date
- Import into your database or software program
- Saves time and increases accuracy

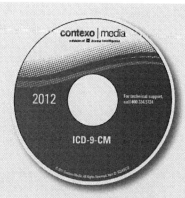

$199.95
Single User
Item ID: ICDASC-12
Available September 2011

$349.95
2-9 Users (Call for 10+ Pricing)
Item ID: ICDASCM-12
Available September 2011

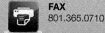
Contexo Media
P.O. Box 25128
SLC, UT 84125-0128

FAX
801.365.0710

PHONE
800.334.5724

ONLINE
www.codingbooks.com

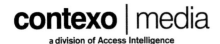

2012 Publications

ICD-9-CM
Volumes 1, 2 & 3 Expert for Hospitals & Payers

Choosing the right diagnosis and procedure codes is the key to reducing denials. Hospital coding and billing staff can rely on this resource to help find the right code quickly, comply with HIPAA and reduce claims denials.

- Detailed, full-page anatomy illustrations plus over 400 code-specific illustrations that have been integrated into the book—allows better interpretation of clinical notes to help you code with more specificity

- Alert icons for POA and HAC indications—aids in reducing risk of upcoding audits and potential fines

- ICD-9-CM Official Coding Guidelines integrated into tabular listing with the affected code(s)—one-stop code and guideline look-up

- All 2012 new and revised codes with a summary of all code changes plus official ICD-9-CM Appendixes—using official and updated information is essential to complying with HIPAA and getting paid

- Intuitive icons for age and sex edits, new or revised text and 4th and 5th digit requirements—helps ensure specificity and validity

- V Code designation icons—recognize when V codes can be used only as primary or additional diagnoses

- *AHA Coding Clinic®* for *ICD-9-CM* references noted with applicable codes—lets you know exactly where to look for more guidance

- Valid three-digit list—identify a condition or disease when an additional digit is not available

- Color icons for "Valid O.R." and "Non O.R." procedures—helps you see important information at a glance

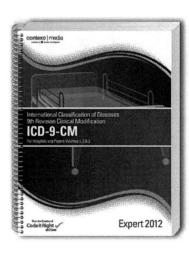

$109.95
Item ID: ICDHP-12
ISBN: 978-1-58383-733-7
Spiralbound
Available September 2011
Promo Code: FOBA12

Ready to order?
Call today—our friendly representatives are waiting to assist you.
800.334.5724

Contexto Media
P.O. Box 25128
SLC, UT 84125-0128

FAX
801.365.0710

PHONE
800.334.5724

ONLINE
www.codingbooks.com

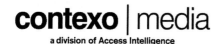
contexo | media
a division of Access Intelligence

2012 Publications

HCPCS
Level II Expert

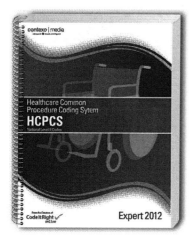

$107.95

Item ID: HCPCS-12
ISBN: 978-1-58383-734-4
Spiralbound
Available December 2011
Promo Code: FOBA12

Do you bill for durable medical equipment (DME), injections, Medicare services, drugs, and other medical supplies? Keep this book close and use it to help reduce claims denials, comply with HIPAA and get paid quicker. Don't settle for less reimbursement than you deserve.

- Added! More Definitions and Brand Names – assists in clarifying documentation in the medical record
- G Codes for PQRI – complete listing of G codes to help with your PQRI program
- Full tabular and alphabetical code lists of all valid 2012 HCPCS Level II codes and modifiers – gives you multiple ways to find a drug, device, or supply quickly
- HCPCS Level II modifiers and a Deleted Codes Crosswalk – helps you code more appropriately to reduce delays and denials
- Medicare Pub. 100 information – reference included with associated code and full descriptions in Appendix in the back of the book
- Age and sex edit icons – see at a glance codes with restrictions based on age or sex of the patient to help reduce claims denials
- APC and ASC edits – determine quickly which codes are payable under Outpatient Prospective Payment System (OPPS) and which codes can use ASC groupings to improve reimbursement
- Key references and excerpts from the National Coverage Determinations Manual – find out the regulations and guidelines for Medicare's covered services
- *AHA Coding Clinic® for HCPCS* – identifies where to find critical guidance on challenging HCPCS Level II codes or sections

HCPCS ASCII File

- Two sets of descriptions: short (28 characters) and full (unabbreviated)
- Pub 100 references along with HCPCS Level II modifiers
- Keep computer systems current and up-to-date
- Import into your database or software program
- Saves time and increases accuracy
- Fixed-width and tab-delimited file formats available

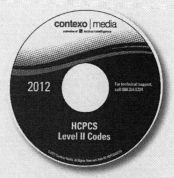

$199.95
Single User
Item ID: HCPCSASC-12
Available December 2011

$299.95
2-9 Users
(Call for 10+ User Pricing)
Item ID: HCPCSASCM-12
Available December 2011

Contexo Media
P.O. Box 25128
SLC, UT 84125-0128

FAX
801.365.0710

PHONE
800.334.5724

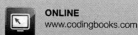
ONLINE
www.codingbooks.com

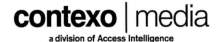

2012 Publications

Procedural Coding Expert

Contexo Media has designed the *Procedural Coding Expert* to be the best resource in its class to make CPT® coding as accurate as possible. Elegant in design and loaded with the help on Medicare coverage, modifier and global billing information needed to code on a daily basis.

- Best in Class Index—helps the user find codes faster than any other CPT reference

- Detailed Table of Contents—an exhaustive listing of every chapter, section, table and illustration so you can locate important information quickly

- Full codes and descriptions—all new 2012 new and revised CPT codes with entire code description listed so you can avoid any confusion

- The most illustrations—more than 800 illustrations to provide greater insight to specific procedures and help interpret clinical notes more effectively

- Detailed introduction—loaded with essential information such as CPT coding fundamentals, listing and description of modifiers, common medical abbreviations, prefixes, suffixes and roots, coding terms glossary, detailed explanation of all icons and data elements and multiple summary tables

- Coding tips—valuable information on CPT and HCPCS Level II codes integrated throughout the book to help code more efficiently

- Additional assistance on new, revised and deleted codes—unique symbols identify new procedure codes and substantially altered procedure descriptions have a second icon to alert you. Deleted codes are highlighted with a strikethrough and a valid cross-reference, if available

- Hundreds of references for guidance from the AMA's CPT Assistant and Medicare's Pub 100 manuals integrated with the relevant codes—helps you validate code choices

- PQRI designation—code-level icons denote those codes and services subject to the Physician Quality Reporting Initiative

- Relative Value Units (RVUs) and Medicare global follow-up days for each code, age and sex edit icons and icons—alert you to potential unbundling errors

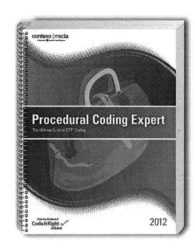

$107.95

Item ID: PCE-12
ISBN: 978-1-58383-731-3
Spiralbound
Available December 2011

Promo Code: FOBA12

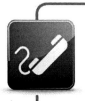

Ready to order?
Call today—our friendly representatives are waiting to assist you.
800.334.5724

CPT® is a registered trademark of the American Medical Association.

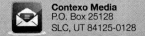
Contexo Media
P.O. Box 25128
SLC, UT 84125-0128

FAX
801.365.0710

PHONE
800.334.5724

ONLINE
www.codingbooks.com

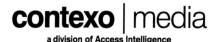

2012 Publications

Plain English Descriptions for ICD-9-CM

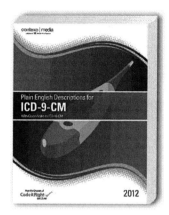

$107.95

Item ID: CDAICD-12
ISBN: 978-1-58383-718-4
Perfectbound
Available September 2011
Promo Code: FOBA12

The *Plain English Descriptions for ICD-9-CM* is a handy reference tool for any coder, biller or other medical staffer who works with ICD-9-CM codes. Each code is defined by the actual description and the plain English description. This tool is a must for any coder.

- Added! More ICD-10-CM Mappings—see how the ICD-9-CM codes map to new ICD-10-CM codes
- ICD-9-CM Official Coding Guidelines—understand the rules of how to code for ICD-9-CM
- Over 13,000 ICD-9-CM codes and categories—provides coders, medical staff, payers and health care professionals with comprehensive clinical, coding and documentation guidance
- Detailed, full-page anatomy illustrations—helps you interpret clinical notes to code with more specificity
- Numerically arranged just like the official ICD-9-CM book—easy identification and look-up
- *AHA Coding Clinic©* for ICD-9-CM references—helps you validate code choices

Plain English Descriptions for Pharmacology Coding

When reviewing a patient's medical record, there may be drugs listed that are not be readily familiar to you or do not have a diagnosis or procedure associated with them. The *Plain English Descriptions for Pharmacology Coding* reference book will increase your knowledge of drug names – brand and generic – as well as the conditions for which those drugs may be used. In addition, coding information that is associated with the drugs is provided, specifically ICD-9-CM diagnostic and HCPCS Level II coding information.

- Brand and Generic Names—find information you need on pharmaceuticals by either the brand or generic name
- Alphabetized—makes it easy and convenient for drug look-up
- ICD-9-CM Codes—assists the user in understanding and refining diagnostic code selection
- HCPCS Level II Codes—find updated codes for HCPCS Level II codes, if applicable
- Drug Coding Assistance—get answers to questions about coding for drugs for Medicare and other payers

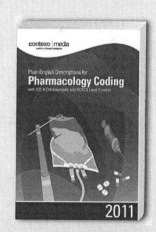

$107.95

Item ID: PHARM-11
ISBN: 978-1-58383-730-6
Compact Perfectbound 6 x 9
Available Now
Promo Code: FOBA12

Contexo Media
P.O. Box 25128
SLC, UT 84125-0128

FAX
801.365.0710

PHONE
800.334.5724

ONLINE
www.codingbooks.com

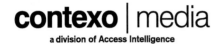

contexo | media
a division of Access Intelligence

2012 Publications

Plain English Descriptions for Procedures

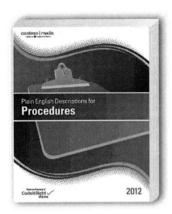

$107.95
Item ID: CDA-12
ISBN: 978-1-58383-714-6
Perfectbound
Available November 2011
Promo Code: FOBA12

The *Plain English Descriptions for Procedures* is a handy reference tool for any coder, biller or other medical staffer who works with CPT® codes. Each code/code range is defined by the actual description and the plain English description. This tool is a must for any coder.

- Over 8,000 codes—provides coders, medical staff, payers and health care professionals with comprehensive clinical, coding and documentation guidance
- Detailed, full-page anatomy illustrations plus hundreds of code-specific illustrations that have been integrated into the book—helps you interpret clinical notes to code with more specificity
- Plain English descriptions of procedures—compare wording on operative reports and medical records with plain English descriptions to determine the appropriate code quickly
- Listing of prefixes and suffixes—understand the parts of medical terminology that are included in medical procedures
- Numerically arranged just like the official CPT procedure book—easy identification and look-up

Plain English Descriptions for Coding Terms

The *Plain English Descriptions for Coding Terms* is a handy reference tool for any coder, biller or other medical staffer who works with medical documentation and translates it into codes. Each term is defined and most codes include an ICD-9-CM, HCPCS Level II, and/or CPT code. This tool is a must for any healthcare professional that uses codes.

- Updated! Code sets—updated CPT, ICD-9-CM and HCPCS Level II codes for 2012!
- A to Z Format—makes finding information easy and quick
- Over 7,500 codes defined—provides coders, medical staff, payers and health care professionals with comprehensive clinical, coding and documentation guidance
- Detailed, full-page anatomy illustrations helps to crosswalk the illustrations to the plain English description for anatomy
- Coding term crosswalk—many terms are cross-referenced to the applicable CPT, and ICD-9-CM diagnostic and procedural codes, updated for 2012
- Clarification of medical documentation for acronyms, eponyms, common abbreviations and suffixes/prefixes—decipher clinical notes and improve coding knowledge

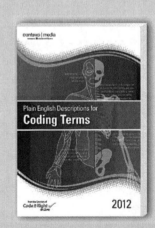

$107.95
Item ID: CDAT-12
ISBN: 978-1-58383-723-8
Compact Perfectbound 6 x 9
Available December 2011
Promo Code: FOBA12

CPT® is a registered trademark of the American Medical Association.

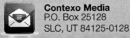
Contexo Media
P.O. Box 25128
SLC, UT 84125-0128

FAX
801.365.0710

PHONE
800.334.5724

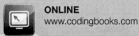
ONLINE
www.codingbooks.com

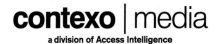

2012 Publications

Illustrated Coding and Billing Experts for Specialties

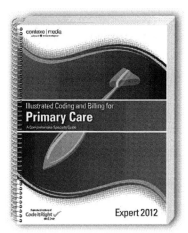

Primary Care
MEDPC-12

$169.95 Each

Spiralbound
Available December 2011

Promo Code: FOBA12

This all-in-one resource contains all the coding information you need for your specialty. Plain English descriptions of each CPT® code, coding tips, CPT to ICD-9-CM crosswalks and other valuable information to make specialty coding easier and more efficient than ever. This is the code book you'll be reaching for again and again for use on a daily basis.

- The most illustrations of any specialty reference—nearly one for every CPT code/code range—gives visual clarification for coding

- CPT Alphabetic Index—find the right tabular section quickly

- Comprehensive coding tips—one for every CPT® code/code range

- Powerful crosswalks—identify medical necessity with CPT to ICD-9-CM crosswalks

- 2012 CPT, ICD-9-CM and HCPCS Level II codes relevant to each respective specialty—speeds up coding

- Plain English descriptions of the most common CPT codes for each specialty—guides code selection and verification and explains associated conditions or medical indications

- Code-specific RVUs—determine fees, global days, assistant-at-surgery and prior approval at a glance

- Pub 100 references—find out the regulations and guidelines for Medicare's covered services

- Modifiers that are appropriate for each code from the MPFS—know which modifiers can or cannot be used with each procedure

MEDANEST-12	2012 Illustrated Coding and Billing Expert for Anesthesia/Pain Management
MEDCARD-12	2012 Illustrated Coding and Billing Expert for Cardiology/Cardiothoracic Surgery/Vascular Surgery
MEDENT-12	2012 Illustrated Coding and Billing Expert for ENT/Allergy/Pulmonology
MEDSURG-12	2012 Illustrated Coding and Billing Expert for General Surgery/Gastroenterology
MEDOB-12	2012 Illustrated Coding and Billing Expert for OB/GYN
MEDOPT-12	2012 Illustrated Coding and Billing Expert for Ophthalmology
MEDORTL-12	2012 Illustrated Coding and Billing Expert for Orthopaedics, Lower
MEDORTU-12	2012 Illustrated Coding and Billing Expert for Orthopaedics, Upper
MEDPLAS-12	2012 Illustrated Coding and Billing Expert for Plastic Surgery/Dermatology
MEDPC-12	2012 Illustrated Coding and Billing Expert for Primary Care
MEDURO-12	2012 Illustrated Coding and Billing Expert for Urology/Nephrology

CPT® is a registered trademark of the American Medical Association.

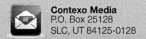

Contexo Media
P.O. Box 25128
SLC, UT 84125-0128

FAX
801.365.0710

PHONE
800.334.5724

ONLINE
www.codingbooks.com

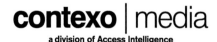

contexo | media
a division of Access Intelligence

2012 Publications

Medicare Coverage Sourcebook

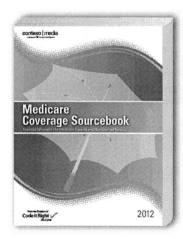

$179.95

Item ID: COVER-12
ISBN: 978-1-58383-739-9
Perfectbound
Available November 2011
Promo Code: FOBA12

The *Medicare Coverage Sourcebook* provides the Medicare coder and biller with the most up-to-date coverage information from the Pub. 100 Internet Only Manuals (IOMs). This book has been organized according to general guidelines, regulations, and other relevant coverage information pertaining to Medicare.

- Extensive alphabetical index—helps you locate the exact policy you need quickly
- An icon noting any new policy implemented within the past year—quickly locate this year's policies that could impact you financially
- Preventive service coverage—for all types of screenings covered by Medicare
- DME, prosthetic and orthotic guidelines—find out how and where to bill for these services, along with reimbursement data for specific items
- Billing information for non-physician practitioners and payment methodologies—helps you bill appropriately
- Specialty-specific guidelines and regulations for Medicare coverage—identify rules targeted at your specialty
- Alert icons—easily identify services that fall under medical review policies or fraud alerts
- Listing of Part A Fiscal Intermediaries and Part B Carriers by state—allows you to quickly locate and contact your intermediaries and carriers

Medicare RBRVS Sourcebook

This book will help build a systematic approach to fee-setting with the Medicare Physician Fee Schedule data. The straight-forward instructions, examples and formulas in this well-organized resource will help clarify the fee-setting process. Included are the code changes for the upcoming year and much of the Medicare information that is required for Medicare coding and billing, such as modifier usage.

- 2012 CPT® and HCPCS Level II code RVU changes—using updated information is key to getting the reimbursement you deserve
- Gap-fill code data (RVUs not provided by Medicare) are included—helps complete the reimbursement picture
- Instructions on conducting cost analysis and comparing fees by payer—know the reimbursement mix for your practice
- Modifier information integrated throughout—see at-a-glance which modifiers can or cannot be used with each CPT code
- Professional component and/or technical component guidance—identifies which service or procedures have only one or both
- Facility and Non-facility totals are both included, as well as work, practice expense and malpractice breakdowns for each CPT and HCPCS Level II code

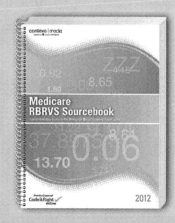

$179.95

Item ID: RBRVS-12
ISBN: 978-1-58383-743-6
Spiralbound
Available December 2011
Promo Code: FOBA12

CPT® is a registered trademark of the American Medical Association.

 Contexo Media
P.O. Box 25128
SLC, UT 84125-0128

 FAX
801.365.0710

 PHONE
800.334.5724

 ONLINE
www.codingbooks.com

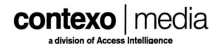

2012 Publications

ICD-9-CM Compact Coders

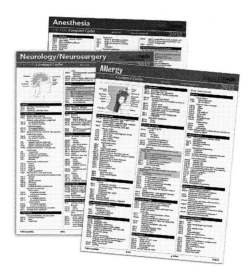

Each specialty *ICD-9-CM Compact Coder* is a double-sided sheet containing the top reported ICD-9-CM diagnoses codes for each specialty. With shortened descriptions and instructional notes, these are fast, convenient and reliable.

- 200-300 commonly-used codes with smart groupings by diagnosis—helps you code faster for your specialty
- Organized alphabetically—makes code look-up easier
- Durable enough not to get bent, and double-sided—incredibly user-friendly for specialty coding
- Fits in the ICD-9-CM book—get one for every office and/or specialty
- Additional 5th digits clearly indicated—easy to choose the right code

$25.95 Each
Available September 2011
Promo Code: FOBA12

Get your ICD-9-CM cheat sheet today for just $25.95!

ICCALL-12	2012 ICD-9-CM Compact Coder for Allergy	ICCNEU-12	2012 ICD-9-CM Compact Coder for Neurology/Neurosurgery
ICCANE-12	2012 ICD-9-CM Compact Coder for Anesthesia	ICCOBG-12	2012 ICD-9-CM Compact Coder for OB/GYN
ICCBH-12	2012 ICD-9-CM Compact Coder for Behavioral Health	ICCONC-12	2012 ICD-9-CM Compact Coder for Oncology
ICCCAR-12	2012 ICD-9-CM Compact Coder for Cardiology	ICCOPH-12	2012 ICD-9-CM Compact Coder for Ophthalmology
ICCDER-12	2012 ICD-9-CM Compact Coder for Dermatology	ICCORT-12	2012 ICD-9-CM Compact Coder for Orthopaedics
ICCEMR-12	2012 ICD-9-CM Compact Coder for Emergency Medicine	ICCPM-12	2012 ICD-9-CM Compact Coder for Pain Management
ICCEND-12	2012 ICD-9-CM Compact Coder for Endocrinology	ICCPED-12	2012 ICD-9-CM Compact Coder for Pediatrics
ICCOTO-12	2012 ICD-9-CM Compact Coder for ENT	ICCPT-12	2012 ICD-9-CM Compact Coder for Physical Therapy/Physical Medicine
ICCFAM-12	2012 ICD-9-CM Compact Coder for Family Practice	ICCPLA-12	2012 ICD-9-CM Compact Coder for Plastic Surgery
ICCGAS-12	2012 ICD-9-CM Compact Coder for Gastroenterology	ICCPUL-12	2012 ICD-9-CM Compact Coder for Pulmonology
ICCGEN-12	2012 ICD-9-CM Compact Coder for General Surgery	ICCRHE-12	2012 ICD-9-CM Compact Coder for Rheumatology
ICCINT-12	2012 ICD-9-CM Compact Coder for Internal Medicine	ICCURO-12	2012 ICD-9-CM Compact Coder for Urology

Contexo Media
P.O. Box 25128
SLC, UT 84125-0128

FAX 801.365.0710

PHONE 800.334.5724

ONLINE www.codingbooks.com

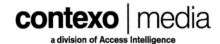

contexo | media
a division of Access Intelligence

2012 Publications

Coding CrossWalks for Laboratory/Pathology Services

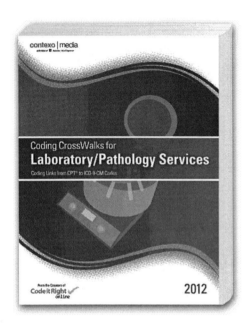

This highly-targeted specialty crosswalk links CPT® codes to common ICD-9-CM codes used to define medical necessity. This publication contains full CPT and ICD-9-CM code descriptions, and icons that identify gender and age edits and new, revised and deleted codes, available for Laboratory and Pathology services.

- Organized by CPT code for easy look-up, commonly used ICD-9-CM diagnostic codes are listed for each specialty right on the same page—saves you time

- Full CPT and ICD-9-CM descriptions—helps you choose the appropriate code(s) based on medical record documentation

- Straight-forward icons for new and revised codes and codes with Age and Sex Edits—helps you self-audit coding at a glance

- Built from Local Carrier Determinations (LCDs) as well as clinical assumptions by a highly experienced clinical and coding staff—helps you code more appropriately

$169.95

Item ID: CXWLAB-12
ISBN: 978-1-58383-697-2
Perfectbound
Available December 2011
Promo Code: FOBA12

CPT® is a registered trademark of the American Medical Association.

Contexo Media
P.O. Box 25128
SLC, UT 84125-0128

FAX
801.365.0710

PHONE
800.334.5724

ONLINE
www.codingbooks.com

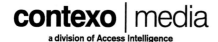

2012 Publications

Medicare National Correct Coding Sourcebook - Physicians

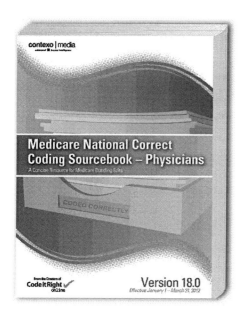

The *Medicare National Correct Coding Sourcebook – Physicians* assists the user in understanding CPT® bundling issues, prevent claim denial, and still get the reimbursement that you deserve. With a year subscription, customers receive a book quarterly, complete with the updates. Also included are the official guidelines as put forth by the Centers for Medicare and Medicaid Services (CMS).

- All published NCCI tables and code pairs—including Column 1, Column 2 and Mutually Exclusive codes
- Anesthesia codes included in every quarterly edition—no need to look these up elsewhere
- CMS policy narratives that describe the principles used to develop edits—understand the reasons behind the guidelines and regulations
- New book each quarter—no more wasting time replacing binder pages—keep the outdated editions to ensure older denied claims are accurately resubmitted and adjudicated properly
- Supplemental chapters—identify NCCI edits for HCPCS Level II codes and CPT Level I Category III codes

$249.95

Item ID: NATSUB-12 – 1 year subscription
Published Quarterly
Perfectbound
Updates in October, January, April, and July
Promo Code: FOBA12

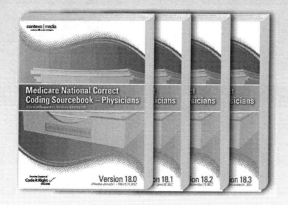

You'll get a new book delivered each quarter with full updates.

CPT® is a registered trademark of the American Medical Association.

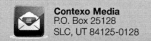
Contexo Media
P.O. Box 25128
SLC, UT 84125-0128

FAX
801.365.0710

PHONE
800.334.5724

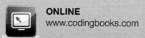
ONLINE
www.codingbooks.com

2012 Publications

contexo | media

CPT® Professional Edition

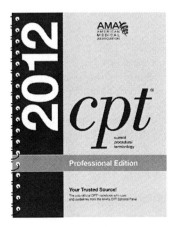

$109.95
Item ID: PCPT-12
ISBN: 978-1-60359-568-1
Spiralbound
Available October 2011
Promo Code: FOBA12

Correctly interpreting and reporting medical procedures and services begins with *CPT® Professional Edition*. Straight from the American Medical Association (AMA), this is the only CPT codebook with the official CPT coding rules and guidelines developed by the CPT Editorial Panel. This publication covers hundreds of code, guideline and text changes.

- E/M reference tables—summarize the requirements for reporting E/M services and help to select and validate proper E/M coding
- Coding tips added throughout—a select group of helpful tips added throughout each section to aid in better understanding
- Section-specific table of contents—provide users with an efficient tool to navigate information relevant to the codes listed in each section
- Anatomical and procedural illustrations incorporated within the code sections—help users accurately code procedures
- Reference tables for quick identification of the codes—assist in understanding the definition and differentiation of key parameters in large families of codes
- Clinical examples for E/M services codes—learn how to use and report services
- Summary of additions, deletions and revisions provide a quick reference to 2012 changes without having to refer to previous editions
- Place-of-service codes with facility name and description

CPT® Standard Edition

Correctly interpreting and reporting medical procedures and services begins with *CPT Standard Edition*. Straight from the American Medical Association (AMA), this is the only CPT codebook with the official CPT coding rules and guidelines developed by the CPT Editorial Panel. Covers hundreds of code, guideline and text changes.

- Anatomical illustrations—a limited number of anatomical illustrations added to aid coders in properly assigning CPT codes
- Summary of additions, deletions and revisions provide a quick reference to 2012 changes without having to refer to previous editions
- Clinical examples for E/M services codes—learn how to use and report services
- Extensive index—helps you locate codes by procedure/service, organ/other anatomic site, condition, synonyms/eponyms, and abbreviations

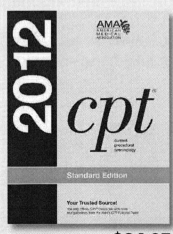

$84.95
Item ID: CPT4-12
ISBN: 978-1-60359-567-4
Perfectbound
Available October 2011
Promo Code: FOBA12

CPT® is a registered trademark of the American Medical Association.

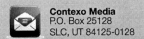 Contexo Media
P.O. Box 25128
SLC, UT 84125-0128

 FAX 801.365.0710

 PHONE 800.334.5724

 ONLINE www.codingbooks.com

Order Form

contexo | media

Call Today! 800.334.5724 or visit www.codingbooks.com

ITEM #	PRODUCT	PRICE	QTY	TOTAL

Thank you for your order.

Subtotal _____
Sales Tax _____
(Sales tax applies to CA, CO, MD, NJ, NY PA, TX, UT, & VA)
Shipping _____
GRAND TOTAL _____

Shipping Chart

Qty	1	2-4	5-7	8-10	11+
Price	$13.95	$18.95	$23.95	$28.95	$33.95 + $3.00 each additional book

---

Customer/Payment Information   Source Code: FOBA12

4 Easy Ways to Order

 Contexo Media
P.O. Box 25128
SLC, UT 84125-0128

 FAX
801.365.0710

 PHONE
800.334.5724

 ONLINE
www.codingbooks.com

Company Name: _____

Ordered By: _____

Ship to Attn: _____

Address: _____
(No PO boxes)

City: _____ State: _____ ZIP: _____

Phone: (____) _____ - _____ *Fax: (____) _____ - _____

*Email: _____
Required for confirmations

❑ Check # _____ Amount Enclosed $ _____

❑ CC Card # _____ Exp. ____ / ____

Authorization: _____

❑ Invoice Me   PO# _____

Health Care Setting:

❑ Physician Office/Clinic _____# of Coders   ❑ Payer   ❑ ASC/Lab/Home Health/SNF/Hospice
❑ Hospital/Medical Center _____# of Beds   ❑ Business/Government   ❑ Student
Specialty _____

* "I understand that by providing a fax number or email above, I am giving Contexo Media express permission to notify me of upcoming programs and/or useful products via facsimile or email."

contexo | media
a division of Access Intelligence

Anatomy & Terminology For Coders

Liver

Stomach

Kidney

Adductor brevis

Rectus femoris

Adductor magnus

Femoral vein

Femoral artery

4th Edition

Anatomy & Terminology for Coders, 4th Edition

Published by Contexo | Media, a division of Access Intelligence
P.O. Box 25128
Salt Lake City, UT 84125-0128
800.334.5724

Copyright © 2011 Contexo Media
All rights reserved

Printed in the United States of America

Item ID: WSAT4

DISCLAIMER

No part of this publication may be reproduced, stored in a retrieval system, or transmitted, in any form or by any means, electronic, mechanical, photocopy, recording, or otherwise, without the prior written permission of the publisher. Any five-digit numeric *Physicians' Current Procedural Terminology, Fourth Edition* (CPT®) codes, service descriptions, instructions and/or guidelines are Copyright 2010 American Medical Association (AMA). All rights reserved. CPT is a trademark of the American Medical Association. This notice applies to all CPT codes in this manual. This presentation includes only CPT codes and descriptions selected by Contexo Media for inclusion in this publication. The AMA assumes no responsibility for the consequences attributable to, related to any use or interpretation of any information or views contained in, or not contained in this publication. This publication is sold with the understanding that the publisher is not engaged in rendering legal, medical, accounting, or other professional service in specific situations. Although prepared for professionals, this publication should not be utilized as a substitute for professional service in specific situations. If legal or medical advice is required, the services of a professional should be sought.

Contents

Chapter 1
Introduction to Anatomy 1
The Anatomical Position 1
Anatomical Planes 2
Anatomical Movements 4
Practice Quiz 6

Chapter 2
Integumentary System 7
Structures of the Integument 9
Practice Quiz 11

Chapter 3
Musculoskeletal System 15
The Skeletal System 15
The Skeletal Division 21
The Muscle System 23
Practice Quiz 28

Chapter 4
Respiratory System 47
Practice Quiz 51

Chapter 5
Cardiovascular System and Lymphatic System .. 55
The Heart 55
Blood Vessels 57
Lymphatic System 59
Practice Quiz 60

Chapter 6
Digestive System 65
Practice System 67

Chapter 7
Urinary System 71
Practice Quiz 74

Chapter 8
Male Genital System 77
Practice Quiz 78

Chapter 9
Female Genital System 81
Practice Quiz 83

Chapter 10
Endocrine System 87
Practice Quiz 88

Chapter 11
Nervous System 89
Structure of the Nervous System 90
Practice Quiz 94

Chapter 12
Immune System 99
Immune Response 99
Types of Immunity 99
Practice Quiz 100

Chapter 13
Root Words 101
Practice Quiz 106

Chapter 14
Prefixes and Suffixes 107
Practice Quiz 111

Chapter 15
Abbreviations 113
Practice Quiz 135

Chapter 16
Terms to Know 137
Practice Quiz 155

Chapter 17
Practice Quiz Answers 157

Chapter 1

INTRODUCTION TO ANATOMY

Anatomy is the science of the structure and function of the body. As a medical coder, you will see many of these terms repeat themselves over and over throughout your career. As a result, being familiar with these terms is of the utmost importance, and is in fact, key to becoming successful.

There are two kinds of anatomy: gross anatomy and microscopic anatomy. Microscopic anatomy is the study of the body's cells (cytology) and tissues (histology) that must be viewed with the use of a microscope. Gross anatomy is the study of the parts of the body that we can see with our eyes. In this section and the section to follow, we will focus on gross anatomy.

The Anatomical Position

All descriptions of the human body start in the anatomical position. When physicians describe the location or position of a patient's body part, they always describe it as if the patient were in the position known as the anatomical position. In this position, the subject's palms are always facing upward, with thumbs extended.

Anatomical Position

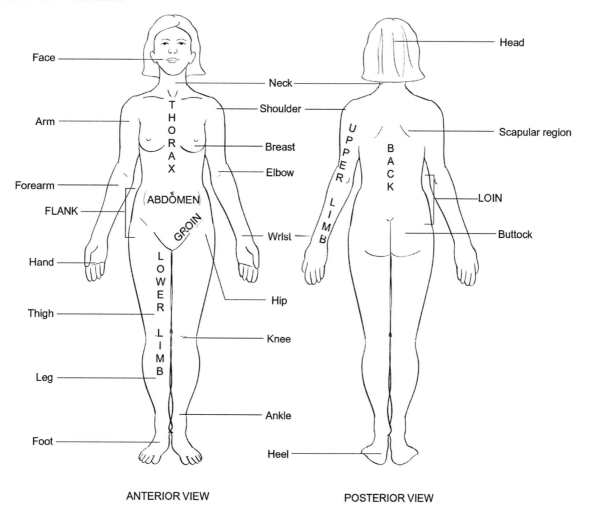

ANTERIOR VIEW POSTERIOR VIEW

Introduction to Anatomy

Anatomical Planes

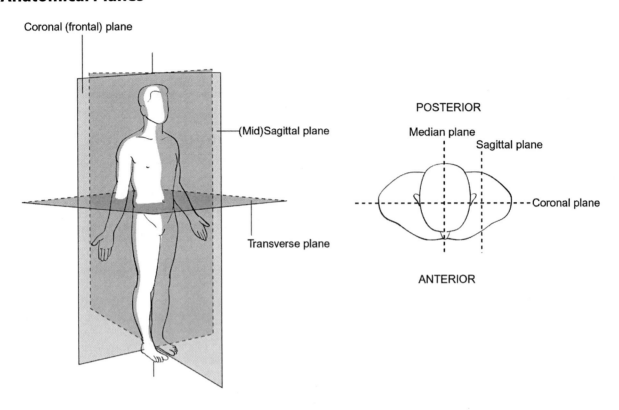

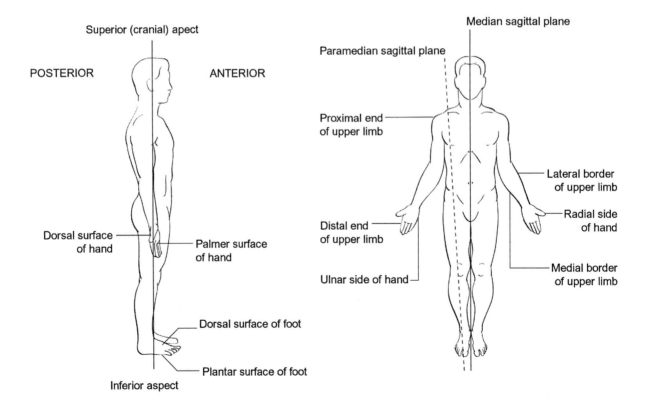

Term	Meaning	Usage
Superior (cranial)	Nearer to head	The heart is superior to the stomach
Inferior (caudal)	Nearer to feet	The stomach is inferior to the heart
Anterior (ventral)	Nearer to front	The sternum is anterior to the heart
Posterior (dorsal)	Nearer to back	The kidneys are posterior to the intestines
Medial	Nearer to the median plane	The fifth digit (little finger) is on the medial side of the hand
Lateral	Farther from the median plane	The first digit (thumb) is on the lateral
Proximal	Nearer to trunk or point of origin	The elbow is proximal to the wrist
Distal	Farther from the trunk or point of origin	The wrist is distal to the elbow
Superficial	Nearer to, or on the surface	The muscles of the arm are superficial to its bone
Deep	Farther from surface	The humerus is deep to the arm muscle

Anatomical Planes Terms

Anatomical descriptions are based on anatomical planes that pass through the body in the anatomical position:

Median plane (midsagittal plane) is the vertical plane passing longitudinally through the body, dividing it into right and left halves.

Sagittal planes are vertical planes passing through the body parallel to the median plane, bisecting the coronal plane.

Transverse planes are planes passing through the body at right angles to the median and coronal planes; a horizontal plane divides the body into superior (upper) and inferior (lower) parts (it is helpful to give a reference point such as a horizontal plane through the umbilicus).

Anatomical Movement Terms

Various terms are used to describe movements of the body (e.g., flexion of the limbs). Movements take place at joints where two or more bones or cartilages articulate with one another. They are described as pairs of opposites (e.g., flexion and extension).

Flexion — Bending of a part or decreasing the angle between body parts.

Extension — Straightening a part or increasing the angle between body parts.

Abduction — Moving away from the median plane of the body in the coronal plane.

Adduction — Moving toward the median plane of the body in the coronal plane. In the digits (fingers and toes), abduction means spreading them, and adduction refers to drawing them together.

Rotation — Moving a part of the body around its long axis. Medial rotation turns the anterior surface medially and lateral rotation turns this surface laterally.

Circumduction — The circular movement of the limbs, or parts of them, combining in sequence the movements of flexion, extension, abduction, and adduction.

Pronation — A medial rotation of the forearm and hand so that the palm faces posteriorly.

Supination — A lateral rotation of the forearm and hand so that the palm faces anteriorly, as in the anatomical position.

Eversion — Turning sole of foot outward.

Inversion — Turning sole of foot inward.

Protrusion (protraction) — To move the jaw anteriorly.

Retrusion (retraction) — To move the jaw posteriorly.

Introduction to Anatomy

Anatomical Movements

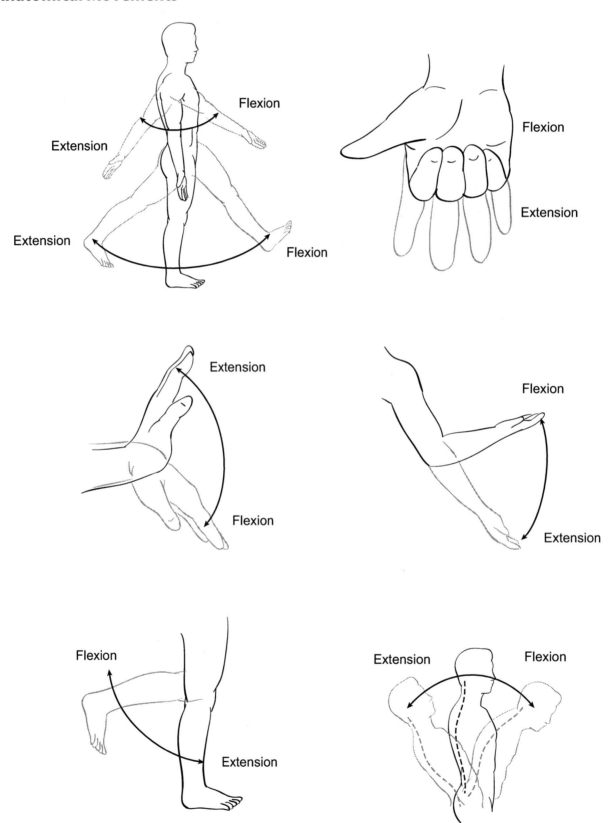

Anatomical Movements

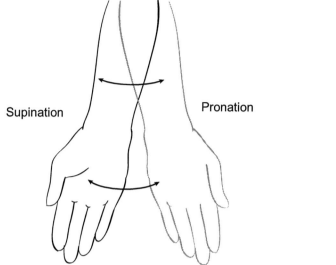
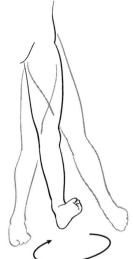
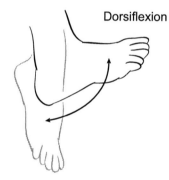
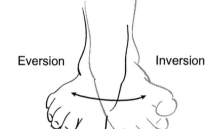
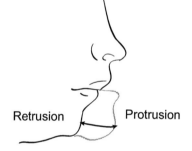

Introduction to Anatomy

Practice Quiz

1. The median plane is also known as the _____.

2. Physicians describe all body parts in relationship to the _____ position.

3. The three primary anatomical planes are _____, _____, and _____.

Chapter 2

INTEGUMENTARY SYSTEM

The skin (integument) and the appendages that develop from the skin, such as hair, nails, and glands, make up the integumentary system. The integument is a protective organ that covers the entire surface of the body. Another name for the integument is the cutaneous membrane. A membrane is defined as being a thin, pliable layer of tissue that lines a tube or cavity, covers an organ or structure, or separates one part from another. Therefore, the cutaneous membrane might be described as a layer of tissues that cover the organ known as the skin.

Types of Cutaneous Membranes

Mucous membranes — These membranes line the digestive, urinary, reproductive, and respiratory systems. These membranes are composed of goblet cells that secrete mucus, which serves as a protective coating that prevents bacteria and viruses from attacking the organs.

Serous membranes — These membranes line the ventral body cavity and cover the surfaces of the organs contained in that cavity. Serous membranes secrete a watery, serous fluid that moistens their surfaces and serves to reduce friction as the organs move.

Synovial Membranes — These membranes line joint cavities and synovial fluid lubricates the joint to reduce friction.

Functions of the Integument

The integumentary system is responsible for performing important functions, five of which are listed below:

Protection — Skin protects humans from dangers in the external environment such as abrasion, dehydration, ultraviolet radiation, and bacterial invasion.

Excretion — Skin helps rid the body of organic wastes, such as salt and water, by sweating.

Temperature Regulation — When the body is exposed to excessive heat, the evaporation that occurs as a result of the skin's perspiration lowers body temperature. On the other hand, when the body is exposed to heat loss, blood vessels near the body's surface constrict to keep it warmer.

Sensory Perception — Skin contains nerve endings and receptors that help detect stimuli associated with touch, pressure, temperature, and pain.

Vitamin D Production — When skin is exposed to ultraviolet radiation, certain molecules in the skin are converted to Vitamin D.

Layers of the Integument

The integument consists of two layers: the epidermis and the dermis. The epidermis is the outermost, superficial cellular layer of skin. The dermis is the deeper, inner layer that is composed of dense connective tissue. Where the epidermis and the dermis connect there are numerous dermal papillae. Dermal papillae are cone-like projections that fit into the crevices caused by the shape of the epidermis. The epidermal grooves and ridges that produce fingerprints result from the pattern of dermal papillae. Beneath the dermis lies the subcutaneous layer. The subcutaneous layer is not a part of the skin. It attaches the skin to underlying tissues and organs. It functions to conserve body heat and works to lower the penetration of external heat into the body.

The epidermis is the portion of the skin that is responsible for protecting the body from external influences such as ultraviolet radiation and bacterial invasion. The epidermis also protects the body from excessive water loss.

The dermis is the portion of the skin that contains both collagen and elastic fibers. Collagen provides the dermis with strength and toughness, while elastic fibers provide flexibility and elasticity. The dermis also contains sensory receptors which make it possible for humans to distinguish touch, pressure, and temperature.

Each layer of skin consists of its own layers. The following figure illustrates the components of both the epidermis and the dermis.

© 2011 Contexo Media

Integumentary System

The Integument (Figure 2.1)

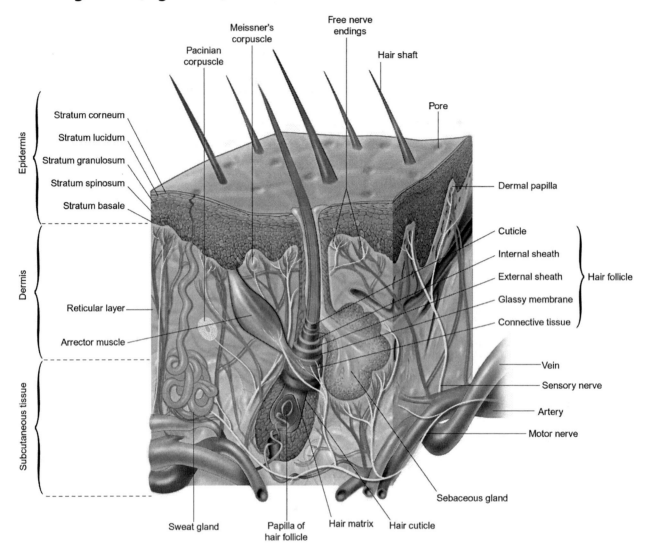

The Epidermis

The epidermis is comprised of five different layers. The innermost layer, the stratum basale, is the layer where most of the new cells are produced. Cells are created and they divide into new cells which push into the next layer, the stratum spinosum. The stratum spinosum is several layers thicker than the stratum basale and is comprised of Keratinocytes. Keratinocytes produce a waxy substance called Keratin which is a waterproofing protein that is resistant to abrasion. Both the stratum basale and the stratum spinosum are considered to be the living layers of the epidermis. The stratum granulosum is composed of 3-4 layers of flat keratinocytes. Cells within the stratum granulosum begin to die off as new cells push in from the stratum spinosum. The stratum lucidum is usually only evident in areas where the epidermis is thick, such as the bottom of the feet and palms of the hands, and functions to transition cells from the stratum lucidum to the stratum corneum. The stratum corneum is the outermost layer of the epidermis and it is constantly losing cell layers. Cells that reach the stratum corneum have about 1 month before they flake off.

The Dermis

The dermis is thicker over the palms of the hands and the soles of the feet than in other places on the body, such as the eyelids or wrists. Unlike the epidermis, which consists mostly of thin, flat squamous cells, the dermis consists of blood vessels, nerve endings, collagen, and elastic fibers.

The papillary layer of the dermis is where we would find the dermal papillae, the fingerlike projections that extend into the epidermis, joining the two. In addition to fingerprints, the papillae are responsible for the nerve endings in the dermis that make it possible for humans to feel sensations, such as heat and pain. The reticular layer, the deeper layer of the dermis, is home to skin appendages such as hair follicles, glands, and corpuscles. The two corpuscles depicted in Figure 2.1 are sensory receptors: The Pacinian corpuscle is a sensory receptor which detects deep pressure placed on the skin. The Meissner's corpuscle is associated with light pressure and is found in large numbers on the hands and feet. The dermis also contains phagocytes, which are cells that ward off infection by destroying, or ingesting, dead bacteria and debris.

Structures of the Integument

The skin has certain accessory structures (hair, glands, and nails) which develop from within the epidermis. They are located in the dermis, and sometimes the subcutaneous layer, due to the fact that they originate from inward growths of the epidermis.

Hair

A hair is formed of keratinized cells and consists of both a shaft and a root. The shaft projects above the skin's surface while the root lies below in a hair follicle. The hair follicle extends into the dermis from the epidermis. Cells are continuously reproduced in the stratum basale. As cells go through the process of becoming keratinized, and die, new cells that are produced result in hair growth. The hair follicle is comprised of several layers. The cuticle consists of a single layer of flattened keratinized cells, which function to protect the hair. This glassy membrane separates the inner and outer sheaths from the connective tissue. The outer sheath surrounds the inner sheath and is the base for attachment of the arrector muscle which holds the hair up. The inner sheath of the hair follicle disintegrates and mixes with sebum secreted from the sebaceous gland, which sometimes hardens to form what is commonly known as a blackhead. The connective tissue provides physical support for the hair follicle.

Hair Follicle (Figure 2.2)

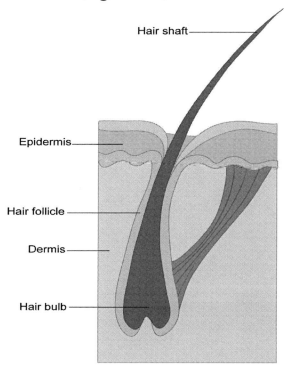
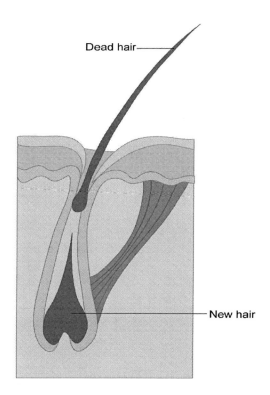

Nails

Nails are formed of extremely keratinized epidermal cells. Nails are composed of a body and a root. The body is the visible portion, and the root is the portion that is inserted into the dermis. Nails are actually colorless. The blood vessels in the underlying nail bed are responsible for the varying shades of pink that are manifest. Nails can be used to quickly determine if a person is suffering from severe anemia or lack of oxygen. These disorders result in a bluish tinge (cyanosis) of the nail.

Nails (Figure 2.3)

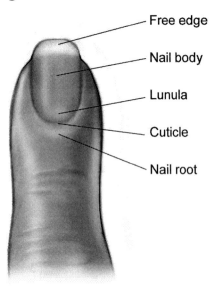

Glands

Glands that develop in the skin are known as exocrine glands. Exocrine refers to external secretion. In this case, it is the secretion of oil, sweat, and wax. The following outlines the three types of exocrine glands associated with the skin.

Sebaceous Glands — These glands are located in the dermis and produce an oily substance (sebum), which is emptied into hair follicles. Sebum keeps the hair and skin soft, smooth, and pliant, and it inhibits the growth of some bacteria.

Sudoriferous Glands — Otherwise known as sweat glands, sudoriferous glands are located in the dermis and are responsible for regulating the body's temperature. When the body heats up, the sudoriferous glands kick into action, causing the body to sweat through the holes in our skin known as pores. The evaporation of this sweat is what actually causes our bodies to cool down.

Ceruminous Glands — Ceruminous glands are modified sweat glands. These glands produce a waxy secretion called cerumen. These coiled, tubular glands are located in the external auditory canal. The sticky, waxy cerumen (ear wax), produced by these glands, helps to protect the inner ear from foreign particles, objects, and insects.

Practice Quiz: Integumentary System

Please complete this exercise to be sure that this portion of the lesson is fully understood before moving on. Answers for this section can be found in the back of the book.

1. Another term for skin is:

    a. cutaneous membrane

    b. serous membrane

    c. integument

    d. both a and c

    e. all of the above

2. Please list and define the two layers of the integument:

    a. _____

    b. _____

3. The _____ connects the epidermis to the dermis.

4. _____ is defined as a waterproof protein that is resistant to abrasion.

5. On which parts of the body is the dermis the thickest? _____

6. _____ are cells that ward off infection by ingesting dead bacteria and debris.

7. Please list the three accessory structures of the integument:

    a. _____

    b. _____

    c. _____

8. Please match the following glands with the substances they produce:

    _____ Sudoriferous glands   a. Oil

    _____ Ceruminous glands   b. Sweat

    _____ Sebaceous glands   c. Wax

Integumentary System

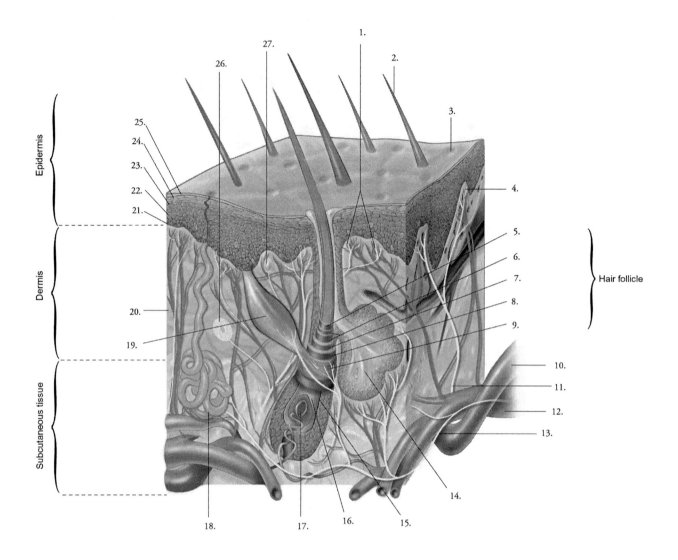

9. Figure 2.1

Fill in the blanks below with the corresponding numbers in the diagram above.

1. _____
2. _____
3. _____
4. _____
5. _____
6. _____
7. _____
8. _____
9. _____
10. _____
11. _____
12. _____
13. _____
14. _____
15. _____
16. _____
17. _____
18. _____
19. _____
20. _____
21. _____
22. _____
23. _____
24. _____
25. _____
26. _____
27. _____

Integumentary System

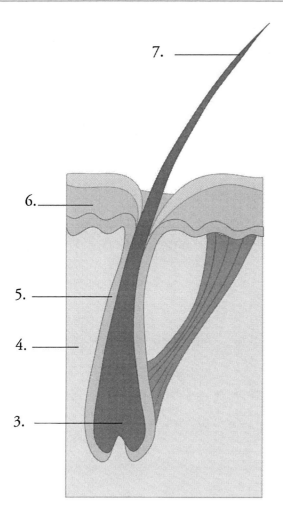
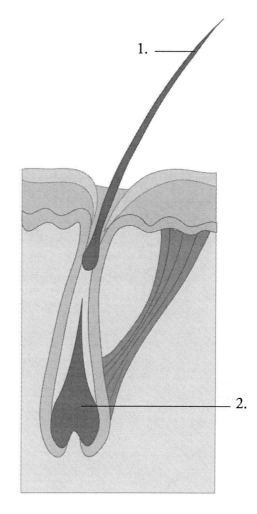

10. Figure 2.2

Fill in the blanks below with the corresponding numbers in the diagram above.

1. _____
2. _____
3. _____
4. _____
5. _____
6. _____
7. _____

Integumentary System

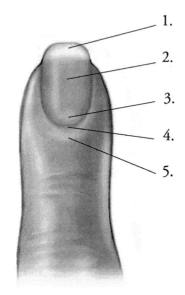

11. Figure 2.3

Fill in the blanks below with the corresponding numbers in the diagram in the first column.

1. _____

2. _____

3. _____

4. _____

5. _____

Chapter 3

MUSCULOSKELETAL SYSTEM

The musculoskeletal system is a combination of the skeletal system and the muscle system. These sections have been combined in the CPT® book because of the close interrelated nature of the two systems.

The Skeletal System

The main function of the skeletal system is to support the framework of the body. In addition to providing support, the skeletal system maintains shape, protects vital organs, and provides a system of muscle levers that allow body movement. The following are some of the major functions of the skeletal system:

Protection — The way in which the bones are arranged in the body result in the protection of the internal organs that are housed within.

Muscle Attachment Sites — Bones also serve as attachment sites for muscles. Skeletal muscles attach to bones and span across joints between bones. When skeletal muscles contract, bones function as levers, enabling movement at bone joints.

Blood Cell Production — The red marrow in bones produces red and white blood cells, and platelets.

Mineral Storage — Bones store vast amounts of calcium phosphate, to be used in other parts of the body when needed.

The skeletal system is made up of three types of supportive connective tissue: cartilage, ligaments, and bone.

Cartilage

The major functions of cartilage are support and protection. There are three types of cartilage in the human body. They are:

Hyaline Cartilage — Forms a protective covering for bones at joints, attaches ribs to the sternum, and supports the nose.

Elastic Cartilage — Provides support for the ears and forms part of the voicebox (larynx).

Fibrocartilage — A very resilient tissue that forms the intervertebral disks that are located between vertebrae, provides padding in the knee joints, and furnishes the pelvic bones with a protective cushion.

Ligaments

Ligaments, strong bands of fibrous tissue, work to connect one bone to another at the joints and provide them with strength or support. Ligaments have a very wide range of motion. They can either limit movement or make movement easier.

Bone Tissue

Bone tissue, or osseous tissue, is the most rigid of all supportive connective tissues. Bone tissue provides the strength necessary for bones in the skeletal system to support the body.

Bone tissue is termed compact bone when it is formed of tightly packed tissue. Compact bone, also known as dense bone, provides support and strength to long bones. When bone tissue contains spaces that appear to be small, needle-like holes, it is known as spongy bone. Spongy bone sounds soft, but in actuality its design allows it to reduce the weight of a bone without losing strength. The open spaces in spongy bone are filled with red marrow, which is essential for red blood cell production. Compact bone is filled with yellow marrow, which consists of fat cells.

Except for any areas that may be covered by cartilage, the entire bone is covered by the periosteum. Blood vessels from the periosteum provide nourishment for bone cells.

Bone Formation

Each bone is an organ that is composed of many tissues. Bone tissue forms the bulk of each bone and consists of living cells and a nonliving matrix that consists primarily of calcium salts.

The process of bone formation is known as ossification. There are two types of ossification: intramembranous ossification and endochondrical ossification. During the process of ossification, connective tissue cells turn into bone forming cells referred to as osteoblasts. Osteoblasts deposit bone matrix around themselves and become imprisoned in lacunae, the space occupied by cells. Once they have become incarcerated they are called, osteocytes, or bone cells.

During development, some bone must be removed and/or reformed to produce the correct shape of the developing bone as it grows. Cells that remove bone matrix as opposed to depositing it are known as osteoclasts. The shape of the mature bone is a direct result of the corresponding actions of the osteoblasts and the osteoclasts.

Bone Classification

Bones are classified according to their shape. The classification of bones is outlined below.

Cuboidal (Short bones) — Cuboidal bones are also referred to as short bones. They are found in the bones of the wrist and ankle.

© 2011 Contexo Media

15

Musculoskeletal System

Flat — Flat bones can be found in the skull and serve to protect the brain. Flat bones also make up the ribs and the shoulder girdle.

Sesamoid — Sesamoid bones are usually small and protect tendons from wear and tear. The patella, or kneecap, is a sesamoid bone.

Tubular (long bones) — Tubular bones are usually long bones, such as the femur, commonly known as the thigh bone. Long bones are found in the upper and lower extremities. Some long bones are the humerus, tibia, ulna, and metacarpals.

Irregular — Irregular bones are those that do not fit into any of the categories listed above. Zygomatic bones, or facial bones, are irregular bones, along with vertebrae and some of the bones of the skull.

Bone Shapes (Figure 3.1)

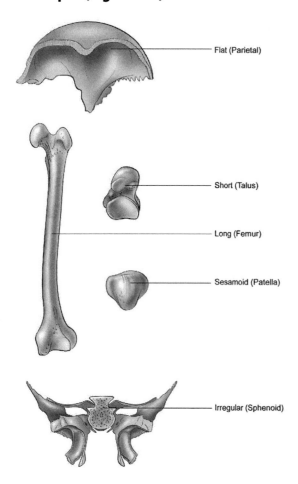

Joints

The mechanism that allows these bones to function together despite their variances in shape is joints. A joint, or articulation, is the junction between two bones that allow varying degrees of movement. Joints are classified as immovable, slightly movable, or freely movable.

Immovable (Fibrous joints) — Bones that form immovable joints are tightly joined. The articulations (sutures) that join the skull bones, with the exception of the mandible (lower jawbone), are immovable. Teeth in their socket are also considered immovable joints.

Slightly movable (Cartilagenous joints) — Bones that form slightly movable joints have limited flexibility. The limited flexibility of intervertebral disks allows for slight movement between adjacent vertebrae.

Freely movable — Freely movable joints account for most articulations and are by far the more complex of the three types of joints. Freely movable joints are further categorized by their movement and structure below.

Ball and socket joints — Ball and socket joints are the most flexible of the freely movable joint types. An example of a ball and socket joint is the shoulder joint. Shoulder movement may be rotational or in any plane may move back and forth or side to side.

Condyloid joints — Condyloid joints move in two planes: from side to side and back and forth. These joints can be found between the metacarpals (bones of the hand).

Gliding joints — Gliding joint movements are either side to side or back and forth (without angular or rotational motion). An example of this type of movement can be found in the joints between the clavicle (collarbone) and scapula (shoulderblade).

Hinge joints — The movements of hinge joints is only in one plane, just like a hinge. The knee, elbow, and phalanges are hinge joints.

Pivot joints — Pivot joints move rotationally in a single plane. The movement of the head is possible as a result of pivot joints that are located in the cervical vertebrae.

Saddle joints — Saddle joints move side to side and back and forth. A saddle joint movement occurs between the bones of the hand and the metacarpal bone of the thumb.

As described in Chapter 1, there are several classifications of joint movements. Some of these types of movements are described below:

- Abduction – Movement away from the midline of the body
- Adduction – Movement toward the midline of the body
- Circumduction – Circular movement
- Extension – Increase in the angle between the bones forming a joint
- Flexion – Decrease in the angle between the bones forming a joint

Musculoskeletal System

Skeletal System (Anterior View) (Figure 3.2)

Figure 3.23.2

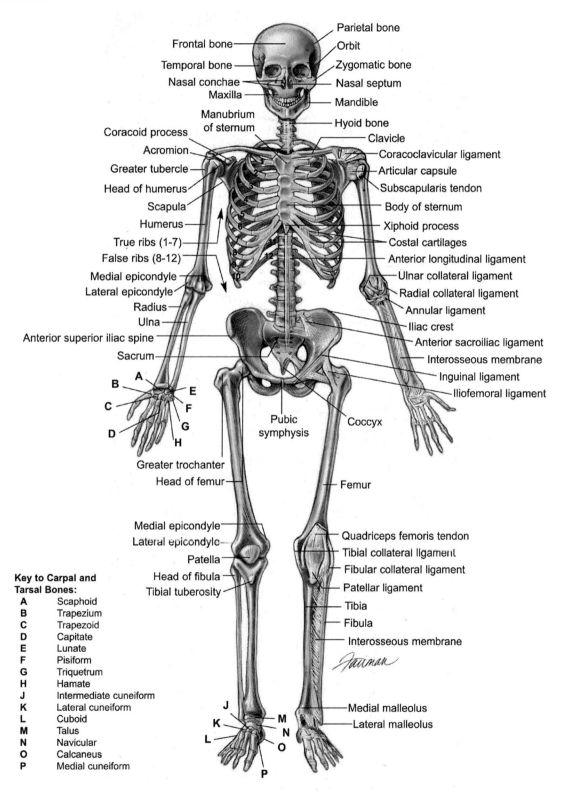

Key to Carpal and Tarsal Bones:
- A   Scaphoid
- B   Trapezium
- C   Trapezoid
- D   Capitate
- E   Lunate
- F   Pisiform
- G   Triquetrum
- H   Hamate
- J   Intermediate cuneiform
- K   Lateral cuneiform
- L   Cuboid
- M   Talus
- N   Navicular
- O   Calcaneus
- P   Medial cuneiform

Musculoskeletal System

Skeletal System (Posterior View) (Figure 3.3)

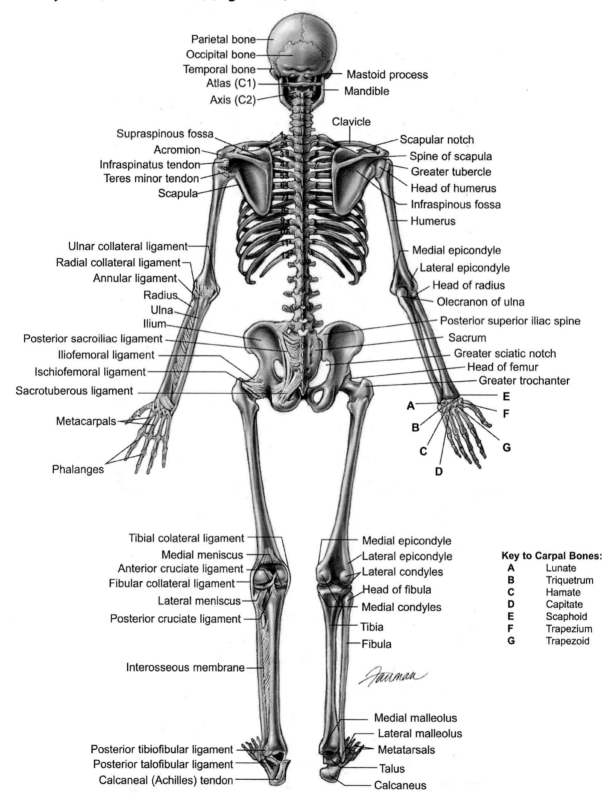

Musculoskeletal System

Shoulder and Elbow (Anterior and Posterior View) (Figure 3.4)

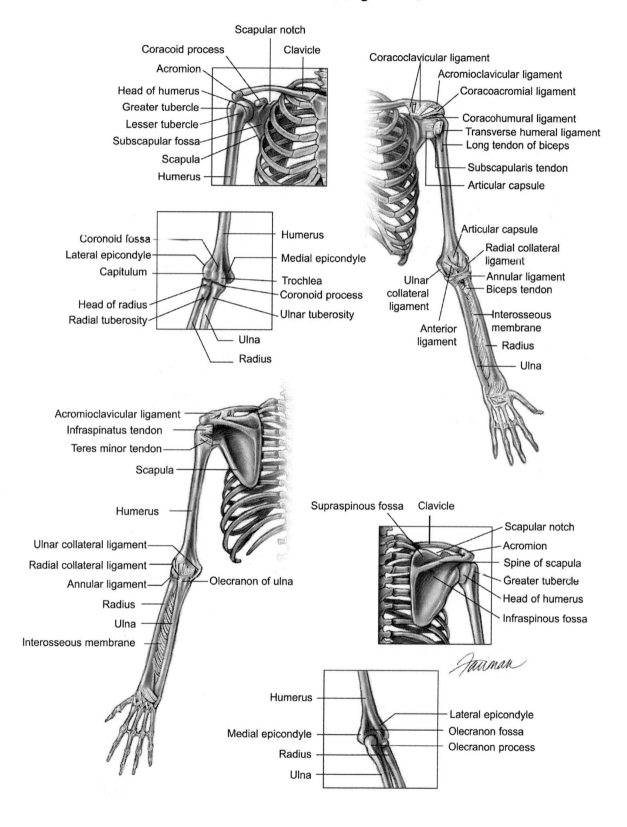

Musculoskeletal System

Hip and Knee (Anterior and Posterior Views) (Figure 3.5)

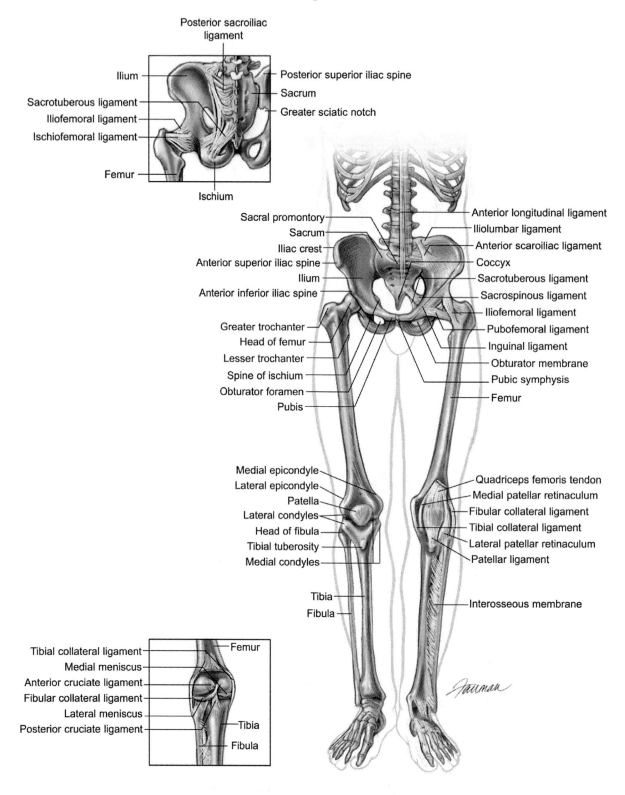

The Skeletal Division

The skeleton is divided into two sections: the Axial skeleton and the Appedicular skeleton.

The Axial Skeleton

The major components of the axial skeleton, or the bones in the long axis (trunk) of the body are: the skull, facial bones, vertebral column, and thoracic cage.

Brain and Skull (Figure 3.6)

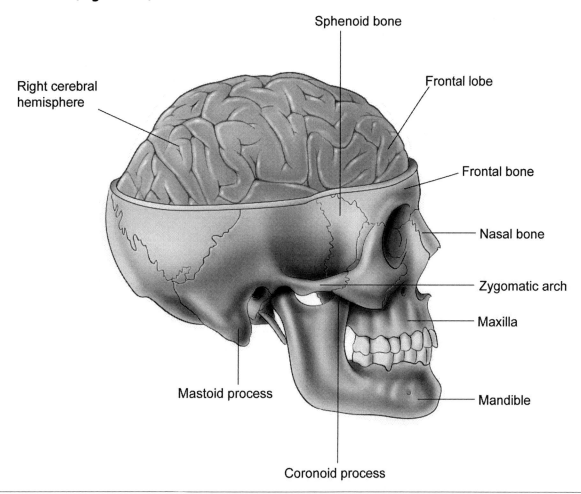

The skull is a combination of the cranium and the facial bones. The cranium is made up of 8 flat bones. The frontal bone forms the forehead, the eye orbits (sockets), and the roof of the nasal cavity. Two parietal bones form the sides and roof of the cranium. A temporal bone lies beneath and is joined to each parietal bone. The occipital bone forms the posterior portion of the cranium. The occipital bone has a large opening through which the brain stem extends to join with the spinal cord. This opening is referred to as the foramen magnum. The sphenoid bone forms the floor of the cranium and the walls of the eye sockets. The ethmoid bone forms the roof of the nasal cavity and the medial surface of the eye.

Several bones in the skull contain sinuses, air-filled spaces that reduce the weight of the skull. The sinuses are named in relation to their position in the skull. They are the frontal, ethmoidal, sphenoidal, and maxillary sinuses.

The facial bones consist of 13 fused bones and the movable lower jaw. The fused bones are bound together by immovable joints that resemble stitches. These stitch-like joints of the skull are known as sutures. The maxillae form the upper jaw. The maxillae is actually formed of two maxilla that join together during our embryonic development. The zygomatic bones form the cheek bones. The nasal bones form the bridge of the nose. The mandible is the lower jawbone. The hyoid bone is an independent, small, U-shaped bone that lies inferior to the mandible. The hyoid bone does not articulate with other bones, but rather serves as an attachment for muscles of the tongue.

Musculoskeletal System

The Vertebral Column

The vertebral column is commonly known as the spine. The spine extends from the skull to the pelvis and provides support for the skeleton so that we may stand upright. It also protects the spinal cord, which runs from the brain to the sacrum. The spinal cord transmits impulses between the brain and spinal nerves. The semi-flexible spine is formed of twenty four movable vertebrae, the sacrum, and the coccyx. The vertebrae are separated from each other by intervertebral disks. These disks serve as protective cushions that allow spinal flexibility.

The vertebrae are divided into three groups according to their location in the body. The groups are: cervical, thoracic, and lumbar.

Vertebral Column (Left Lateral View) (Figure 3.7)

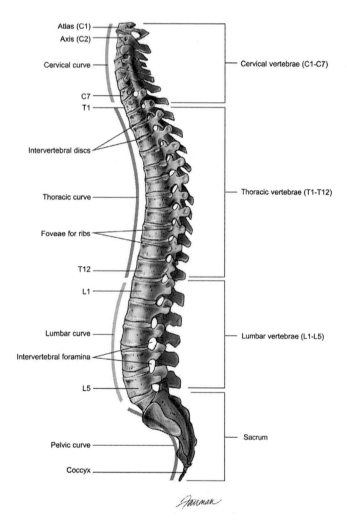

Cervical Vertebrae — The first seven of the vertebrae make up the cervical vertebrae (C1-C7). The main function of the cervical vertebrae is to support the neck, hence its name is derived from cervic/o, meaning neck. The first two cervical vertebrae, the atlas and axis, allow for movement of the head. When we turn our heads, the atlas is actually rotating on the axis.

Thoracic Vertebrae — These twelve vertebrae are located in the thorax, or chest, region (T1-T12). Thoracic vertebrae serve as the site of attachment for our ribs, which in turn, protect the thoracic organs such as the heart and liver.

Lumbar Vertebrae — The next five vertebrae in the vertebral column are known as lumbar vertebrae (L1-L5). They are named for their location in the lumbus, or lower back. These vertebrae are very strong, made to support the larger amount of weight that would be placed on this region from our everyday activities of lifting and bending.

The Sacrum

The sacum is a large, flat bone that is developed from the fusion of five vertebrae. The sacrum has no intervertebral disks and is the most inferior weight bearing bone in the spine. The sacrum forms the posterior wall of the pelvic girdle and articulates with the fifth lumbar vertebrae.

The Coccyx

The coccyx, or the tailbone, is composed of fused vertebrae that bear no weight. These fused vertebrae are the smallest of the spine.

The Thoracic Cage

The thoracic cage is formed of the thoracic vertebrae, ribs, costal cartilages, and sternum. In addition to providing protection to the internal organs, it also provides support for the upper body.

Sternum

The sternum, or breast bone, actually consists of three bones: the manubrium, the body, and the xiphoid process. This flat, elongated bone serves as an attachment for the ribs.

Ribs

There are twelve pairs of ribs attached to the thoracic vertebrae. Costal cartilage keeps the upper seven pairs of ribs attached to the sternum. The remaining pairs of ribs are called false ribs. The first three of the false ribs are attached by other cartilages to the costal cartilage rather than being attached directly. The last two pairs of false ribs are known as floating ribs since they lack cartilage and are not attached to the sternum at all.

The Appendicular Skeleton

The appendicular skeleton is composed of the pectoral girdle, the pelvic girdle, and bones that make up the upper and lower extremities.

The pectoral girdle is also known as the shoulder girdle. The shoulder girdle is made up of two clavicles and two scapulae. The shoulder girdle attaches the upper extremities to the axial skeleton.

The upper extremities are the bones of the arms which includes the forearms, upper arms, wrists, and hands. The bones of the forearm and upper arms are called long bones. The forearm is composed of two bones: the radius and the ulna. The ulna is the medial bone of the forearm (the pinkie side) while the radius is the lateral bone (the thumb side). Of the two bones, the ulna is the largest.

Speaking of the pinkie and the thumb, the bones in the hand consist of the carpus, metacarpus, and phalanges. The carpus are wrist bones. They consist of eight small (carpal) bones that are joined together by ligaments that allow gliding movement. Five metacarpal bones make up the palm of the hand. They are numbered 1 to 5 starting with the thumb. The bones of the fingers are called phalanges. Each finger consists of three phalanges: proximal, middle, and distal. The thumb, however, has only proximal and distal phalanges.

The pelvic girdle consists of two hip bones or coxal bones. The coxal bones articulate with the sacrum to form the pelvis. Each of the two coxal bones is formed by the fusion of three bones: the ilium, the ischium, and the pubis. The ilium forms the upper part of the hip bone, the ischium forms the inferior part, and the pubis is the central front most part. The pelvic girdle forms strong support for the attaching of limbs. It is an attachment point for the strong muscles of the back, legs, and buttocks.

The bones in the lower extremities are the femur (thigh bone), patella (knee bone), tibia (shin bone), and fibula (lower leg bone). The femur is the longest bone in the body. The patella is a small, triangular, flat bone which develops on the tendon of the thigh muscle and is attached by ligaments to the tibia. This enables movement in the knee joint. The tibia is the larger of the lower leg bones and extends from the knee to the ankle. The tarsus, metatarsus, and phalanges are the bones of the foot. There are 7 tarsals, 5 metatarsals, and 14 phalanges in each foot. These bones interact together to make it possible for the body to walk, to support the human frame, and to bear its own weight.

The Muscle System

The movements of the body and the production of heat energy are possible as a result of the contraction (shortening) of muscle tissue. There are three types of muscle tissue in the body: smooth, cardiac, and skeletal.

Smooth muscle tissue — Smooth muscle tissue is made up of thin-elongated muscle cells. Smooth muscle is involuntary tissue, i.e. it is not controlled by the brain. Smooth muscle controls slow, involuntary movements such as the contraction of the smooth muscle tissue in the walls of the stomach and intestines. The muscle of the arteries contracts and relaxes to regulate blood pressure and the flow of blood. Smooth muscle forms the muscle layers in the walls of hollow organs such as the digestive tract (lower part of the esophagus, stomach, and intestines), the walls of the bladder, the uterus, various ducts of glands, and the walls of blood vessels.

Cardiac muscle tissue — This is a unique tissue found only in the walls of the heart. Cardiac (heart) muscle tissue shows some of the characteristics of smooth muscle and some of skeletal muscle tissue. Its fibers, like those of skeletal muscle, have cross-striations and contain numerous nuclei. However, like smooth muscle tissue, it is an involuntary muscle. Cardiac muscle tissue plays the most important role in the contraction of the atria and ventricles of the heart. The contractions cause the rhythmical beating of the heart, thereby circulating the blood and its contents throughout the body.

Skeletal muscle tissue — Skeletal muscle is the most abundant tissue in the body. These muscles are attached to, and bring about, the movement of the various bones of the skeleton, hence the name skeletal muscles. They are attached to bone by bands of tissue called tendons. These muscle tissues, unlike others, are controlled voluntarily. Voluntary contractions occur as a result of conscious control. Skeletal muscles function in pairs to bring about the coordinated movements of the limbs, trunk, jaws, eyeballs, etc. They are also directly related to the breathing process.

Skeletal muscles

Skeletal muscles are composed of primarily skeletal tissue. Skeletal muscles are considered to be the organ of the muscle system. Each skeletal muscle contains many individual muscle fibers, or muscle cells. Muscle fibers are arranged into groups called fasciculi (fah-sik-oo-lee). The perimysium keeps fasciculi divided into separate groups. The separate groups of fasciculi are then bound together by the epimysium. The epimysium is covered by a layer of dense connective tissue known as the deep fascia. The deep fascia extends to the end of the muscle where it forms tendons or aponeuroses. Tendons attach the muscle to bone. Where some tendons and bones connect, there is a fibrous sac called a bursa, which secretes fluid that serves as a cushion when there is movement at the site of connection.

Skeletal muscles are usually attached to the bone on each side of a joint. The type of movement the body is capable of producing depends largely upon the type of joint that the skeletal muscle is attached to, and where it is attached.

When muscles contract, one end of the joint that the muscle is attached to will move while the other will not. The part that moves is called the insertion. The immovable attachment of a muscle is called the origin. The insertion is pulled toward the origin when the muscle contracts.

Muscles function in groups. These groups are designed to provide opposing movements. A group of muscles producing an action are known as agonists. Opposing groups of muscles are called antagonists. In order for movement to occur, these muscles must oppose each other. For example, if an antagonists contracts, the agonist must relax. If muscle groups try to contract at the same time, the movable body part will become rigid. This is what would occur if an individual were to have a seizure.

Musculoskeletal System

Muscular System (Anterior View) (Figure 3.8)

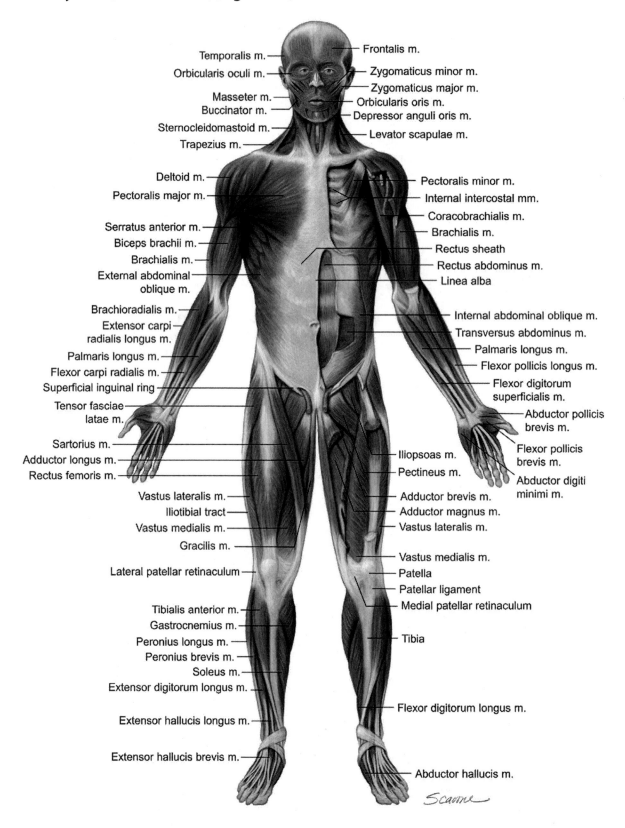

Musculoskeletal System

Muscular System (Posterior View) (Figure 3.9)

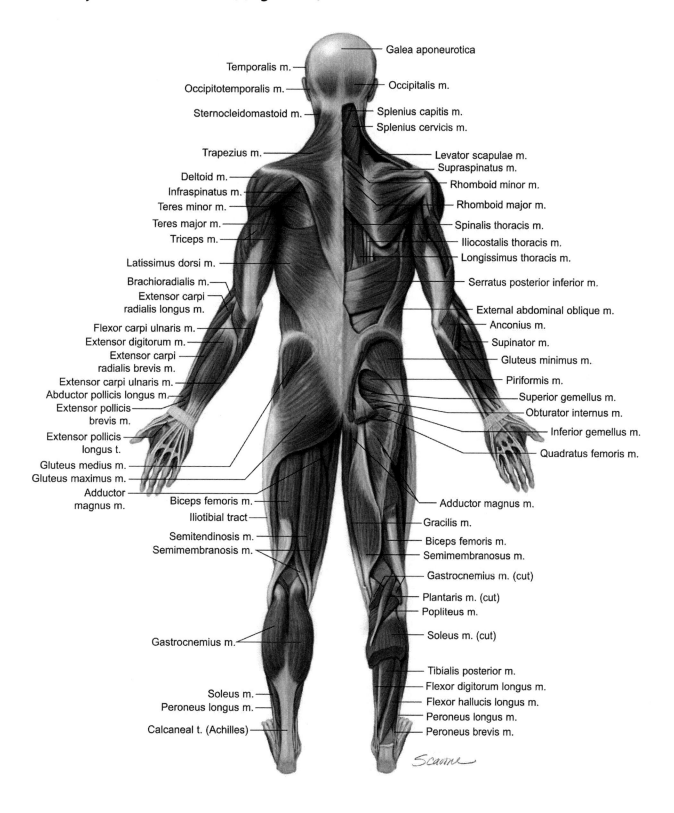

© 2011 Contexo Media

25

Musculoskeletal System

Hand and Wrist (Dorsal and Palmar views) (Figure 3.10)

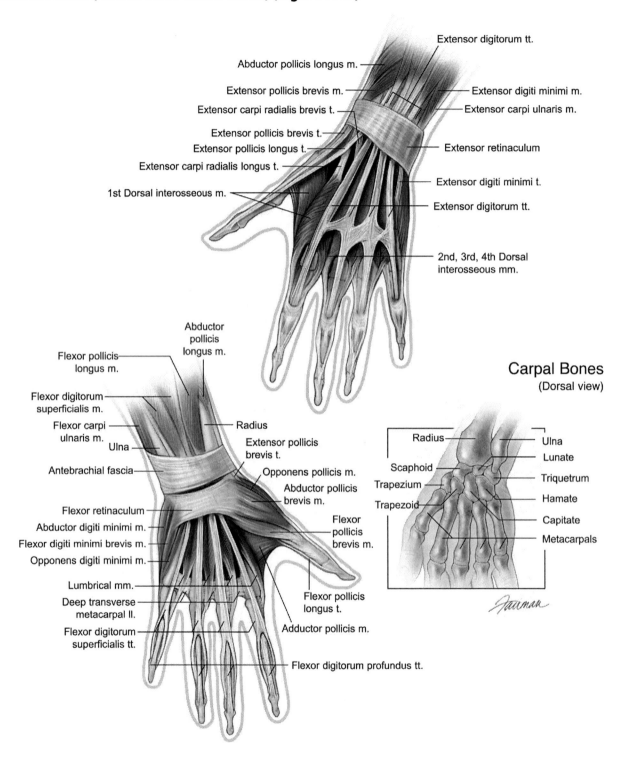

Muscle Names

The names of muscles can be complex and confusing. Sometimes information in the name of the muscle can provide information about the muscle even if the meaning is not known. Below are some examples of how muscles names may be categorized:

- Size: vastus (huge); maximus (large); longus (long); minimus (small); brevis (short).
- Shape: deltoid (triangular); rhomboid (like a rhombus with equal and parallel sides); latissimus (wide); teres (round); trapezius (like a trapezoid, a four-sided figure with two sides parallel).
- Direction of fibers: rectus (straight); transverse (across); oblique (diagonally); orbicularis (circular).
- Location: pectoralis (chest); gluteus (buttock or rump); brachii (arm); supra- (above); infra- (below); sub- (under or beneath); lateralis (lateral).
- Number of origins: biceps (two heads); triceps (three heads); quadriceps (four heads).
- Origin and insertion: sternocleidomastoideus (origin on the sternum and clavicle, insertion on the mastoid process); brachioradialis (origin on the brachium or arm, insertion on the radius).
- Action: abductor (to abduct a structure); adductor (to adduct a structure); flexor (to flex a structure); extensor (to extend a structure); levator (to lift or elevate a structure); masseter (a chewer).

Muscle Groups by Location/Function

There are over 600 types of muscles present in the human body. The following categorizes just a few of the major muscle groups by their location on the body and their function.

Facial Expression

Buccinator	Moves cheeks inward
Orbicularis oculi	Closes eye
Orbicularis oris	Shapes lips for speech
Zygomaticus	Pulls corner of mouth upward
Frontalis	Raises eye brows
Platysma	Opens mouth

Chewing

Masseter	Raises mandible
Temporalis	Raises mandible

Movement of the Head

Splenius capitus	Extends head
Sternoceidomastoid	Flexes head toward chest

Breathing

Diaphragm	Inspiration (breathing in)
External intercostals	Raises ribs for inspiration
Internal intercostals	Draws ribs for expiration (breathing out)

Pectoral girdle

Trapezius	Elevates clavicle
Levator scapulae	Elevates scapula
Serratus anterior	Pulls scapula downward

Upper arm

Deltoid	Extends humerus
Pectoralis major	Draws humerus forward across the chest
Supraspinatus	Rotates humerus laterally
Latissimus dorsi	Rotates humerus medially

Forearm

Triceps brachii	Extends forearm
Brachialis	Flexes forearm
Biceps brachii	Flexes and rotates forearm laterally

Fingers and Wrist

Palmaris longus	Flexes wrist
Extensor digitorum	Extends fingers

Thigh

Iliopsoas	Flexes thigh
Gluteus maximus	Extends and rotates thigh laterally
Gluteus medius	Abducts and rotates thigh medially

Leg

Rectus femoris	Extends leg and flexes thigh
Vastus lateralis	Extends leg
Biceps femoris	Flexes and rotates leg laterally
Sartorius	Assists in performing the action of crossing legs

Feet and Toes

Gastrocnemius	Extends foot
Peroneus longus	Supports arch
Tibialis interior	Flexes and inverts foot
Extensor digitorum	Extends toes

Practice Quiz: Musculoskeletal System

1. Please list four functions of the skeletal system

    a.   c.

    b.   d.

2. What type of tissues are cartilage, ligaments, and bone tissue?

3. Osseous tissue is another term for_____?

4. The process of bone formation is known as _____?

5. Please list five classifications of bones.

    a.   d.

    b.   e.

    c.

6. An articulation is also a _____?

7. The skeleton is divided into two sections. They are the _____ and the _____.

8. _____ are air filled spaces that reduce the weight of the skull.

9. The vertebral column is commonly known as the _____.

10. The vertebrae are divided into three groups. They are the:

    a.

    b.

    c.

11. Please list the three types of muscle tissue.

    a.

    b.

    c.

12. What does it mean when a muscle contracts:

    Voluntarily –

    Involuntarily –

13. What happens if muscle groups try to contract at the same time?

Please match the following bones to the skeletal division in which they belong.

a. Appendicular Skeleton

b. Axial Skeleton

14. ___skull

15. ___humerus

16. ___coccyx

17. ___sacrum

18. ___radius

19. ___patella

20. ___sternum

21. ___thoracic cage

22. ___femur

23. ___ulna

24. ___pectoral girdle

25. ___ribs

26. ___shoulder girdle

27. ___coxal bones

28. ___vertebrae

29. The red marrow in bones produce

    a. red blood cells

    b. fatty tissue cells

    c. white blood cells

    d. a and c

    e. red marrow does not produce anything

30. Blood vessels from the _____ provide nourishment for bone cells.

    a. compact bone

    b. yellow marrow

    c. periosteum

    d. cartilage

31. The shape of mature bone is a result of the corresponding actions of the:

    a. yellow marrow and the red marrow

    b. osteoblasts and osteoclasts

    c. osteocytes and osteoclasts

    d. osteocytes and osteoblasts

32. The junction between two bones is called:
    a. an articulation
    b. an adduction
    c. an abduction
    d. an atlas

33. _____ are the most flexible of the freely moving joints.
    a. gliding joints
    b. pivot joints
    c. hinge joints
    d. ball and socket joints

34. Figure 3.1

Fill in the blanks below with the corresponding numbers in the diagram in the previous column.

1. _____

2. _____

3. _____

4. _____

5. _____

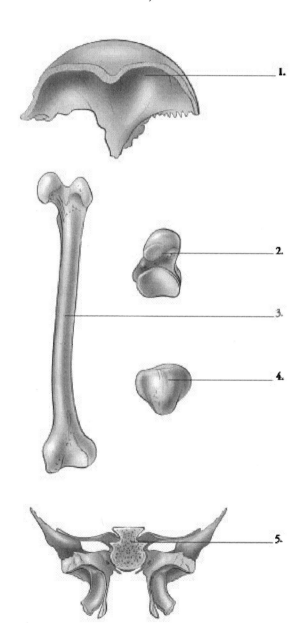

Musculoskeletal System

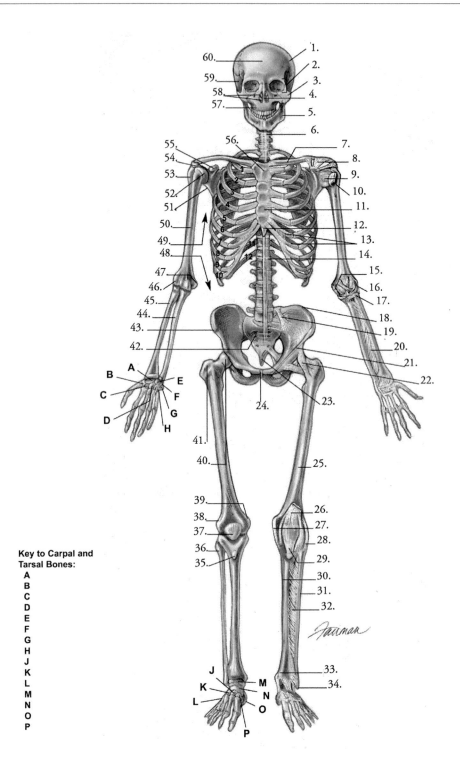

Key to Carpal and Tarsal Bones:
A
B
C
D
E
F
G
H
J
K
L
M
N
O
P

30

Musculoskeletal System

35. Figure 3.2

Fill in the blanks below with the corresponding numbers in the diagram on the previous page.

1. _____
2. _____
3. _____
4. _____
5. _____
6. _____
7. _____
8. _____
9. _____
10. _____
11. _____
12. _____
13. _____
14. _____
15. _____
16. _____
17. _____
18. _____
19. _____
20. _____
21. _____
22. _____
23. _____
24. _____
25. _____
26. _____
27. _____
28. _____
29. _____
30. _____
31. _____
32. _____
33. _____
34. _____
35. _____
36. _____
37. _____

38. _____
39. _____
40. _____
41. _____
42. _____
43. _____
44. _____
45. _____
46. _____
47. _____
48. _____
49. _____
50. _____
51. _____
52. _____
53. _____
54. _____
55. _____
56. _____
57. _____
58. _____
59. _____
60. _____
A. _____
B. _____
C. _____
D. _____
E. _____
F. _____
G. _____
H. _____
J. _____
K. _____
L. _____
M. _____
N. _____
O. _____
P. _____

Musculoskeletal System

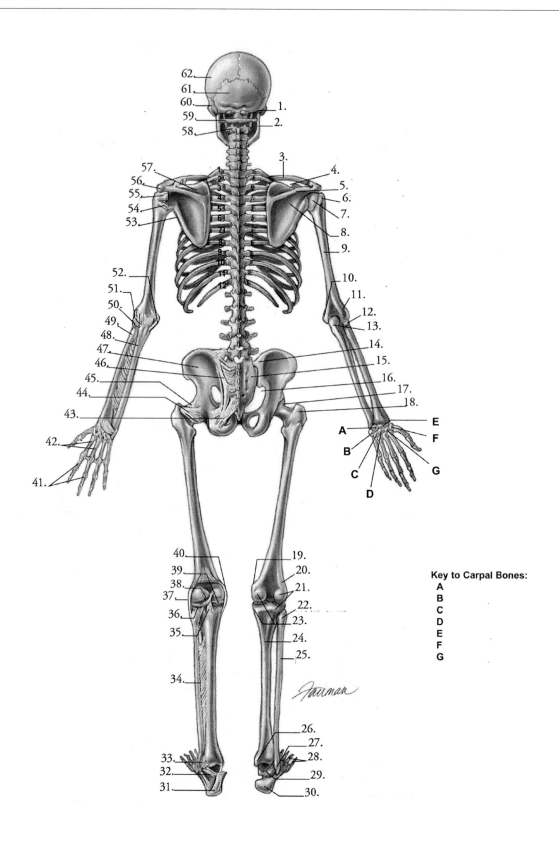

Key to Carpal Bones:
A
B
C
D
E
F
G

32 © 2011 Contexo Media

Musculoskeletal System

36. Figure 3.3

Fill in the blanks below with the corresponding numbers in the diagram on the previous page.

1. _____
2. _____
3. _____
4. _____
5. _____
6. _____
7. _____
8. _____
9. _____
10. _____
11. _____
12. _____
13. _____
14. _____
15. _____
16. _____
17. _____
18. _____
19. _____
20. _____
21. _____
22. _____
23. _____
24. _____
25. _____
26. _____
27. _____
28. _____
29. _____
30. _____
31. _____
32. _____
33. _____

34. _____
35. _____
36. _____
37. _____
38. _____
39. _____
40. _____
41. _____
42. _____
43. _____
44. _____
45. _____
46. _____
47. _____
48. _____
49. _____
50. _____
51. _____
52. _____
53. _____
54. _____
55. _____
56. _____
57. _____
58. _____
59. _____
60. _____
61. _____
62. _____
A. _____
B. _____
C. _____
D. _____
E. _____
F. _____
G. _____

© 2011 Contexo Media

Musculoskeletal System

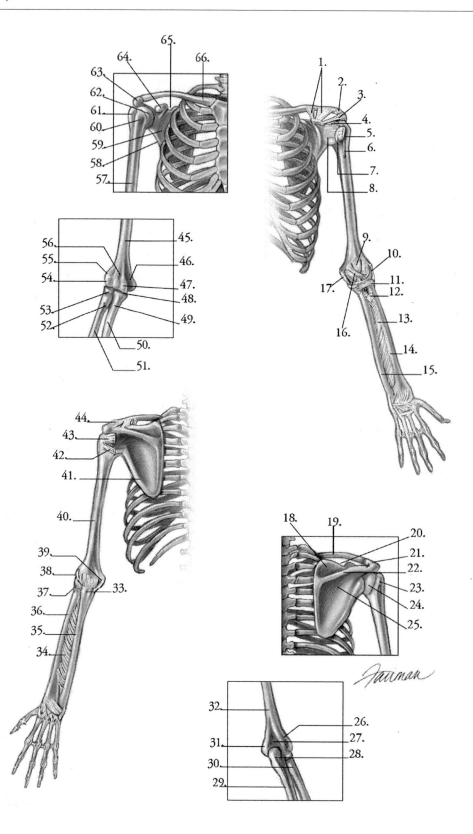

34

Musculoskeletal System

37. Figure 3.4

Fill in the blanks below with the corresponding numbers in the diagram on the previous page.

1. _____

2. _____

3. _____

4. _____

5. _____

6. _____

7. _____

8. _____

9. _____

10. _____

11. _____

12. _____

13. _____

14. _____

15. _____

16. _____

17. _____

18. _____

19. _____

20. _____

21. _____

22. _____

23. _____

24. _____

25. _____

26. _____

27. _____

28. _____

29. _____

30. _____

31. _____

32. _____

33. _____

34. _____

35. _____

36. _____

37. _____

38. _____

39. _____

40. _____

41. _____

42. _____

43. _____

44. _____

45. _____

46. _____

47. _____

48. _____

49. _____

50. _____

51. _____

52. _____

53. _____

54. _____

55. _____

56. _____

57. _____

58. _____

59. _____

60. _____

61. _____

62. _____

63. _____

64. _____

65. _____

66. _____

Musculoskeletal System

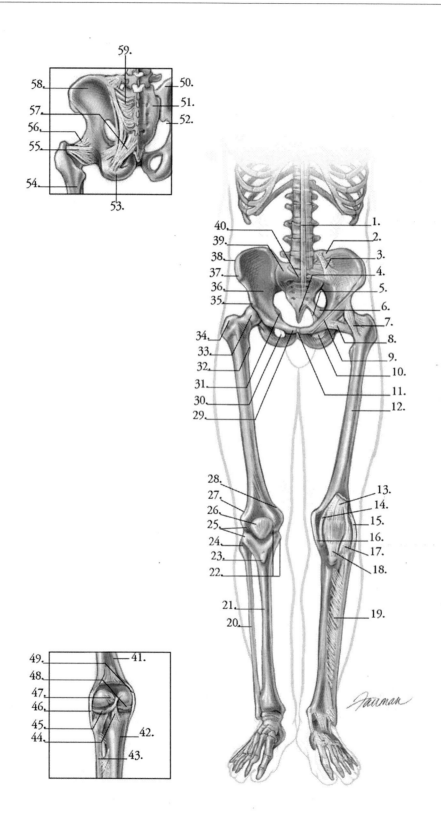

36

Musculoskeletal System

38. Figure 3.5

Fill in the blanks below with the corresponding numbers in the diagram on the previous page.

1. _____

2. _____

3. _____

4. _____

5. _____

6. _____

7. _____

8. _____

9. _____

10. _____

11. _____

12. _____

13. _____

14. _____

15. _____

16. _____

17. _____

18. _____

19. _____

20. _____

21. _____

22. _____

23. _____

24. _____

25. _____

26. _____

27. _____

28. _____

29. _____

30. _____

31. _____

32. _____

33. _____

34. _____

35. _____

36. _____

37. _____

38. _____

39. _____

40. _____

41. _____

42. _____

43. _____

44. _____

45. _____

46. _____

47. _____

48. _____

49. _____

50. _____

51. _____

52. _____

53. _____

54. _____

55. _____

56. _____

57. _____

58. _____

59. _____

Musculoskeletal System

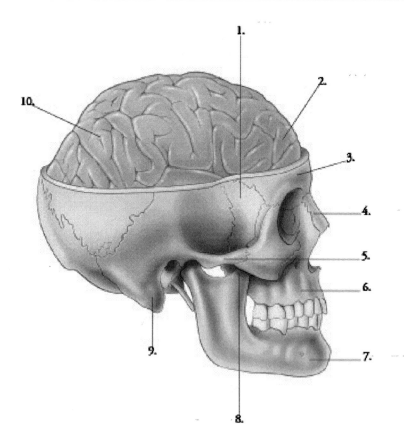

39. Figure 3.6

Fill in the blanks below with the corresponding numbers in the diagram above.

1. _____
2. _____
3. _____
4. _____
5. _____
6. _____
7. _____
8. _____
9. _____
10. _____

Musculoskeletal System

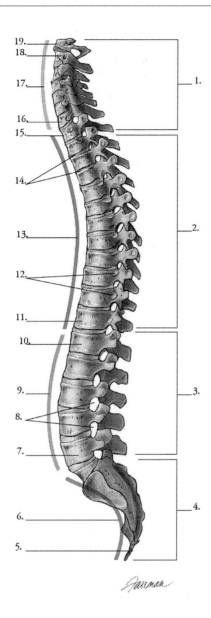

40. Figure 3.7

Fill in the blanks below with the corresponding numbers in the diagram in the previous column.

1. _____
2. _____
3. _____
4. _____
5. _____
6. _____
7. _____
8. _____
9. _____
10. _____
11. _____
12. _____
13. _____
14. _____
15. _____
16. _____
17. _____
18. _____
19. _____

© 2011 Contexo Media

Musculoskeletal System

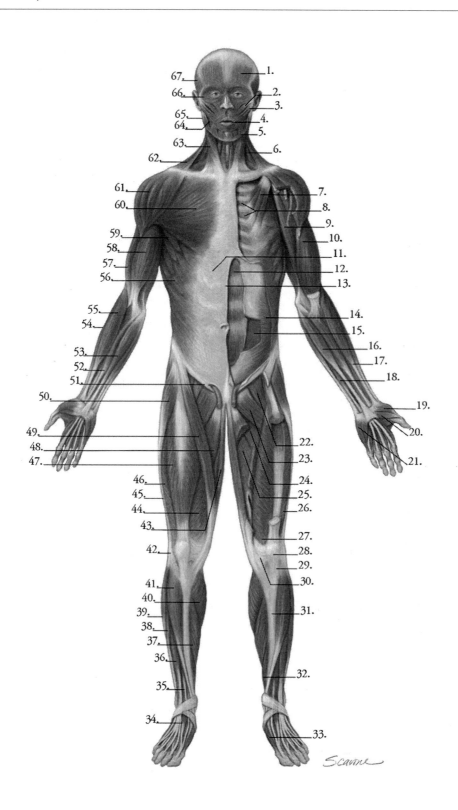

40

Musculoskeletal System

41. Figure 3.8

Fill in the blanks below with the corresponding numbers in the diagram above.

1. _____

2. _____

3. _____

4. _____

5. _____

6. _____

7. _____

8. _____

9. _____

10. _____

11. _____

12. _____

13. _____

14. _____

15. _____

16. _____

17. _____

18. _____

19. _____

20. _____

21. _____

22. _____

23. _____

24. _____

25. _____

26. _____

27. _____

28. _____

29. _____

30. _____

31. _____

32. _____

33. _____

34. _____

35. _____

36. _____

37. _____

38. _____

39. _____

40. _____

41. _____

42. _____

43. _____

44. _____

45. _____

46. _____

47. _____

48. _____

49. _____

50. _____

51. _____

52. _____

53. _____

54. _____

55. _____

56. _____

57. _____

58. _____

59. _____

60. _____

61. _____

62. _____

63. _____

64. _____

65. _____

66. _____

67. _____

Musculoskeletal System

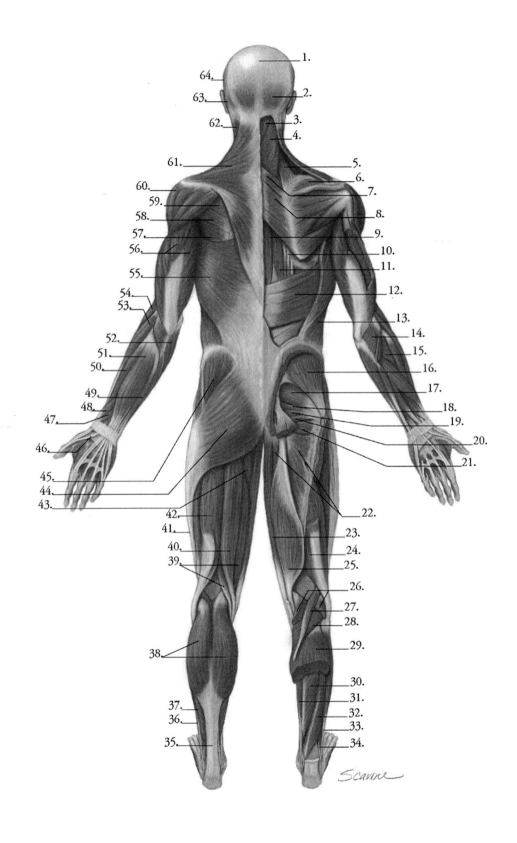

42

Musculoskeletal System

42. Figure 3.9

Fill in the blanks below with the corresponding numbers in the diagram on the previous page.

1. _____

2. _____

3. _____

4. _____

5. _____

6. _____

7. _____

8. _____

9. _____

10. _____

11. _____

12. _____

13. _____

14. _____

15. _____

16. _____

17. _____

18. _____

19. _____

20. _____

21. _____

22. _____

23. _____

24. _____

25. _____

26. _____

27. _____

28. _____

29. _____

30. _____

31. _____

32. _____

33. _____

34. _____

35. _____

36. _____

37. _____

38. _____

39. _____

40. _____

41. _____

42. _____

43. _____

44. _____

45. _____

46. _____

47. _____

48. _____

49. _____

50. _____

51. _____

52. _____

53. _____

54. _____

55. _____

56. _____

57. _____

58. _____

59. _____

60. _____

61. _____

62. _____

63. _____

64. _____

Musculoskeletal System

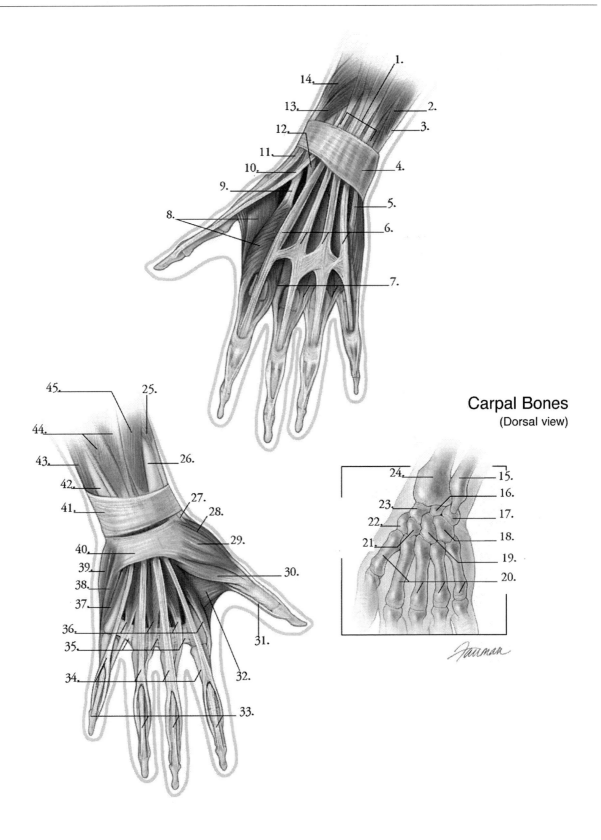

Carpal Bones
(Dorsal view)

Musculoskeletal System

43. Figure 3.10

Fill in the blanks below with the corresponding numbers in the diagram on the previous page.

1. _____

2. _____

3. _____

4. _____

5. _____

6. _____

7. _____

8. _____

9. _____

10. _____

11. _____

12. _____

13. _____

14. _____

15. _____

16. _____

17. _____

18. _____

19. _____

20. _____

21. _____

22. _____

23. _____

24. _____

25. _____

26. _____

27. _____

28. _____

29. _____

30. _____

31. _____

32. _____

33. _____

34. _____

35. _____

36. _____

37. _____

38. _____

39. _____

40. _____

41. _____

42. _____

43. _____

44. _____

45. _____

Chapter 4

Respiratory System

The respiratory system is comprised of six organs: the nose, pharynx, larynx, trachea, bronchial tree, and lungs. All of these organs work together to supply the body with oxygen while also removing carbon dioxide from the body.

Respiratory System (Figure 4.1)

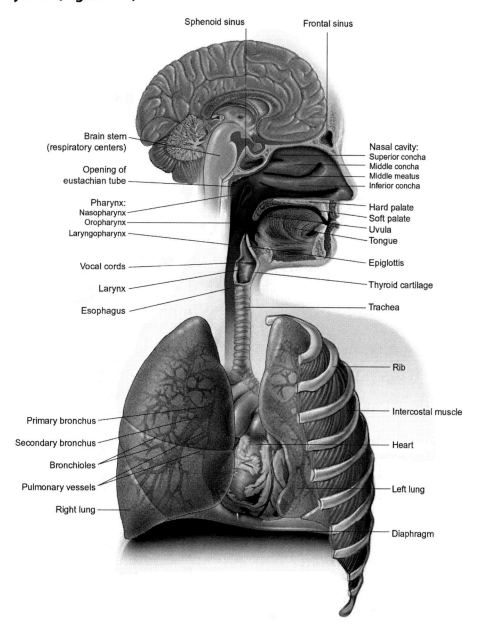

Respiratory System

Each organ of the respiratory system contributes to the process of supplying the body's cells with oxygen in its own special way. Each organ's individual function is an integral part of the respiratory process. Please read how each organ of the respiratory system functions.

The Nose

The nose consists of two openings called nostrils. These nostrils allow air to enter the nasal cavity. The nasal cavity behind the nose is a hollow space lined with mucous membranes. These membranes, along with stiff surface hairs, called cilia, filter out debris and any other foreign airborne particles that are inhaled. The nose functions to prep the air for entry into the pharynx by cleaning, moistening, and warming it. Various types of cartilage are used to protect the nasal opening and they also determine the shape of the nose.

Nose (Figure 4.2)

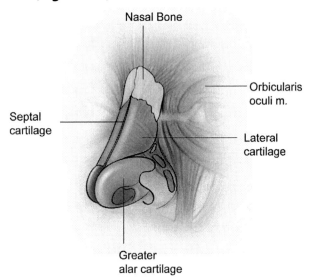

The Pharynx

The pharynx is also known as the throat. It leads a double life since it functions as both a respiratory organ and an organ of the digestive system. The pharynx double checks the work of the nose by, again, filtering the air, cleaning it and warming it. The pharynx houses auditory tubes and provides air to these tubes in an effort to equalize the air pressure on either side of the eardrum.

The Larynx

The larynx, or voicebox, is the organ of sound. This organ of the respiratory system contains our vocal cords (Fig 4.3). Vocal cords function by producing sounds as air passes over them upon expiration. There are four vocal cords: two false vocal cords and two true vocal cords. The upper two vocal cords, which are actually folds in the larynx, are called false cords because they do not actually produce sound. The lower two cords are the true cords that enable humans to produce sound and speak. There is an opening between the vocal cords called the glottis. The glottis is the opening that leads to the trachea.

Larynx (Figure 4.3)

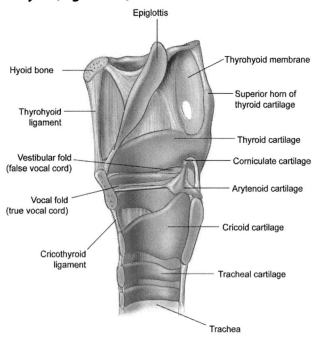

The Trachea

The trachea, or windpipe, is a direct passageway to the lungs. The trachea, as it descends downward, actually divides to form bronchi, which are the main couriers of air into the lungs. Bronchi are large branches that carry air to and from the lung via the trachea. In the lungs, bronchi branch off into many progressively smaller branches known as the bronchial tree. Various types of cartilage such as the thyroid, cricoid, and arytenoid cartilage serve a protective function within the trachea by shielding the vocal cord from harm. Another very important piece of cartilage is the epiglottis. The epiglottis is a yellow leaf-shaped piece of cartilage that folds down during swallowing to block the entrance to the pharynx. Air moves from the trachea into the lungs where it is processed by the alveoli.

The Bronchial Tree

The bronchial tree is named as such due to its many branches or bronchioles. The bronchioles extend from the bronchi, thereby causing it to look much like an upside down tree that is housed in the lung. The bronchioles continue to branch off until they form alveolar ducts, which are microscopic. These ducts end in the air sacs of the lung known as alveoli. The bronchial tree functions to provide air to these alveoli.

Gaseous Exchange (Figure 4.4)

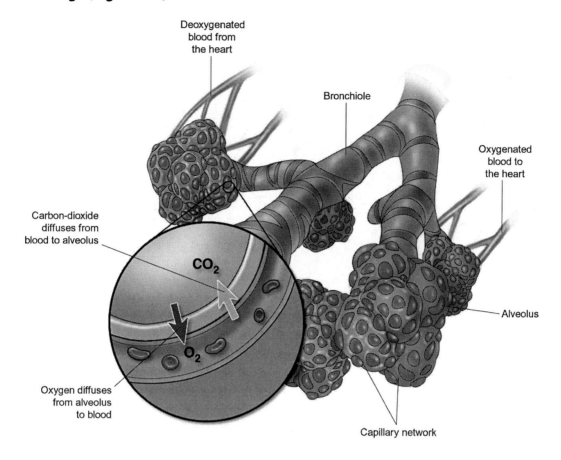

The Lungs

Deoxygenated blood travels from the heart to the lungs via arteries. These arteries become smaller as they enter the lungs where they eventually branch off into millions of capillaries. Each lung is supplied with air by the trachea and is divided into lobes which contain millions of alveoli. The alveoli are tiny air sacs where the actual exchange of deoxygenated blood and oxygenated blood takes place. From Figure 4.4 note that the alveoli is where the carbon-dioxide (CO_2) in the deoxygenated blood moves out into the lungs and in turn, oxygen (O_2) diffuses into the bloodstream through the capillaries providing oxygenated blood which is then circulated through the body until it returns to the lungs where the process repeats. This process is generally referred to as gaseous exchange and is a function of what is commonly termed "breathing." When breathing out, carbon dioxide is exhaled from the lungs. When breathing in, oxygen is inhaled into the lungs. Breathing is therefore the way to introduce the needed component (oxygen) and eliminate the waste product (carbon-dioxide).

Respiratory System

Lungs (Figure 4.5)

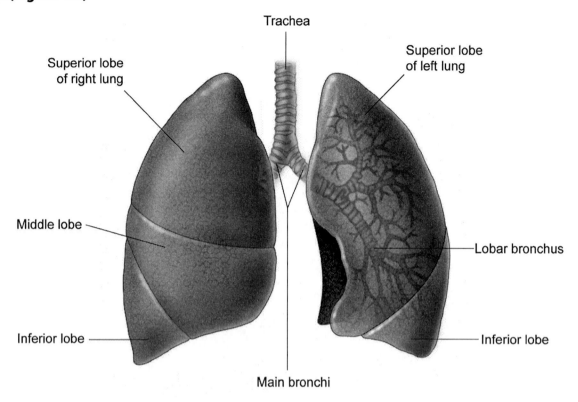

Practice Quiz: Respiratory System

1. The process of respiration consists of two actions. They are
    a.
    b.

2. When air is exhaled out of the body, it is mostly composed of _____.

3. What is the function of the respiratory system?

4. Besides the respiratory system, what other body system does the pharynx belong to?

5. In which organ of the respiratory system does gas exchange occur?

6. What is the common name for the trachea?

7. The hair in the nose are called _____.

8. Figure. 4.1
Fill in the blank areas below with the appropriate term from each figure.

1. _____
2. _____
3. _____
4. _____
5. _____
6. _____
7. _____
8. _____
9. _____
10. _____
11. _____
12. _____
13. _____
14. _____
15. _____
16. _____
17. _____
18. _____
19. _____
20. _____
21. _____
22. _____
23. _____
24. _____
25. _____
26. _____
27. _____
28. _____
29. _____
30. _____
31. _____

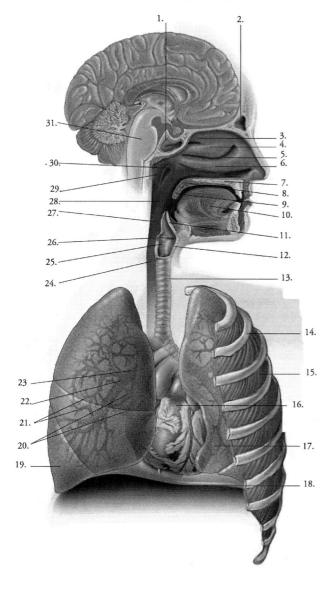

© 2011 Contexo Media

Respiratory System

51

Respiratory System

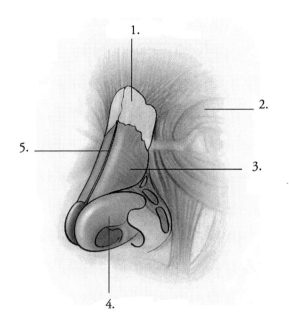

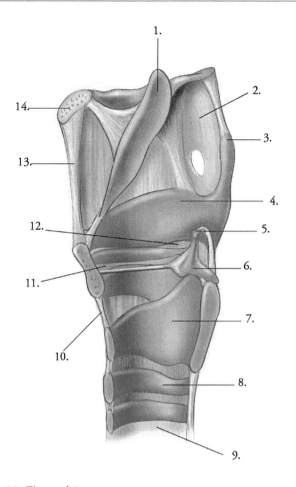

9. Figure 4.2

Fill in the blanks below with the corresponding numbers in the diagram above.

1. _____
2. _____
3. _____
4. _____
5. _____

10. Figure 4.3

Fill in the blanks below with the corresponding numbers in the diagram above.

1. _____
2. _____
3. _____
4. _____
5. _____
6. _____
7. _____
8. _____
9. _____
10. _____
11. _____
12. _____
13. _____
14. _____

Respiratory System

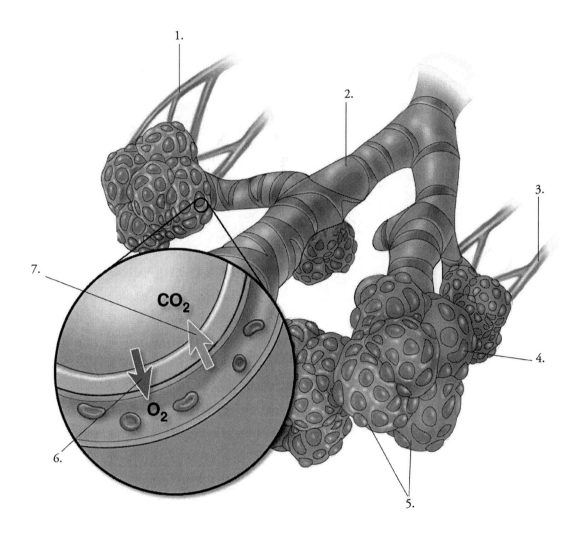

11. Figure 4.4

Fill in the blanks below with the corresponding numbers in the diagram above.

1. _____
2. _____
3. _____
4. _____
5. _____
6. _____
7. _____

Respiratory System

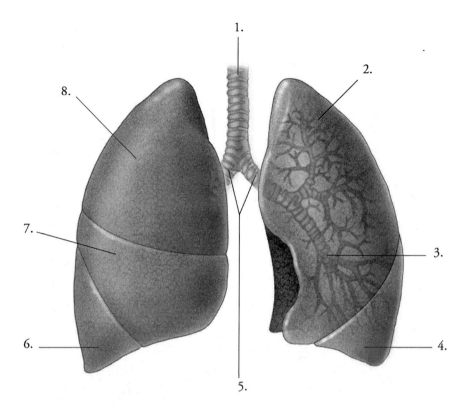

12. Figure 4.5

Fill in the blanks below with the corresponding numbers in the diagram above.

1. _____
2. _____
3. _____
4. _____
5. _____
6. _____
7. _____
8. _____

Chapter 5

CARDIOVASCULAR SYSTEM AND LYMPHATIC SYSTEM

The cardiovascular system consists of a muscular pump (the heart) and a very intricate system of vessels. The function of the cardiovascular system is to circulate blood within the body to sites where it can be oxygenated, and where any wastes can be disposed of. This system also brings, through the process of circulation, nutrients such as glucose, amino acids, and hormones to all of the body's cells. As blood travels through the body, it transports nutrients while also serving to eliminate wastes and other unwanted substances.

Please read this section which describes in more detail, how each component of the cardiovascular system functions in the circulatory process.

The Heart

The human heart is approximately the size of a fist. There are four cavities, or open spaces, inside the heart that fill with blood. Two of these cavities are called atria. The other two are called ventricles. The two atria form the curved top of the heart. The ventricles meet at the bottom of the heart to form a pointed base which points toward the left side of your chest. The forceful contractions of the left ventricle can be felt pumping on the left side of the chest.

The left side of the heart houses one atrium and one ventricle. The right side of the heart also houses one atrium and one ventricle. A wall, called the septum, separates the right and left sides of the heart. A valve connects each atrium to the ventricle below it. The mitral valve connects the left atrium with the left ventricle. The tricuspid valve connects the right atrium with the right ventricle.

Each atrium is responsible for receiving the blood that flows from the body to the heart. When the atria contract, they pump blood into the lower chamber. The ventricles in the lower chamber function to push blood away from the heart. They have very thick walls which they need in order to be able to pump blood so forcefully that it goes away from the heart yet eventually comes back around to the heart.

Between the atria and the ventricles are valves which allow blood to flow in only one direction. These valves allow blood to flow from the atrium into the ventricle, and also prevents a backflow of blood back into the atrium. These particular valves are known as atrioventricular valves. There are two types: tricuspid and bicuspid valves. The tricuspid valve, located between the right atrium and right ventricle, has three flaps of tissue (cusps). The bicuspid valves, also known as the mitral valve and the aortic valve, are located between the left atrium and the left ventricle

The average heart's muscle, called cardiac muscle, contracts and relaxes about 70 to 80 times per minute without a person ever having to think about it. As the cardiac muscle contracts, it pushes blood through the chambers and into the vessels. Nerves connected to the heart regulate the speed with which the muscle contracts. The average adult heart is about the size of a clenched fist and weighs about 11 ounces (310 grams). Located in the middle of the chest behind the breastbone and between the lungs, the heart rests in a moistened chamber called the pericardial cavity which is surrounded by the ribcage.

© 2011 Contexo Media

Cardiovascular System and Lymphatic System

Heart (External and Internal views) (Figure 5.1)

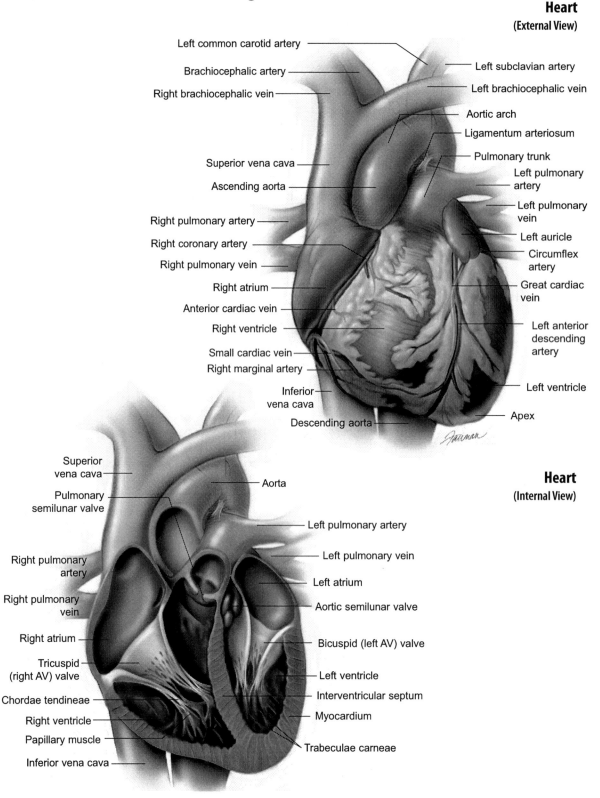

Cardiovascular System and Lymphatic System

Blood Vessels

The cardiovascular system contains an elaborate network of vessels that are designed to carry blood to and from the heart. There are, essentially, three types of blood vessels present in the cardiovascular system: arteries, veins, and capillaries.

Vascular System (Figure 5.2)

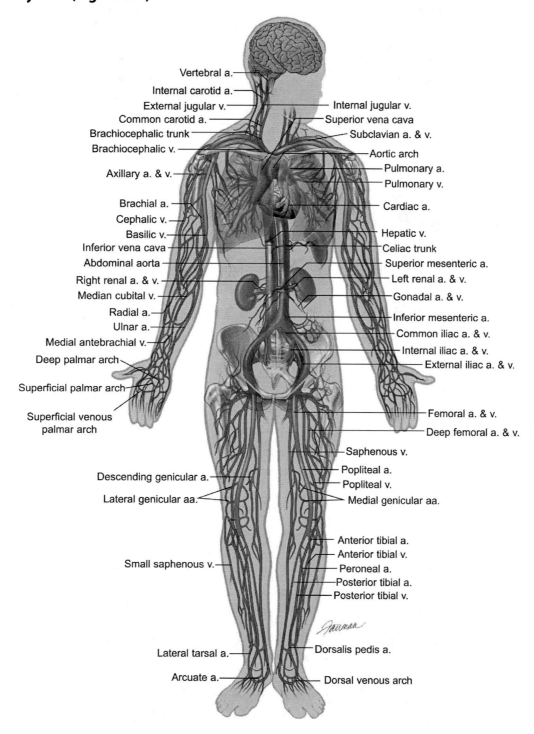

© 2011 Contexo Media

Arteries

Simply put, arteries carry blood away from the heart. Most arteries transport oxygen-rich (oxygenated) blood. Arteries branch off from the main artery, the aorta, which extends from the heart. Arteries branch off repeatedly into smaller and smaller branches until they are microscopic. These microscopic arteries are called arterioles and will be discussed in detail later. The aorta functions to carry oxygenated blood from the left ventricle of the heart to all parts of the body, with the exception of the lungs. The pulmonary artery is the only artery that carries deoxygenated blood.

All of the arteries that branch off of the aorta are known as systemic arteries. Below is a list of the major branches of aortic arteries as well as arteries found in other parts of the body.

Coronary Arteries — Coronary arteries are the first arteries to branch off of the aorta. There are left and right coronary arteries. These arteries directly supply blood to the heart.

Arteries of the Aortic Arch — The aorta ascends from the heart and arches to the left and right. These arches form the coronary arteries. Between those arteries lie the arteries of the aortic arch.

Brachiocephalic artery — supply blood to right side of head and neck, right shoulder, and right arm

Left Common Carotid Artery — pronounced (kuh-rot-id), supplies blood to the left side of the head and neck

Left Subclavian Artery — supplies blood to left shoulder and left arm

Intercostal Arteries — These arteries supply blood to organs located in the thoracic cavity as well as the intercostal muscles between the ribs.

Abdominal Aortic Arteries — As the aorta ascends through the abdominal region, many arteries branch off to supply blood to the abdominal wall and organs. The celiac artery is a short abdominal artery that branches off to form three additional arteries.

- **Gastric Artery**: supplies blood to the stomach

- **Splenic Artery**: supplies blood to the spleen

- **Hepatic Artery**: supplies blood to the liver

Superior Mesenteric Arteries — These arteries provide a blood supply for most of the small intestine and the first portion of the large intestine.

Renal Arteries — There is one left and one right renal artery. These arteries supply blood to the kidneys.

Gonadal Arteries — In females, these arteries supply the ovaries. In males the arteries are responsible for supplying to the male testes. Both of these arteries are also paired.

Lumbar Arteries — These arteries supply blood to the walls of the abdomen and the lower back. There are several pairs of lumbar arteries.

Inferior Mesenteric Artery — This artery supplies the inferior (lower) portion of the large intestine with blood.

Common Iliac Arteries — At this portion of the body, below the abdomen, the aorta branches off into two large arteries, similar to the coronary arteries. These arteries, however, branch off into each leg, which form the left and right common iliac arteries.

Arteries of the Head and Neck — The subclavian and carotid arteries branch off into many arteries that supply blood to the head and neck. They are:

- Right common carotid artery

- Right subclavian artery

- Vertebral arteries

- Basilar arteries

- Thyrocervical arteries

Arteries of the Shoulders and Arms — Arteries that branch off from the subclavian artery of the head and neck, branch off to the shoulders and arms. Arteries of the head and neck are:

- Axillary Artery

- Brachial artery

- Radial artery

- Ulnar artery

Arteries of the Pelvis and Legs — The arteries that branch from the common iliac arteries, which branch from the inferior portion of the aorta, supply the pelvis and legs with blood. They are:

- Femoral artery

- Popliteal artery

- Anterior tibial artery

- Dorsal pedis artery

- Posterior tibial artery

- Peroneal artery

Capillaries

As mentioned previously, arteries continue to branch off into smaller and smaller arteries until they become microscopic. These microscopic arteries are called arterioles. Arterioles branch off into even smaller arterioles and eventually these arterioles connect with capillaries. Capillaries continue to branch off, but they branch off and interconnect differently from arteries. In fact, their branch effect has been described as appearing more web-like. A network of capillaries is known as a capillary bed.

Capillaries are the smallest and most narrow of the three types of blood vessels present in the cardiovascular system. They are responsible for carrying blood to bodily tissues as well as linking together arteries and veins. It is in the capillaries that the exchange between the blood and cells actually takes place. During this process, the blood releases carbon dioxide and exchanges it for oxygen, which is distributed throughout the body.

Veins

Capillaries eventually begin to thicken and merge to form venules. Venules are similar to arterioles in the way that they are the smallest branches of veins. Veins function to return blood from the capillaries to the heart.

All veins branch off from two major veins, the superior and inferior vena cavae. The veins that branch from the superior vena cava stem from the arms, head, neck, and shoulders. Veins from the lower trunk and legs stem from the inferior vena cava. All of these veins work to return the blood back to the right atrium of the heart.

Collectively, the veins that branch off of the vena cavae are known as systemic veins. Systemic veins function by "draining" blood from different areas of the body rather than supplying the body with blood as arteries do.

Lymphatic System

The lymphatic system of the human body performs two main functions: it removes excess fluid from tissues and returns it to the blood to be used again, and it works hand in hand with white blood cells to protect the body from organisms that cause disease. The main organs that assist with these processes are lymph nodes, the tonsils, the thymus, and the spleen.

Lymph Nodes

Often referred to as lymph glands, these small, oval shaped nodes function to filter lymph as it passes through the body. Lymph is a transparent, yellow, watery substance that is produced as runoff from the spaces left between cells. It usually consists of white blood cells, water, waste products, dissolved salts and proteins. Lymph nodes are the only organs in the lymphatic system that filter lymph.

Tonsils

Tonsils are located at the back of the mouth, near the entrance to the throat. They function to protect the body from infection by producing disease-fighting white blood cells. They do this by intercepting any bacteria or other pathogens from entering the mouth, nose, or throat cavities.

Thymus

This dual lobed gland is located just above the heart. It functions to produce thymosin, a hormone that stimulates the production of white blood cells which help to fight off illness.

Spleen

The spleen is by far the largest of all the lymphatic organs. It functions to serve as a storage for blood. It is also responsible for removing damaged blood cells from circulating blood. Like the other organs, the spleen also produces white blood cells.

Cardiovascular System and Lymphatic System

Practice Quiz: Cardiovascular System

1. The _____ are responsible for pumping blood away from the heart.
   a.　　arteries
   b.　　veins
   c.　　atria
   d.　　ventricles

2. The _____ are responsible for pushing blood into the lower chamber of the heart.
   a.　　arteries
   b.　　veins
   c.　　atria
   d.　　ventricles

3. The _____ are responsible for carrying blood away from the heart.
   a.　　arteries
   b.　　veins
   c.　　atria
   d.　　ventricles

4. The _____ are responsible for carrying blood toward the heart.
   a.　　arteries

   b.　　veins
   c.　　atria
   d.　　ventricles

5. _____, located in the heart, force blood to move in one direction into and away from the heart, so that there is no backflow of blood into the heart.

6. Microscopic arteries are called_____.

7. Microscopic veins are called _____.

8. The main artery in the human body is known as the _____ _____.

9. The arteries that branch off of the main artery are known as _____.

10. What are the two major veins of the body?

11. What are the veins that branch off of the main veins known as?

12. Which vessels are responsible for linking the arteries and veins together?

13. Which arteries supply blood directly to the heart?

Cardiovascular System and Lymphatic System

14. Figure 5.1

Fill in the blanks below with the corresponding numbers in the diagram below and to the right.

1. _____
2. _____
3. _____
4. _____
5. _____
6. _____
7. _____
1. _____
2. _____
3. _____
4. _____
5. _____
6. _____
7. _____
8. _____
9. _____
10. _____
11. _____
12. _____
13. _____
14. _____
15. _____

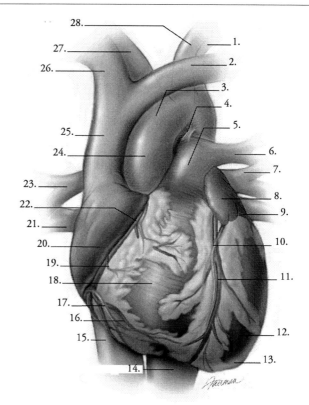

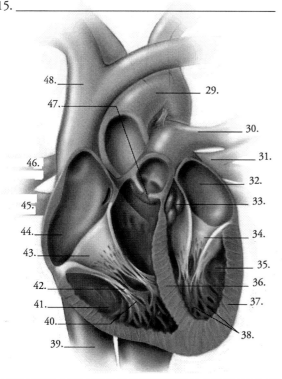

24. _____
25. _____
26. _____
27. _____
28. _____
29. _____
30. _____
31. _____
32. _____
33. _____
34. _____
35. _____
36. _____
37. _____
38. _____
39. _____
40. _____
41. _____
42. _____
43. _____
44. _____
45. _____
46. _____
47. _____
48. _____

© 2011 Contexo Media

Cardiovascular System and Lymphatic System

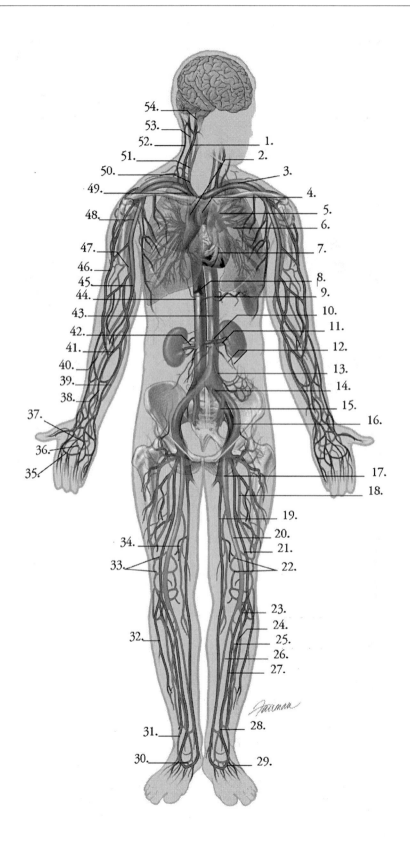

62

15. Figure 5.2

Fill in the blanks below with the corresponding numbers in the diagram on the previous page.

1. _____
2. _____
3. _____
4. _____
5. _____
6. _____
7. _____
8. _____
9. _____
10. _____
11. _____
12. _____
13. _____
14. _____
15. _____
16. _____
17. _____
18. _____
19. _____
20. _____
21. _____
22. _____
23. _____
24. _____
25. _____
26. _____
27. _____
28. _____
29. _____
30. _____
31. _____
32. _____
33. _____
34. _____
35. _____
36. _____
37. _____
38. _____
39. _____
40. _____
41. _____
42. _____
43. _____
44. _____
45. _____
46. _____
47. _____
48. _____
49. _____
50. _____
51. _____
52. _____
53. _____
54. _____

Chapter 6

Digestive System

Digestion is the process by which food is broken down mechanically and chemically in the gastrointestinal tract and converted into absorbable forms. Mechanical breakdown is the act of breaking food down into smaller pieces, which is accomplished by chewing. Chemical breakdown is how all of the foods and liquids that are consumed get divided up into smaller components such as proteins, carbohydrates, vitamins, and minerals. Once the components are broken down they are then distributed to parts of the body that need them or they are stored for future use.

All of the body parts and organs that participate in digestion are located in the alimentary canal. The alimentary canal, or digestive tract, is a long tube about 30 feet in length. This canal extends from the mouth to the anus. The body parts and organs that make up the digestive system are the mouth, pharynx, esophagus, stomach, small intestine, large intestine, anus, teeth, salivary glands, liver, gallbladder, and pancreas.

Each component of the alimentary canal is responsible for performing different digestive functions.

The tube that is the alimentary canal consists of four layers: the serous layer, muscular layer, submucosa, and mucosa. The serous layer is the outermost layer that covers the outside of the tube. Directly underneath the serous layer, lies the muscular layer. The muscular layer consists of two types of smooth muscle whose contractions cause wave-like movements that propel food through the alimentary canal. These movements are known as peristalsis. The two innermost layers are the mucosa and submucosa. The submucosa is the layer closest to the muscular layer. It contains nerves, lymphatic vessels, and blood vessels. The mucosal layer contains cells that produce digestive secretions and mucus. These secretions aid in the digestion of food and the absorption of nutrients.

The Mouth

The mouth, also know as the oral cavity, is directly involved with the digestive process as this is how food initially enters our system. The mouth itself consists of the cheeks, tongue, palate, teeth, and salivary glands. The anterior portions of the cheeks form the lips, which allow movement so that the mouth may open and close. The palate moves upward during swallowing which serves to ensure that the food moves in a downward direction along the alimentary canal. The tongue helps the manipulation of food in the mouth so that chewing can occur.

Digestive System (Figure 6.1)

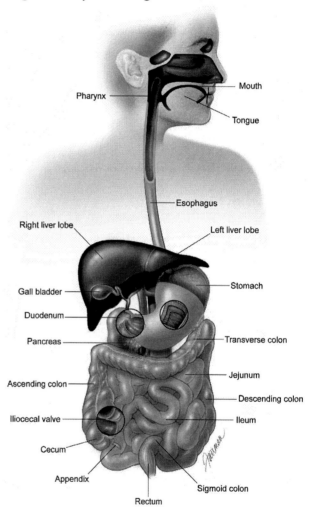

Chewing, or mastication, is the result of our teeth breaking food down into smaller pieces. Movement of the tongue stimulates the production of saliva (produced through the salivary glands) which is an important element in the physical breakdown and swallowing of food. Saliva is secreted from clusters of cells called acini. Saliva is composed primarily of water, electrolytes, mucus, and enzymes which are secreted into ducts which lead to the mouth. Saliva lubricates the masticated food so that it moves through the alimentary canal smoothly.

The Pharynx

The pharynx is one of the organs that leads a double life by functioning both in the respiratory system and the digestive system. In the digestive system it functions to transport food from the mouth to the esophagus while swallowing. When swallowing occurs, the tongue pushes food into the pharynx. The soft palate contracts upward, pushing the food downward into the pharynx, which assists the food into the esophagus.

The Esophagus

The esophagus, the part of the alimentary tube that extends down from the pharynx connects with the stomach. Once food has moved through the pharynx to the esophagus, it is carried to the stomach by peristalsis, the wave-like contractions of the smooth muscle located in the esophageal portion of the alimentary canal. The smooth muscle located at the bottom of the esophagus also helps to keep the food and gastric juices in the stomach from receding back into the esophagus. Failure to prevent the gastric juices from entering the esophagus causes what is commonly known as heartburn.

The Stomach

The stomach is a sac-like organ in which the major chemical breakdown efforts begin. The stomach contains gastric glands which produce highly acidic gastric juices. The gastric juices combine with food to form a semiliquid substance know as chyme. The stomach performs several different functions: It is the primary location for the storage of food as it waits to be digested, in addition, it also provides a mechanical digestive role by mixing the food using the strong muscles in the walls of the stomach. In addition, the acid sterilizes unhealthy food particles. From the stomach, food then moves into the small intestine.

The Small Intestine

The small intestine is divided into three parts: the duodenum, the jejunum, and the ileum. The duodenum is the part of the small intestine that is attached to the stomach. Chyme is passed into the duodenum from the stomach, and begins to digest here. The jejunum is the area where most of the nutrients from the food are absorbed into the body. The process of absorption occurs as thousands of cells in the intestines which contain tiny microvilli enrich the blood with nutrients that are necessary for the body to survive. The ileum's main function is to absorb vitamin B_{12}, some salts, carbohydrates and proteins. Most digestive efforts along with the absorption of food occur within the small intestine. Once food has gone through the digestion and absorption process, the residue passes from the ileum to the large intestine.

The Pancreas and the Liver

The pancreas is a gland that lies behind the stomach and connects to the duodenum. It functions primarily to secrete enzymes which assist with the breaking down of food into fats, nucleic acids, carbohydrates, and proteins. The pancreas also produces the hormone insulin. Insulin is a key factor in determining metabolic rate, which is the rate at which energy is consumed in the body.

The liver is a gland that is located just below the diaphragm. This reddish-brown gland is divided into two lobes known as the left lobe and the right lobe. The left lobe is considerably smaller than the right lobe. The liver regulates, synthesizes, stores, and secretes several nutrients and proteins that are essential to the body. The liver synthesizes and stores most blood proteins including albumin and several proteins associated with the coagulation of blood.

Bile is a yellow-greenish liquid that is both a waste product of the liver as well as a major contributor in the digestion of fats. Bile is stored in the gallbladder, which is a pear-shaped sac located just below the liver. The liver continuously produces bile, it is then transported to the gall bladder until it is needed, in which case, it will leave from the gall bladder and make its way into the small intestine to assist in the absorption of fatty acids, cholesterol, and fat soluble vitamins by the small intestine.

The Large Intestine

The large intestine and its accessories are the last components of the alimentary canal, or digestive tract. By the time chyme gets to the large intestine, it will have already been depleted of any nutrients. Unlike the other parts of the digestive system, those of the large intestine do not function to "digest" food. The large intestine primarily functions to absorb water, minerals, and vitamins. The products that are unabsorbed or undigested are then expelled from the body in the form of feces.

The large intestine consists of the cecum, colon, and rectum. The cecum is a little pouch that lies at the junction of the large and small intestine. This junction is known as the ileocecal sphincter. There is a short, worm-like tube attached to the cecum. This appendage is known as the appendix. Although attached to a digestive organ, the appendix has no known function, digestive or otherwise.

The bulk of the large intestine is comprised of the colon. The colon's primary function is to absorb water into the body. It is divided into four sections. In anatomical order, they are: ascending colon, transverse colon, descending colon, and sigmoid colon. The ascending colon moves from the cecum up to the transverse colon which connects to the descending colon in the upper left-hand quadrant of the abdomen.

As food is being absorbed, it moves slowly through the colon. Most absorption by the colon will have already taken place once it reaches the descending portion.

The latter portion of the large intestine is known as the rectum. The rectum contains muscles that help to propel feces through the anal canal to be released from the body through the anus.

Practice Quiz: Digestive System

1. Another name for the digestive tract is the _____.

2. The wave-like movements that propel food through the digestive tract are called _____.

3. The oral cavity is located in which part of the body?

4. When gastric juices combine with food they form a semiliquid substance known as _____.

5. The small intestine is divided into three parts. They are:
   a.
   b.
   c.

6. What is the waste product of the liver?

7. What is the function of the gall bladder?

8. What is the short, worm-like tube attached to the cecum?

9. The _____ is the primary section of the intestines that absorbs water.

Digestive System

10. Figure 6.1

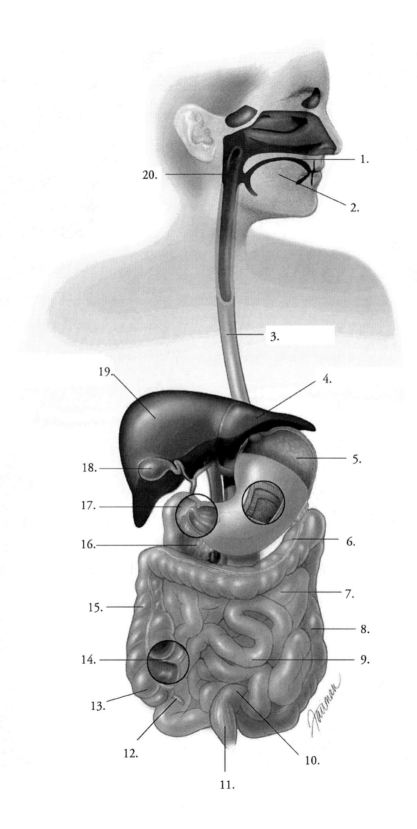

Digestive System

Fill in the blanks below with the corresponding numbers in the diagram on the previous page.

1. _____

2. _____

3. _____

4. _____

5. _____

6. _____

7. _____

8. _____

9. _____

10. _____

11. _____

12. _____

13. _____

14. _____

15. _____

16. _____

17. _____

18. _____

19. _____

20. _____

Chapter 7

Urinary System

The urinary system is also known as the urinary tract. The urinary tract is comprised of two kidneys, two ureters, a bladder, and urethra. The main function of the urinary system is to remove waste and excess fluids from the body. The process by which these wastes are removed is urination. Urination begins in the kidneys. There, waste products are filtered from the blood to be expelled in the form of urine. Once filtered, the waste product flows through the ureters to the bladder. Urine is stored in the bladder until it is voluntarily expelled through the urethra.

Please read this section which describes each of the organs of the urinary tract and their function in the urinary process in more detail.

Urinary System (Figure 7.1)

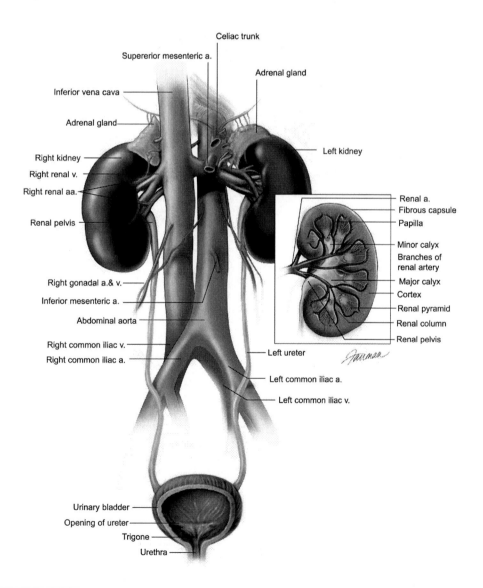

Urinary System

Urine Formation

The kidneys are bean shaped organs that lie on either side of the spine. The kidneys are supported by connective tissue. This connective tissue creates a protective layer around the kidneys. This layer is known as the renal capsule. Beneath the renal capsule the kidney has three distinct regions: the renal cortex, the renal medulla, and the renal pelvis.

The renal cortex is a thin layer of tissue that lies directly beneath the renal capsule. Beneath that lies the renal medulla, often referred to as renal pyramids due to their triangular shape.

Both the renal cortex and the renal medulla house millions of nephrons, which are the functional units of the kidneys. Nephrons are responsible for the production of urine.

The renal pelvis of the kidney is a flattened cavity that forms ducts which branch off from the renal medullae. These ducts are known as calyces. Urine is released into the renal cortex through calyces, which connect to form the ureter. It is through this tube that urine travels to the bladder.

Kidney (internal) (Figure 7.2)

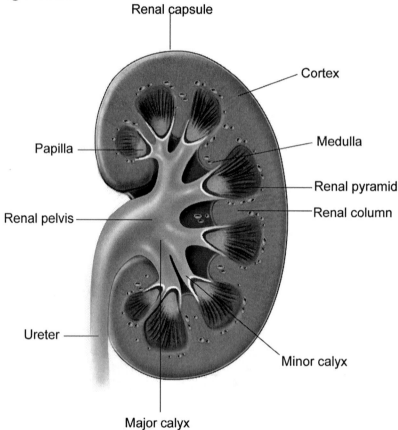

Urinary System

Kidney (midsagital) (Figure 7.3)

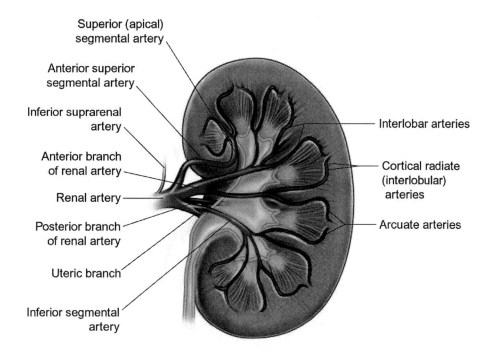

Urine Excretion

The ureters, urethra, and bladder are responsible for urine excretion. The ureters provide a means for the urine to travel from the kidneys into the bladder.

The bladder provides temporary storage for urine. The shape of the bladder changes to accommodate the amount of urine it stores. Once the bladder is full, nerves signal the brain that it needs to be emptied. Urine can be highly toxic – holding it in too long can cause an overgrowth of bacteria which could lead to infection or irritation.

The urethra is a thin tube through which urine leaves the body. The female urethra is quite short, approximately 1.5 inches long. Because of this, females are more inclined to contract urinary tract infections unlike their male counterparts whose urethra is approximately 8 inches long.

Practice Quiz: Urinary System

1. The process by which wastes are removed through the urinary system is called _____.

2. The protective layer around the kidneys is called the _____.

3. The three distinct regions of the kidney are:
   a.
   b.
   c.

4. In which organ of the urinary system is urine stored?

5. Why are females more inclined to contract urinary tract infections than men?

6. Figure 7.1

   Fill in the blanks on the following page with the corresponding numbers in the diagram below.

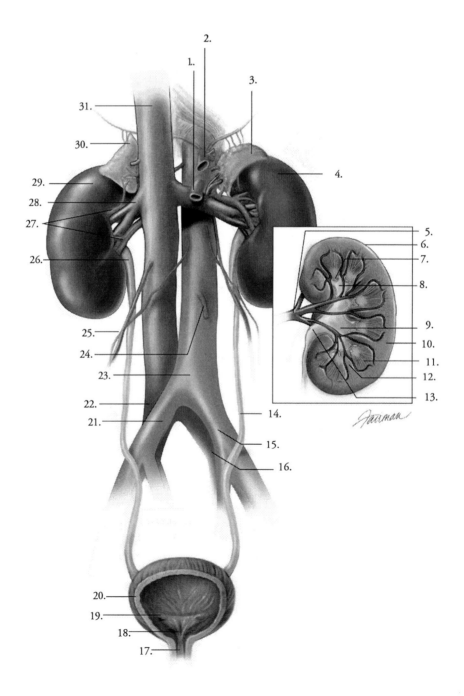

Urinary System

1. _____
2. _____
3. _____
4. _____
5. _____
6. _____
7. _____
8. _____
9. _____
10. _____
11. _____
12. _____
13. _____
14. _____
15. _____
16. _____
17. _____
18. _____
19. _____
20. _____
21. _____
22. _____
23. _____
24. _____
25. _____
26. _____
27. _____
28. _____
29. _____
30. _____
31. _____

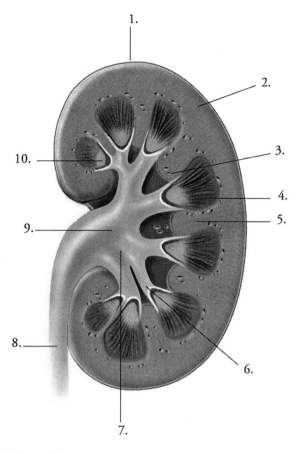

7. Figure 7.2

Fill in the blanks below with the corresponding numbers in the diagram above.

1. _____
2. _____
3. _____
4. _____
5. _____
6. _____
7. _____
8. _____
9. _____
10. _____

Urinary System

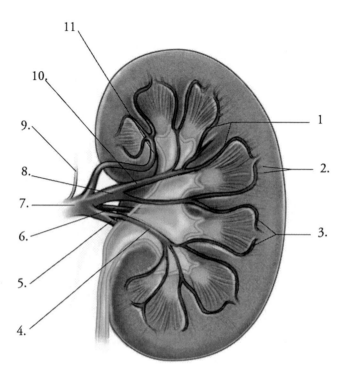

8. Figure 7.3

Fill in the blanks below with the corresponding numbers in the diagram above.

1. _____
2. _____
3. _____
4. _____
5. _____
6. _____
7. _____
8. _____
9. _____
10. _____
11. _____

Chapter 8

MALE GENITAL SYSTEM

The male genital system is comprised of the penis, testes, glands, and the scrotum. The primary function of the male genital system is to create and dispense hormones and sperm for the purpose of reproduction. Please read this section on the male genital system and the accessories which make up the male reproductive system.

Penis (Figure 8.1) and Testicle (Figure 8.2)

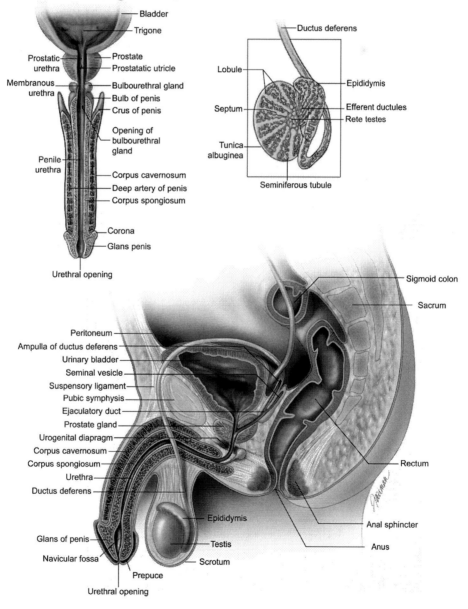

© 2011 Contexo Media

Testes

The paired testes, often termed testicles, are the male's sex glands. The testes are referred to as the sex glands because it is there that sperm and the male hormone, testosterone, are produced.

A capsule of fibrous tissue surrounds each testicle, providing both support and protection. This connective tissue forms to branch inward dividing the testes into many lobules. Each lobule contains a network of extremely coiled seminiferous tubules. The seminiferous tubules are where spermatogenisis, or sperm production occurs. Cells produced in the tubules continuously divide until they form what is commonly known as sperm or spermatozoa. The seminiferous tubules join to form ducts that connect to the epididymis, a massive, coiled tube that lies directly on top of the outer surface of the testes. The epididymis is divided into 3 regions. First the sperm enter into the caput, or head of the epididymis. Here they progress to the corpus, or body of the epididymis and finally to the cauda, or tail. As the sperm move through the 3 regions they mature and gain the ability to move independently. The mature sperm are then moved via the efferent ductules and stored inside the epididymis in preparation for ejaculation. When ejaculation occurs, the seminal vesicle, the bulbourethral glands, and the prostate gland add alkaline fluids which nourish the sperm and lubricate the urethra in preparation for ejaculation. The sperm travels from the epididymis through a muscular tube known as the ductus deferens or more commonly, the vas deferens. In the pelvic cavity, this tube connects to the urethra by way of an ejaculatory duct. Sperm travels through this pathway to be ejected from the body via the urethra. Interestingly enough, the vas deferens moves sperm by peristalsis, the same wave-like movement that occurs in the muscles of the digestive system.

The testes are housed in a sac of skin external to the body. This sac is known as the scrotum. The testes are actually located outside of the body due to the fact that sperm production requires a lower temperature than the body provides. Adequate sperm production and sustenance usually occurs in an environment of around 96.6 degrees, or an average of two to three degrees lower than normal body temperature. To facilitate this need, the scrotum contains muscles that function to help maintain an ideal testicular temperature. The muscles contained within the scrotum contract and relax in response to temperature change. For example, when the scrotum senses cooler temperatures, the muscles contract to bring the testis closer to the body to be warmed. Adversely, in warmer temperatures, the scrotum relaxes to allow testes to hang further away from the body to remain cool.

Penis

The penis is the male reproductive organ which functions to deposit the sperm needed for reproduction into the female vagina. The penis is composed of erectile tissues which enable it to become erect during copulation, as opposed to its normal relaxed, or flaccid state.

The penis is comprised of three columns of erectile tissue. The two separate columns that lie side by side are known as the corpora cavernosa (dorsal) while the third is known as the corpus spongiosum (ventral). The corpora cavernosa expands at the tip to form the glans penis, commonly known as the "head" of the penis, the rim of the glans is know as the corona.

During sexual arousal an erection occurs when the erectile tissues of the penis become engorged with blood. As a result of erection, the penis swells and becomes rigid. Ejaculation occurs from continuous stimulation of the penis, such as the result of sexual intercourse.

Male Hormones

The secondary function of the male reproductive system is the production of hormones to maintain reproductive control. The primary male hormone is known as testosterone. Testosterone is produced by leydig cells in the testes and is responsible for the maturation of male reproductive organs at puberty as well as the development of male secondary sexual characteristics such as the growth of body hair, voice changes, and increased muscular development.

Practice Quiz: Male Genital System

1. What is the primary male sex hormone?

2. What is the vas deferens?

3. To become erect _____ flows into the penis.
   a. Urine
   b. Blood
   c. Water

4. The vas deferens moves the semen and sperm via _____.

5. The sac of skin surrounding the testicles is called the _____.

Fill in the blanks on the following page with the corresponding numbers in the diagrams below.

6. Figure 8.1

7. Figure 8.2

8. Figure 8.3

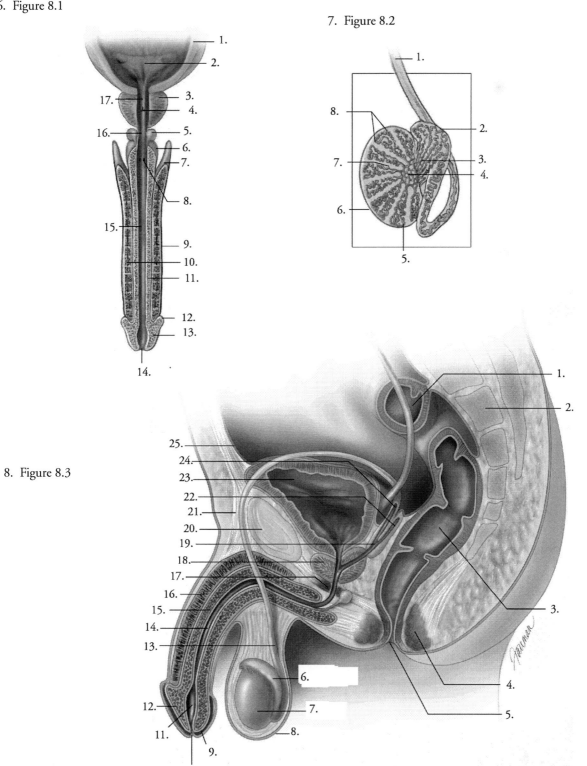

Male Genital System

6. Figure. 8.1

1. _____
2. _____
3. _____
4. _____
5. _____
6. _____
7. _____
8. _____
9. _____
10. _____
11. _____
12. _____
13. _____
14. _____
15. _____
16. _____
17. _____

7. Figure 8.2

1. _____
2. _____
3. _____
4. _____
5. _____
6. _____
7. _____
8. _____

8. Figure 8.3

1. _____
2. _____
3. _____
4. _____
5. _____
6. _____
7. _____
8. _____
9. _____
10. _____
11. _____
12. _____
13. _____
14. _____
15. _____
16. _____
17. _____
18. _____
19. _____
20. _____
21. _____
22. _____
23. _____
24. _____
25. _____

Chapter 9

Female Genital System

The female genital system is comprised of a pair of ovaries, a pair of fallopian tubes, uterus, vagina, as well as accessory glands, and external organs. The purpose of the female genital, or reproductive system, is to create and dispense hormones and eggs for the purpose of reproduction. The female reproductive system is also responsible for providing an environment for a developing fetus until it is ready to be born.

Female Genital (anterior) (Figure 9.1)

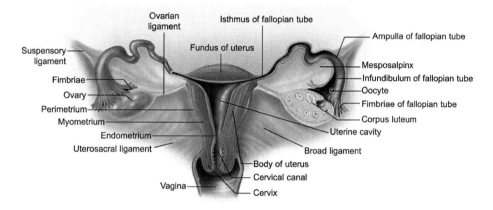

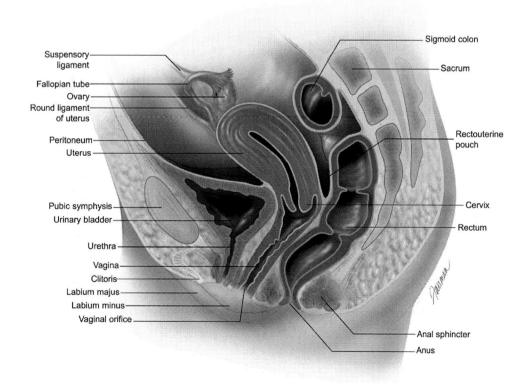

Ovaries

The ovaries are located on either side of the uterus in the pelvic cavity. They are held in place by various ligaments including the ovarian ligament, extending from the uterus to the ovary, and the suspensory ligament, extending from the ovary to the pelvic wall. The main function of the ovary is to produce eggs, and various feminine hormones. Inside the ovaries are multiple follicles that are the "birth place" of the eggs, and they also nurture the eggs until maturation. The brain produces FSH, follicle-stimulating hormones, that trigger an increase in the production of the female hormone estrogen. As estrogen levels continue to rise, they will eventually stop the production of FSH limiting the number of follicles that can reach maturation. As a type of natural selection, the dominant follicle will cause the others to die, and will continue to produce estrogen and progesterone. Progesterone is a hormone that will inhibit the development of new follicles, inhibit contractions of the uterus, and also prepare the endometrium for a possible pregnancy. Once the egg has matured, it is released into the fallopian tube, and the follicle develops into a small mass of tissue known as the corpus luteum, which will continue to produce estrogen and progesterone.

Fallopian Tubes

The fallopian tubes are hollow tubes that connect the ovaries to the uterus, and are an average of five inches in length. They are made mostly of concentric layers of smooth muscle that open into a funnel-like structure called the infundibulum that envelops the ovary. The infundibulum divides into finger-like projections called the fimbrae that hold the ovary. Once a mature egg has been released, the fimbrae move in swinging, pendulum-like movements to assist in guiding it into the fallopian tube from the ovary. The tubes are lined with small hair-like projections called cilia that move the egg down into the intramural portion of the fallopian tube. This is the area where the tube passes through the uterine wall and deposits the egg into the uterus.

The fallopian tubes are the most common location for fertilization to occur. If the cilia are damaged in any way, scar tissue is present, an infection occurs, or any type of blockage is present, the egg may not pass into the uterus. If the fertilized egg remains in the fallopian tube, it can attach to the wall of the tube and an ectopic pregnancy may occur.

Uterus

The uterus is a hollow muscular organ whose main function is to hold and protect a baby during pregnancy, and to push the baby out during delivery. The uterus is an average of three inches long, two inches wide, and has three distinct layers. The first layer is the endometrium, the innermost layer of the uterus. As the ovarian follicles produce estrogen and progesterone the endometrium will thicken in preparation for a fertilized egg. If an egg is present, it will attach to the endometrium and a placenta will form around the egg to supply it with oxygen and nourishment. If fertilization does not occur, the endometrium lining will break down and shed. The uterus will periodically contract to help expel the lining in a process called menstruation. These contractions can sometimes be painful and are commonly referred to as cramps. The next layer of the uterus is the myometrium. This layer is responsible for supporting the vascular tissue of the uterus and is made of smooth muscle cells. After a pregnancy and delivery has occurred, the myometrium will contract and expel the placenta. The third layer of the uterus is the perimetrium. This is the serous layer composed mainly of loose connective tissue, and it also contains a large number of lymphatic vessels. Because of its proximity to the bladder, infection often causes uterine symptoms, especially during pregnancy. The cervix is located at the base of the uterus joining it to the vagina.

Vagina

The vagina, also known as the birth canal, is a tubular canal about four inches long and one inch in diameter. It extends from the cervix to the vaginal opening that exits the body. The main functions of the vagina are: to receive the penis for intercourse, provide sexual pleasure for the female, provide a path for menstrual flow and other secretions, and also to provide safe passage for the exit of the baby during birth. The vagina can expand up to two to three times its average size for sexual intercourse and child birth. There are glands located near the vaginal opening and near the cervix that secrete lubrication for intercourse. There are no glands actually located in the vagina, but rather, their secretions seep through the vaginal wall. Just before the vaginal opening is the opening of the urethra. This is a hollow tube that extends from the urinary bladder to the vaginal opening allowing the expulsion of urine.

Located outside the vaginal opening are the exterior genital organs. All of these exterior structures are collectively known as the vulva. The largest structures outside of the vaginal orifice are the labium minora and majora. These are the smaller and larger skin folds that resemble lips and are homologous to the male's scrotum. Above the labium majora is an area called the mons pubis, which is an elevation of adipose tissue covered by skin and course pubic hair. The purpose of the mons pubis is to cushion the pubic symphysis, the area between the left and right pubic bones, from impact during intercourse. Directly below the mons pubis, and between the folds of the labium majora, is the clitoris. The clitoris is a small mass of erectile tissue homologous to the male penis.

Female Hormones

Hormone production is another function of the female genital system. The two major hormones produced by the female body are progesterone and estrogen. Estrogen is produced by the ovaries and is responsible for the development of female secondary sexual characteristics which include development of the mammary glands and breasts, broadening of the pelvis, pubic hair, as well as the increase of blood supply to the skin.

Progesterone, also produced by the ovarian follicles, is responsible for the monthly breakdown of the uterine lining. It also stimulates contractions and dilation of the cervix.

Practice Quiz: Female Genital System

1. Once an ovarian follicle releases an egg, it then develops into a small mass of tissue known as the _____.

2. The end of a fallopian tube graduates into a funnel shaped extension known as _____.

3. _____, finger like projections, assist in guiding the egg into the fallopian tubes.

4. The endometrium, myometrium, and perimetrium are three distinct layers of the _____.

5. The accessory organs of the vagina are collectively known as _____.

6. The two major hormones produced by the female body are:

    a. _____

    b. _____

Female Genital System

Figure 9.1

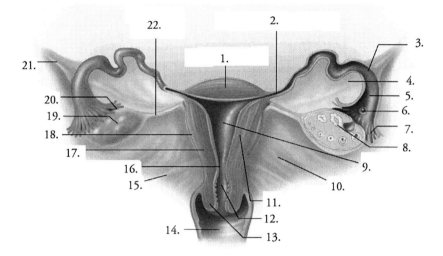

Figure 9.2

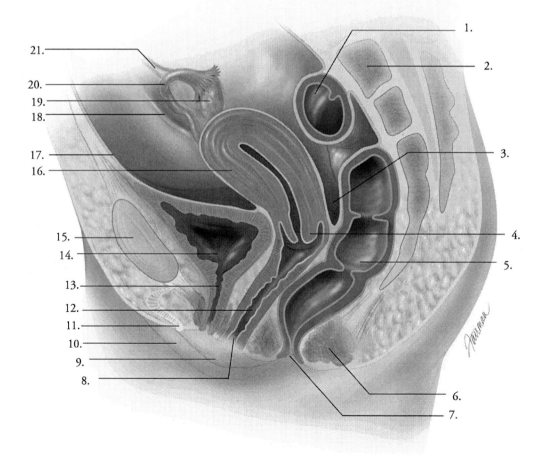

Female Genital System

7. Figure 9.1

Fill in the blanks below with the corresponding numbers in the diagram on the previous page.

1. _____

2. _____

3. _____

4. _____

5. _____

6. _____

7. _____

8. _____

9. _____

10. _____

11. _____

12. _____

13. _____

14. _____

15. _____

16. _____

17. _____

18. _____

19. _____

20. _____

21. _____

22. _____

8. Figure 9.2

Fill in the blanks below with the corresponding numbers in the diagram on the previous page.

1. _____

2. _____

3. _____

4. _____

5. _____

6. _____

7. _____

8. _____

9. _____

10. _____

11. _____

12. _____

13. _____

14. _____

15. _____

16. _____

17. _____

18. _____

19. _____

20. _____

21. _____

Chapter 10

ENDOCRINE SYSTEM

The endocrine system is the body's method of maintaining chemical balance through the secretion of hormones. A hormone is a substance that is conveyed by an organ, gland, or body part, to chemically stimulate that part to increase or decrease functional activity, or to increase or decrease the secretion/production of another hormone. Glands and tissues that secrete hormones are prevalent in many sections of the body. Please read the section below concerning the many endocrine glands and tissues, their location in the human body, and how the release of hormones effects the body.

Brain

There are three types of hormone producing glands in the brain. They are the hypothalamus, pineal, and pituitary glands.

The hypothalamus produces hormones that stimulate other glands to produce their own hormones. This process is integral for maintaining homeostasis. Homeostasis describes the physical and chemical confines that the body must operate within to maintain correct functioning of its parts. The hypothalamus regulates blood pressure, thirst, hunger, and body temperature.

The pineal gland is a tiny gland that secretes melatonin. Melatonin is responsible for influencing circadian rhythm. Circadian rhythm is commonly known as the "internal body clock." This process governs biological cycles in the body such as sleep-wake cycles.

The pituitary gland is often referred to as the "master gland." This gland (no larger than the size of a pea) is responsible for controlling many other endocrine glands. This little gland is divided into two lobes, each part being responsible for separate actions. The anterior lobe produces hormones that stimulate growth, activates milk production in breastfeeding women, and stimulates both the thyroid gland and the adrenal gland to produce their hormones. The posterior lobe of the pituitary gland maintains control over water, balance, and the release of oxytocin (the hormone which triggers contractions in the female uterus during labor).

The pituitary also secretes chemicals that interact with the nervous system in order to minimize sensitivity to pain. It also ensures that the ovaries and testes are producing sex hormones.

Thyroid

The thyroid gland is located in the neck between the larynx and the trachea. This gland produces thyroxine and triiodothryonine, both of which control metabolism. As discussed earlier, the pituitary gland controls the hormones that the thyroid releases.

Unlike many other glands, the thyroid can store the hormones that it produces.

Attached to the thyroid are four tiny glands known as parathyroid glands. The glands located here are responsible for regulating the amount of calcium found in the blood.

Heart

The heart produces hormones a hormone called atriopeptin which regulates blood pressure and the amount of blood produced.

Adrenal

Adrenal glands, of which there are two, are located directly on top of each kidney. These triangular glands have two parts, each of which produces hormones that perform different functions. The adrenal cortex produces corticosteroids which are responsible for regulating the amount of salt in relation to water in the body. It also influences the body's reaction to stress, the rate of metabolism, as well as sexual and immune function. The adrenal medulla produces adrenaline, the body's "fight or flight" hormone. This hormone is released when the body experiences stress, fear, or extreme urgency.

Kidney

The kidneys produce a hormone called erythropoietin, which stimulates the production of red blood cells. The lack of erythropoietin is often responsible for the condition known as anemia.

Pancreas

The pancreas produces hormones that regulate the amount of glucose (sugar) in the blood. This function is important for homeostasis. Higher or lower levels of glucose in the blood can lead to a condition known as diabetes.

Stomach and Intestines

The stomach and the intestines both produce more than 22 different enzymes that aid in the digestion of food. Pepsin is an enzyme that breaks down protein, while gelatinase breaks down gelatin, and amilayse breaks down starch.

Ovaries and Testes

The two female ovaries produce the female sex hormones, estrogen and progesterone. The two male testes produce the male sex hormone testosterone.

© 2011 Contexo Media

Practice Quiz: Endocrine System

Please match up the following functions/hormones with the endocrine gland/body part that performs the function.

1. _____ Brain
2. _____ Thyroid
3. _____ Heart
4. _____ Adrenal
5. _____ Kidney
6. _____ Pancreas
7. _____ Stomach and intestines
8. _____ Ovaries and testes

a. produces female and male sex hormones

b. this gland can store the hormones it produces

c. stimulates the production of red blood cells

d. regulates the amount of sugar (glucose) in the blood

e. has three types of hormone producing glands: hypothalamus, pineal, and pituitary

f. produces enzymes that aid digestion

g. produces atriopeptin which regulates blood pressure

h. produces the "fight or flight" hormones

Chapter 11

NERVOUS SYSTEM

The nervous system is essentially the body's message center. It is, in fact, the most complicated and highly organized of all body systems. Through vast pathways of nerves, neurons, and sensations, the brain communicates with the body, informing it of pain, helping to move any of the voluntary muscles in the body, and controlling what a person thinks and how they feel about those thoughts. The nervous system is an ever watchful eye that carefully scrutinizes actions occurring inside the body as well as those on the outside.

Nervous System (Figure 11.1)

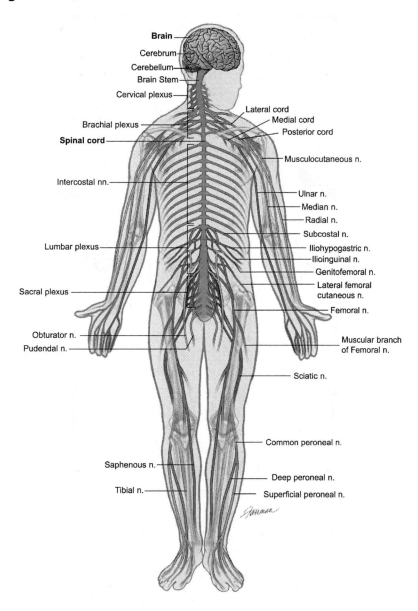

The nervous system is divided into two parts, the central nervous system (CNS) and the peripheral nervous system (PNS). The CNS, which consists of the brain and spinal cord, is the body's command center. It tells the rest of the body what to do. The PNS, which consists of nerves, serves as a liaison between the CNS and the rest of the body. It consists of nerves and sensory receptors which branch from the CNS to connect the CNS with tissues and organs in the body.

The PNS is subdivided into three categories: the autonomic, sensory, and motor nervous system.

Autonomic — The autonomic nervous system controls involuntary actions.

Sensory — The sensory nervous system transports information from the body to the CNS.

Motor — The motor nervous system transports signals from the brain to the rest of the body which facilitates voluntary movement.

Structure of the Nervous System

The nervous system is made of many organs and structures, all of which are designed to sense, pain, happiness, or movement. These structures, which will be described in detail below, are briefly described as the brain, spinal cord, nerves, and sensory receptors.

The following section covers the anatomical structures of the nervous system:

Brain

The brain is one of the most important organs in the human body, not to mention, one of the largest. The brain, which weighs approximately 3 pounds, is responsible for a wide range of activities such as movement, thought, emotions, and feelings.

The brain consists of three parts: the forebrain, the brain stem, and the hindbrain. Of the three parts, the forebrain is the most complex. The forebrain is responsible for a person's ability to feel, learn, and remember.

Brain (Figure 11.2)

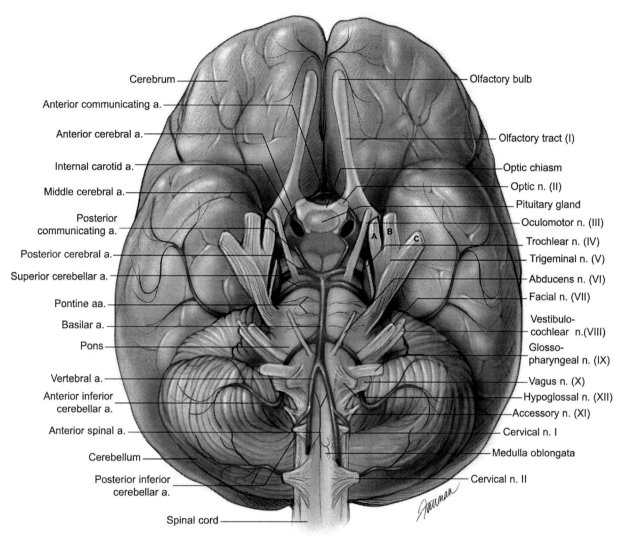

Forebrain

The forebrain is further divided into two parts: the telencephalon and the diencephalon.

Telencephalon

The telencephalon contains the cerebral cortex and the corpus callosum. The cerebral cortex is divided into right and left hemispheres. Both the left and right sides work together to control thinking, reasoning, language apprehension, perception, hearing, sense of smell and vision, as well as voluntary movements. Not surprisingly, the cerebral cortex encompasses at least two-thirds of the entire brain mass due to the fact that it has more responsibility.

The corpus callosum is a thick band of tissue that separates the left and the right regions of the cerebral cortex. The primary function of the corpus callosum is to integrate motor, sensory, and cognitive performances between then two hemispheres of the cerebral cortex.

Diencephalon

The diencephalon consists of the thalamus and hypothalamus. The thalamus is responsible for connecting the areas of the cerebral cortex that are responsible for sensory perception and regulation of motor functions, such as movement, to other parts of the brain and spinal cord that also play a role in those functions. As noted in chapter 10, the hypothalamus has a significant role in daily body maintenance. It is involved in the production and regulation of hormones, emotions, body temperature, appetite, thirst, arousal, heartbeat, fluid balance, and glandular function, to name a few.

Brainstem

The brainstem, which resembles a small branch, consists of the midbrain and the upper portion of the brainstem. The brainstem connects the brain and the spinal cord. It controls many basic voluntary and involuntary functions such as breathing, heart rate, eating, swallowing, and sleeping.

Hindbrain

The hindbrain is the lower portion of the brainstem. It consists of three parts: the medulla oblongata, the pons, and the cerebellum.

Medulla Oblongata — The medulla oblongata controls involuntary functions such as digestion, respiration, and blood pressure.

Pons — This part of the brainstem provides a connection which makes it possible for the medulla oblongata and the thalamus to communicate.

Cerebellum — This cauliflower-shaped portion of the brain is primarily responsible for the coordination of movement. It does not actually initiate movement, rather facilitates the synchronization of voluntary muscular function. The cerebellum is responsible for muscle tone, hand-eye-coordination, and balance.

Spinal Cord

The spinal cord is a thick bundle of nerves that runs down the inside center of the spine, from the brain. It provides a pathway from the brain to the nervous system. The spinal cord is divided into 4 distinct regions the cervical, thoracic, lumbar and sacral regions. The spinal cord is protected from injury by the spinal column. The nerves that occupy each of these regions are responsible for performing different functions within the human body.

Cervical Nerves — Cervical nerves provide sensation to the head, neck, diaphragm, arms, wrists, and hands.

Thoracic Nerves — Thoracic nerves supply impulses to the chest and abdominal muscles.

Lumbar Nerves — Lumbar nerves provide sensation to the muscles of the legs.

Sacral Nerves — Sacral nerves provide impulses that affect movement of the bowel and bladder, as well as stimuli that aid in sexual function.

Nerves

There are two types of nerves that can be found throughout the human body: nerves that carry messages only one way and nerves that carry messages back and forth.

Sensory nerves — Also called motor nerves when they carry signals from the brain, sensory nerves are one-way nerves that carry information to the brain.

Mixed nerves — Motor nerves are two-way nerves that carry information both to the brain from the body and from the body to the brain.

Nerve Structure

Nerves are comprised of nerve tissue and consists of bundles of nerve cells, also called neurons. These nerves branch out from the spinal cord and continue to branch off in different directions to eventually occupy every part of the human body.

Nerve Function

The nervous system serves as the body's message center. These messages are sent through the body in the form of electrical impulses. These electrical impulses inspire the body to perform various voluntary and involuntary functions, such as breathing, eating, sleeping, walking, etc. Nerve cells have to be able to communicate and respond to stimuli immediately. In fact, the body's electrical impulses can travel up to 250 miles per hour. The immediate reaction comes in handy especially if something hot is touched. The body needs to be able to respond to such a thing quickly, or else risk greater injury to the body.

Sensations

Bodies detect many sensations every day. Sensations occur as a result of the body becoming aware of an environmental change either inside or outside of the body. They are produced when nerve impulses reach the cerebral cortex. Sensations are translated by the body by two methods: projection and adaptation.

Projection

When the body is injured, the brain receives a message and pain is felt. The projection of sensations is a survival mechanism to let the brain know when any part of the body is in a state requiring repair in order to function normally.

Adaptation

When adaptation occurs, a person is also aware of changes that have occurred within the body. Once senses become accustomed to this new stimulus, the body no longer notices it. This mechanism keeps a person from overloading the senses and responding unnecessarily to stimuli. For example, when a new ring is placed on a finger, the body feels it for a while, but after wearing it for a period of time, the body becomes accustomed to it because the body no longer needs to send alerts to the fact that it is there.

There are general senses that are distributed throughout the body. These general senses provide the capability to sense changes in temperature, to sense pressure, and to sense pain. These are known as internal senses, along with the ability to sense that one is hungry or thirsty. There are also specialized senses. These are known as the five senses which are described in more detail below.

The Five Senses – External Senses

The five senses are a working part of the nervous system that heighten awareness to surroundings at all times. In fact, they are sometimes referred to as external senses. The body is filled with nerve cells that stimulate each of these senses into action, giving the capability to react to environmental changes. The five senses are as follows:

Sense of Sight

Sense of sight could possibly be the most complex of the senses. Not only do the eyes function to 'see' things, they also help one remember the things that are seen by storing a visual representation in the brain, and this is an intricate process.

Eyes do not actually see things as they are, but rather see reflections of light bouncing off of the objects into eyes. The reflections of light that bounce off of the object into the eyes do so by first passing through the cornea. The cornea is a clear, thick layer that protects the surface of the eye. As light passes through the cornea, it bends.

Once light passes through the cornea, it then travels through the pupil to the lens. The pupil is the opening in the center of the iris, the colored part of the eye. The pupil expands and contracts in size depending upon how much light is present. The pupil will enlarge if there is not enough light to see, and it will shrink if there is too much light.

Once the light passes through the pupil, it will pass through the lens. The lens of the eye functions much as the lens of a camera. It focuses the image produced by the beams of light through the vitreous humor, a jelly-like substance.

Once focused, this image is then reflected onto the retina. The retina is a light sensitive membrane that lines the inside of the eye. It is filled with millions of photoreceptors or light-sensitive, cells. There are two types of photoreceptor cells present in the eye and they are called rods and cones. Even though they are both photoreceptor cells, their functions are quite different.

Rods help identify shapes. They work the best in dim light, so they allow a person to see in black and white. Cones allow one to see in color. Unlike rods, cones work the best in bright light.

Once rods and cones receive the image, with assistance from the optic nerve, they then send the image to the brain. The image that the brain receives is upside down. The brain then takes the upside down image and turns it right side up, which is then translated into sight at a speed of 186,000 miles per second.

Sense of Smell

The primary organs for sense of smell are located in the nose. They are olfactory chemoreceptor cells which are located in the upper nasal cavity. These cells sift through the millions of odor particles that are floating around at every second of every day. Odor particles are the culprits responsible for causing smells. In some cases, these odor particles produce pleasant smells while other times they don't. Either way, if the odor particles are strong enough, they will send a message to the brain and cause the body to react.

Sense of Taste

There are almost 10,000 taste buds inside the mouth, which allow one to experience many variations of taste. Essentially, the taste buds are the taste organs. They are located in large numbers all over the tongue. These taste cells have to be activated by liquid, which is generally saliva. There are four different types of taste receptors present on the tongue; they are simply labeled: sweet, sour, salty, and bitter.

The salty and sweet taste cells are located near the tip and front of the tongue. The sour taste receptors are located on the sides of the tongue, while the bitter taste receptors are on the very back of the tongue.

Nervous System

Sense of Touch

The skin is outfitted with many nerves that provide the brain with information about the body's environment. The cells that provide the sense of touch are called mechanoreceptors and are located deep within the dermis of the skin. Mechanoreceptors are located in all areas covered by skin and respond to stimulation when they are disturbed. This sensation plays a vital role by alerting the body to hot or cold sensations that may threaten the body.

Sense of Hearing

Hearing is not only important as a medium to hear sounds, it also helps to maintain balance and posture. The ears are the hearing organ. All sounds are a result of how the ears translate vibrations. These vibrations are known as sound waves. As sound waves travel through the air, the vibrations travel through the ear canal. The ear canal is a portion of the outer ear. The outer ear consists of three parts: the auricle, ear canal, and tympanic membrane. The auricle is the cartilaginous part of the ear that is visible outside of the body. The ear canal leads to the inner ear, and the tympanic membrane is the eardrum. The tympanic membrane vibrates at the same frequency as the sound waves that vibrate in and out. The eardrum, in turn, vibrates three of the smallest bones in the human body: the anvil, the hammer, and the stirrup. These three bones are collectively known as ear ossicles, which make up the middle ear.

The stirrup of the middle ear passes the vibrations to the cochlea. The cochlea is a coiled, fluid filled tube located within the inner ear. The cochlea literally contains hundreds of nerve endings or, "little hairs", called cilia. When the vibrations pass over these cilia, they report this disturbance to the brain, and the brain then translates the disturbance into sound.

Balance and posture is maintained partially by the ear. At the top of the cochlea, there is a small network of loops. These loops, the semi-circular canals, are also filled with fluid. As the body moves, the liquid moves as well. The fluid movement stimulates the cilia, which in turn sends signals to the brain indicating to the brain that their is movement.

Practice Quiz: Nervous System

1. The nervous system is divided into two parts. They are:

    a. _____

    b. _____

2. Please list the three parts of the brain:

    a. _____

    b. _____

    c. _____

3. The _____ separates the two hemispheres of the cerebral cortex:

    a. telencephalon   c. corpus callosum

    b. diancephalon   d. pons

4. The cauliflower shaped part of brain that is responsible for the coordination of movement is the:

    a. cerebellum   c. corpus callosum

    b. cerebral cortex   d. telencephalon

5. The _____ is a pea-sized portion of the brain that is responsible for many critical bodily functions.

    a. thalamus   c. telencephalon

    b. hypothalamus   d. diancephalon

6. The _____ is a thick bundle of nerves that runs down the inside of the spine.

7. Please list the two types of nerves that can be found throughout the human body:

    a. _____

    b. _____

8. The mechanism that keeps the body from overloading senses and responding to unnecessary stimuli is called:

    a. projection   c. sensation

    b. adaptation   d. communication

9. Please match the following cells to the part of the body in which they are present:

    _____ Olfactory chemoreceptor cells

    _____ Photoreceptor cells

    _____ Mechanoreceptor cells

         a. Eyes

         b. Nose

         c. Skin

Nervous System

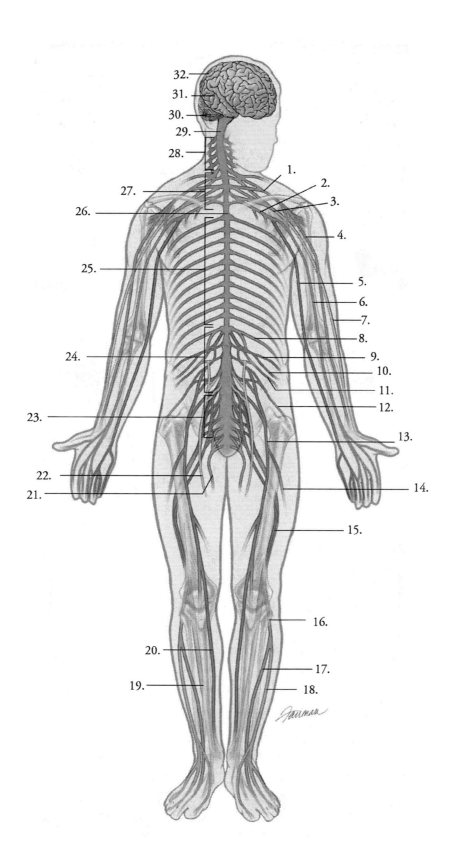

Nervous System

10. Figure 11.1

Fill in the blanks below with the corresponding numbers in the diagram on the previous page.

1. _____
2. _____
3. _____
4. _____
5. _____
6. _____
7. _____
8. _____
9. _____
10. _____
11. _____
12. _____
13. _____
14. _____
15. _____

16. _____
17. _____
18. _____
19. _____
20. _____
21. _____
22. _____
23. _____
24. _____
25. _____
26. _____
27. _____
28. _____
29. _____
30. _____
31. _____
32. _____

Nervous System

Match each number with the corresponding term.

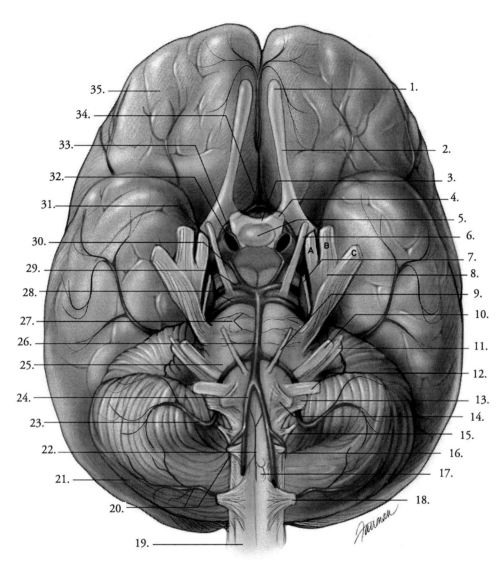

Trigeminal Nerve (V) branches:
A Ophthalmic branch
B Maxillary branch
C Mandibular branch

Nervous System

11. Figure 11.2

Fill in the blanks below with the corresponding numbers in the diagram on the previous page.

1. _____
2. _____
3. _____
4. _____
5. _____
6. _____
7. _____
8. _____
9. _____
10. _____
11. _____
12. _____
13. _____
14. _____
15. _____
16. _____

17. _____
18. _____
19. _____
20. _____
21. _____
22. _____
23. _____
24. _____
25. _____
26. _____
27. _____
28. _____
29. _____
30. _____
31. _____
32. _____
33. _____
34. _____
35. _____

Chapter 12

IMMUNE SYSTEM

The immune system is essentially the body's defense mechanism, designed to protect it from harmful pathogens, such as diseases. When pathogens enter the body, the immune system responds with specific and non-specific resistance.

Immune Response

Non-Specific Resistance

Non-specific resistance serves to protect the body from all pathogens, but it is not directed toward a specific pathogen. Non-specific defense mechanisms manifest themselves as mechanical barriers, chemical actions, phagocytosis, inflammation, and fever.

Mechanical Barriers — Mechanical barriers can be found in the skin and mucous membranes throughout the body. Skin acts a mechanical barrier by attacking bacteria on contact. It contains its own bacteria that prevent foreign pathogens from multiplying once they reach its surface. Other mechanical barriers include tears, saliva, and urine. These fluids assist by flushing out harmful bacteria before they reach bodily tissue.

Chemical Actions — Many areas of the body produce chemicals and enzymes which help attack harmful bacteria. One example is pepsin, a digestive enzyme produced by the stomach. Pepsin works by digesting the proteins of which the microbes are composed.

Phagocytosis — Phagocytosis can be briefly defined as the ingestion of bacteria by phagocytes, which are cells that are designed to be able to break down foreign particles, cell debris, and disease producing microorganisms.

Inflammation — Inflammation is a localized response to cellular injury. When cellular injury occurs, it may become inflamed. Inflammation is recognized as the reddening, swelling, and painfulness of tissues with injured cells.

Fever — Fevers fight off harmful microorganisms by heating them up. The increase in body temperature can inhibit the growth of certain pathogens. Fevers are one of the body's natural defenses that can be quite helpful, yet equally harmful if the body temperature goes too high.

Specific Resistance

Specific resistance, or immunity, occurs when the body directs the immune responses at a specific pathogen. There are two types of immunity: cell-mediated immunity and antibody-mediated immunity.

Types of Immunity

Cell-Mediated Immunity

In this type of immunity, the body's defense cells, lymphocytes, attack pathogens directly. The body contains thousands of different lymphocytes, each of which are capable of responding to different antigens (cells that the body sees as foreign) and pathogens. The type of cell that handles the body's cell-mediated immunity is the T-cell. T-cells keep the body from getting the same infection again. Once they have already acted to protect the body from an antigen or pathogen, T-cells essentially leave behind memory cells which recognize the antigen or pathogen it already conquered. These memory cells function by recognizing the antigen or pathogen to protect the body more quickly. Of course, many viruses, such as the flu, tend to repeat themselves and still cause infection because there are many different strains. If the virus changes even slightly, the body treats it as a new antigen.

As discussed earlier, there are many types of T-cells. All T-cells work together and communicate through chemical secretions. The major types of T-cells and their function are listed below.

Killer T-cells — These cells attach to antigens and release toxins to destroy them

Helper T-cells — These cells release secretions that stimulate immune responses

Suppressor T-cells — Adversely stop immune response

Memory T-cells — Aid in the "remembering" of antigens that have invaded the body so that it can respond very quickly to destroy it.

Antibody-Mediated Immunity

An antibody is a protein produced by plasma cells in response to the presence of an antigen. The cells responsible for antibody-mediated immunity are B-cells. Like T-cells, there are thousands of types of B-Cells. They too respond to specific types of pathogens. When a pathogen enters the system, some make their way to lymph tissue. When they do, the B-cells respond by multiplying. When this occurs, most of the B-cells change into plasma cells. Plasma cells create massive amounts of antibodies to attack the pathogen. These cells also leave behind memory cells to keep the same pathogen from infecting the body again.

Antibodies are also known as immunoglobulins, which is abbreviated as Ig. There are several classes of Ig (immunoglobulins). They are:

IgG — These are the most abundant of all antibodies. They are effective fighters against bacteria and viruses. They are the only type of immunoglobulins that temporarily provide developing fetuses with immunity. They also assist newborns with immunity for the first six months of their life.

IgA — These protect mucous membranes from attack by pathogens. They can be found in tears, mucus, breast milk, and saliva.

IgM — These fight by causing agglugination (clumping of red blood cells) or by attaching themselves to the antigens.

IgE — Stimulates cells to release histamine, which causes allergic reactions.

IgD — Bind to antigens resulting in B-cell activation.

Immune Responses

There are two ways in which the immune system works: through passive and active immune responses. Each type of immune response is categorized as being naturally or artificially induced.

Active Immunity — Active immunity prevents the body from contracting a disease once already present in the system. The body develops natural active immunity from having been exposed to antigens. Artificial active immunity is acquired through vaccination. Vaccines are actually foreign substances in a "dead" state that are injected into the system. The body attacks this virus and, in turn, this pathogen is remembered by memory cells so that if infected by the disease, the body could more readily defend itself.

Passive Immunity — Passive immunity provides temporary defense against disease. This type of immunity is derived from an injection of antibodies actively produced by another organism. Natural passive immunity occurs in newborn infants as they receive the antibodies in the mother's breast milk, which temporarily protects them from disease. Artificial passive immunity is acquired as a result of an individual receiving an injection of gammaglobulins which contain antibodies to, again, temporarily, protect them from the disease.

Practice Quiz: Immune System

1. An immune response that increases body temperature is know as a _____.

2. The most prevalent type of antibody is _____.

3. _____ stimulates cells to release histamine.

4. Saliva and tears are considered _____ barriers.

Chapter 13

ROOT WORDS

Introduction to Medical Terminology

Medical terminology is one of the main key components of medical coding. Medical coders are reviewing medical procedures and diagnoses constantly, so it makes sense that they would need to understand medical terms in order to code properly. When first learning medical terminology, it may appear as if one is attempting to learn a new language! This is undoubtedly so, as medical terms are derived from Latin and Greek, which are not used in everyday language outside the medical profession. In order to understand medical terms and their meanings, it is important that a medical coder be able to dissect the term, analyze the components, and know the associations of the words.

Root Words and Compound Words

Root words are the main components of a word. The root of a word is the basic element used to derive the meaning of the term. Most medical root words refer to a body part, body system, procedure, or disease. The medical term *cystocele* is composed of the word root *cysto-*, meaning bladder (or pouch) and the suffix, which will be discussed later, *–cele*, meaning hernia. Thus, cystocele means a herniation of the urinary bladder. Root words may be at the beginning, middle, or end of a term. Root words may have prefixes attached to the beginning of the term, or suffixes attached to the end of the term (both of these will be discussed later in this lesson).

Table of Common Root Words

Word Component	Meaning	Example
Abdomin(o)-	Abdomen	Abdominalgia - pain in the abdomen.
Acanth-	Spine	Acanthion - a point at the tip of the anterior nasal spine.
Acou-	Hearing	Acoustic - pertaining to sound or to the sense of hearing.
Acro-	Extremity, sharp	Acroesthesia - pain in the extremities.
Aden(o)-	Gland	Adenopathy - glandular disease.
Adipo-	Fat	Adipokinesis - the mobilization of fat in the body.
Aero-	Air	Aerobe - a microorganism that can live and grow in the presence of free oxygen.
Alb-	White	Albino - a person afflicted with albinism.
Algo-	Pain	Algospasm - painful spasm or cramp.
Amnio-	Fetal envelope	Amniocentesis - percutaneous transabdominal puncture of the uterus to obtain amniotic fluid.
Andr(o)-	Male	Androgenic - causing masculinization.
Angi(o)-	Vessel	Angioplasty - any endovascular procedure that reopens narrowed blood vessels and restores forward blood flow.
Ankyl-	Growing together of parts	Ankylocheilia - adhesion of the lips to each other.
Anthro-	Human	Anthropometer - an instrument especially designed for measuring various dimensions of the human body.
Artero-	Artery (vessel carrying blood away from heart)	Arteriolopathy - any disease of the arterioles.

© 2011 Contexo Media

101

Root Words

Word Component	Meaning	Example
Arthr(o)-	Joint	Arthrodesis - the surgical immobilization of a joint.
Artic-	Little joint	Articulated - consisting of separate segments joined as to be movable on each other.
Asthm-	Short of breath	Asthmatiform - resembling asthma.
Atri-	Entry chamber	Atriomegaly - abnormal dilation or enlargement of an atrium of the heart.
Axilla-	Armpit	Axillobifemoral - pertaining to the axillary artery and both femoral arteries.
Bili-	Bile	Biliary - pertaining to bile.
Bleph-	Eyelid	Blepharectomy - excision of a lesion of the eyelids.
Brachi(o)-	Arm	Brachialgia - intense pain in the arm.
Brady-	Slow	Bradykinesia - extreme slowness of movement.
Calc(i)-	Calcium	Calciuria - calcium in the urine.
Calc(o)-	Heel	Calcaneodynia - pain in the heel, or the calcaneus and the fibula.
Carbo-	Charcoal, carbon	Carbonate - any salt of carbonic acid.
Carcin(o)-	Cancer	Carcinogenic - producing cancer.
Cardio(o)-	Heart	Cardiovascular - pertaining to the heart and blood vessels.
Carpo-	Wrist	Carpocarpal - pertaining to two parts of the carpus, especially to the articulations between carpal bones.
Caud-	Tail	Caudad - toward the tail; in a posterior position.
Cephal(o)-	Head	Cephalic - cranial.
Cereb-	Brain	Cerebrifugal - conducting or proceeding away from the brain.
Cerebr(o)-	Cerebrum	Cerebrotomy - incision of the brain to evacuate an abcess.
Cervic(i)(o)-	Neck	Cervical - pertaining to or in the region of the neck.
Chemo-	Chemistry	Chemocautery - destruction of tissue by application of caustic chemical substance.
Chlor(o)-	Green	Chlorophane - a green-yellow pigment in the retina.
Chol(e)-	Bile	Cholangitis - inflammation of the bile ducts.
Chondr(o)	Cartilage	Chondroplasty - plastic or reparative surgery on the cartilage.
Chrom(o)-	Color	Chromatometer - a scale of colors for testing color perception.
Cili-	Eyelash	Ciliarotomy - surgical division of the ciliary zone for glaucoma.
Cost(o)-	Rib	Costectomy - surgical excision or resection of a rib.
Cox-	Hip	Coxalgia - pain in the hip.
Cut-	Skin	Cutaneous - pertaining to the skin.
Cyan(o)-	Blue	Cyanobacteria - blue-green bacteria.
Cyst(i)(o)-	Bladder	Cystalgia - pain in the bladder.
Cyt(o)-	Cell	Cytogenic - producing cells or promoting the production of cells.
Dacry(o)-	Tear	Dacryocele - protrusion of a lacrimal sac.
Dacty-	Fingers, digits	Dactyledema - swelling of the fingers or toes.
Dens/Dent-	Tooth	Dentagra - a forcep or key for extracting teeth.
Derm-	Skin	Dermatopathology - the study of skin diseases.
Dors(i)(o)-	Back	Dorsal - pertaining to the back.
Echin-	Spiny	Echinulate - having small prickles or spines; applied in bacteriology to cultures showing toothed or pointed outgrowths.

102   © 2011 Contexo Media

Root Words

Word Component	Meaning	Example
Enceph-	Brain	Encephalocele - hernia of part of the brain and meninges through a skull defect (cranium bifidum).
Ectasia-	Dilation	Hypostatic ectasia - dilation of a blood vessel from the effect of gravity on the blood.
Enter(o)-	Intestine	Enterology - the study of the intestinal tract.
Erythr(o)-	Red	Erythrocyte - a mature red blood cell.
Febri-	Fever	Febrile - feverish; pertaining to a fever.
Fil-	Threadlike	Filamentous - composed of long, threadlike structures; said of bacterial colonies.
Gastro-	Stomach	Gastratrophia - atrophy of the stomach.
Genu-	Knee	Genucubital - pertaining to the knees and elbows.
Ger(o)- or Geront(o)-	Aging	Gerontophobia - fear of aging.
Gleno-	Shoulder	Glenohumeral joint - shoulder and humor joint.
Gloss(o)-	Tongue	Glossotomy - an incision of the tongue.
Glute-	Buttocks	Glutitis - inflammation of the buttock.
Glyc(o)- or Gluc(o)-	Sweet	Glucokinetic - acting to maintain the blood glucose level.
Gyn(o)-	Woman; female	Gynecology - branch of medicine that treats diseases of the female genital tract.
Heme(a)(o)- or Hemato-	Blood	Hematology - study of blood.
Hepat(o)-	Liver	Hepatic - pertaining to the liver.
Hist(i)(o)-	Tissue	Histology - the study of the microscopic structure of tissue.
Hydro-	Water; Hydrogen	Hydrogenate - to combine with hydrogen.
Hyster-	Uterus	Hysterectomy - surgical removal of the uterus.
Ile(o)-	Ileum	Ileectomy - surgical removal of the ileum.
Ili(o)-	Ilium; flank	Iliometer - an instrument for determining the relative heights of the iliac spines.
Ischi(o)-	Hip	Ischiopagus - conjoined twins fused at the hips.
Kerat(o)-	Cornea	Keratotomy - incision of the cornea.
Kine(t)(o)-	Movement	Kinesiology - the study of movement.
Labio-	Lips	Labioalveolar - pertaining to the lips and tooth sockets.
Lact(o)-	Milk	Lactoprotein - any protein present in milk.
Laryng(o)-	Larynx	Laryngitis - inflammation of the larynx.
Latero-	Side	Lateroduction - movement to one side, especially of the eye.
Leuk(o)-	White	Leukocytes - white blood cells.
Lien-	Spleen	Lienotoxin - splenotoxin.
Lip(o)-	Fat	Liposuction - surgical removal of body fat.
Lith(o)-	Stone	Litholysis - dissolving of stones.
Lymph(o)-	Lymph	Lymphocytopenia - deficiency of lymphocytes in the blood.
Mamm(o)-	Breast	Mammogram - X-ray of breast.
Manu-	Hand	Manual - pretaining to the hand; performed by the hand or hands.
Mast(o)-	Breast	Mastectomy - surgical removal of breast tissue.
Melan(o)-	Black; darkness of hue	Melanuria - black pigment in the urine.
Ment-	Mind	Mentation - mental activity.

© 2011 Contexo Media

Root Words

Word Component	Meaning	Example
Mio-	Less; smaller	Miocardia - decreasing heart volume during systolic contraction.
Mito-	Threadlike	Mitosome - a body formed from the spindle fibers of the preceding mitosis.
Muc(o)- or Myx(o)-	Mucus	Mucosanguineous - containing mucus and blood.
My(o)-	Muscle	Myobradia - slow muscular reaction to stimulation.
Myc(o)-	Fungus	Mycology - the study of fungus.
Narco-	Sleep	Narcolepsy - recurrent, uncontrollable, brief episodes of sleep.
Nas(o)-	Nose	Naso-oral - pertaining to the nose and oral cavities.
Necro-	Dead, decay	Necrocytotoxin - death and decay of cells.
Nephr(o)-	Kidney	Nephritis - inflammation of kidney.
Neuro-	Nerve	Neuroarthropathy - disease of joint structures associated with disease of the central or peripheral nervous system.
Ocul(o)-	Eye	Ocular - pertaining to the eye.
Oma/Onco-	Tumor, lump	Oncology - study of tumors.
Ophthalm(o)-	Eye	Ophthalmology - the study of the eye.
Orchi(o)-	Testes	Orchiotomy - surgical incision of a testicle.
Oro-	Mouth	Orofacial - concerning the mouth and face.
Oss- or Oste(o)-	Bone	Osteoporosis - porous and fragile bones.
Ot(o)-	Ear	Otoncus - a tumor of the ear.
Ox(y)-	Oxygen	Oxidation - the process of a substance combining with oxygen.
Partum-	Birth	Parturifacient - an agent that induces or facilitates childbirth.
Path(o)-	Disease	Pathogen - organism causing disease.
Pect-	Chest	Pectoral muscle - either of two large muscles of the chest.
Ped(o)-	Child	Pediatrician - physician specializing in pediatrics.
Pharmaco-	Medicine	Pharmacology - the study of medicine and perscriptions.
Pharyng(o)-	Pharynx	Pharyngoamygdalitis - inflammation of the phrynx and tonsil.
Phleb(o)-	Vein	Phlebotomy - the surgical incision of a vein to draw blood.
Phot(o)-	Light	Photostable - uninfluenced by exposure to light.
Plantar-	Sole of foot	Plantalgia - a painful condition of the sole of the feet.
Plasm(o)-	Liquid part of the blood	Plasmacyte - a plasma cell.
Pneum(o)-	Lung	Pneumonia - inflammation of the lung.
Pod(o)-	Foot	Podiatrist - physician specializing in the care of the foot.
Proct(o)-	Rectum	Proctologist - physician specializing in diseases of the colon, rectum, and anus.
Prote(o)	Protein	Proteinosis - accumulation of excess protein in the tissues.
Psych(o)-	Mind	Psychologist - physician specializing in the study of the mind.
Pulmo(n)-	Lung	Pulmonology - the study of the lungs.
Pyel(o)-	Pelvis; kidney	Pyelitis - inflammation of the pelvis or kidney.
Pyr(o)-	Heat	Pyrogenic - producing fire.
Ren(o)-	Kidney	Renoprival - pertaining to loss of kidney function.
Rhin(o)-	Nose	Rhinoplasty - plastic surgery of the nose.
Rub(r)-	Red	Rubedo - redness of the skin that may be temporary.

Root Words

Word Component	Meaning	Example
Sangui-	Blood	Sanguicolous - inhibiting the blood, as in a parasite.
Sarc(o)-	Flesh	Sarcoma - malignant tumor comprised of connective tissue cells.
Sclera(o)-	Hard	Slerosis - hardening of tissue.
Scolio-	Crooked	Scoliosis - curvature of the spine.
Sensi-	Feeling	Sensitinogen - the collective of antigens that sensitize the body.
Soma- or Somat(o)-	Body	Somatization - the process of expressing a mental condition as a disturbed bodily function.
Sten(o)-	Narrow	Stenostomia - narrowing of the mouth.
Stom-	Mouth; opening	Stomatomycosis - oral disease due to a fungus.
Tachy-	Rapid	Tachycardia - rapid heart beat.
Therm(o)-	Heat	Thermometer - instrument used to measure temperature.
Thorac(o)-	Chest	Thoracicabdominal - concerning the thorax and abdomen.
Thromb(o)-	Clot	Thrombophilia - the tendency to form blood clots.
Toxi(o)-	Poison	Toxic - poisonous.
Trache(o)-	Trachea	Tracheotomy - incision of the trachea through the skin and muscles of the neck overlying the trachea.
Ur(o)-	Urinary; urine	Urinoma - a cyst containing urine.
Vas(o)-	Vessel	Vascular - pertaining to or containing blood vessels.
Ven(i)(o)-	Vein	Venopuncture - to puncture a vein.
Viscero-	Organs, innards	Viscerotomy - incision of an organ.
Vesic(o)-	Bladder	Vesicoclysis - injection of fluid into the bladder.

A root word may be joined with a combining form to make a **compound word**. In medical terminology, the combining form is usually a vowel. This vowel is called a **combining vowel** which is placed between two root words to make the pronunciation of the term easier. Oftentimes, the combining vowel that is used is the letter "o." Take the word thermometer. *Therm/o*, using the combining form (o), refers to the temperature. The suffix *–meter* means a device used to measure. Another example of compound word is cardiovascular. The two root words are *cardi* and *vascular*.

Compound words using combining forms can be built. For example, if needing a word that meant skimming over the surface of the water, *hydr/o* for water, *-plane* for surface = *hydroplane*. If someone is afraid of water, then *hydrophobia*. For a word that is unknown, such as *photophobia*, separate the words *–phobia* (an unnatural fear of something) and *phot/o* (light). By understanding the meaning of the two root words, it is easier to recognize the meaning "fear of light."

Root Words

Practice Quiz: Root Words

Determine the root word of the following medical terms:

1. Angiography _____

2. Cardiology _____

3. Cyanosis _____

4. Dermatitis _____

5. Hepatomegaly _____

6. Lymphocyte _____

7. Otitis _____

8. Psychosis _____

9. Rhinitis _____

10. Thrombosis _____

Circle the root word for:

11. **Liver:**

    A. Hepat   C. Heparin

    B. Heme   D. Livo

12. **Lung:**

    A. Pnea   C. Pneumon

    B. Pneumonia   D. Pulmonary

13. **Eye:**

    A. Lens   C. Kerat

    B. Opthalmo   D. Macul

14. **Mind:**

    A. Physo   C. Enceph

    B. Pysch   D. Mental

15. **Pain:**

    A. Algo   C. Esthesia

    B. Analgia   D. Algia

Chapter 14

PREFIXES AND SUFFIXES

Prefixes and Suffixes

Prefixes are one or more letters grouped together that are found at the beginning of a word. Prefixes modify the meaning of words. For example, the term anaerobic contains the prefix an-, meaning not. The term anaerobic means "able to live without oxygen." Another example is the term anemia. Anemia contains the prefix an-, meaning not plus the root *hema*, meaning blood. Anemia refers to a reduction in the mass of circulating red blood cells. A table of common prefixes is included on the following pages.

Suffixes are one or more letters grouped together and placed at the end of a word, to modify the meaning. For example, take the term cystocele. The suffix in this example is –*cele*. *Cysto* means bladder (or pouch) and –*cele* means hernia. Therefore, the meaning of cystocele is a herniation of the urinary bladder. It is very common practice to see the letter "y" added to the end of a medical term to indicate that a procedure was performed. Also, the two letters "ly" are often times used as suffixes on medical terms to indicate a process. A table of common suffixes is included on the following pages.

Table of Common Prefixes

Word Component	Meaning	Example
A(n)-	Without	Anorexigenic - causing loss of appetite.
Ab(s)-	From	Abduction - movement of a body part away from the medial plane.
Ad-	Towards	Adhesion - process of uniting two parts or surfaces; opposing surfaces of a wound.
Ambi- or Amphi-	Both	Ambisexual - containing sexual characteristics, or structures, found in both sexes.
Ana-	Up to; move from	Anabiosis - resuscitation after apparent death; to be moved from death.
Aniso-	Unequal	Anisotropic - not having properties that are the same in all directions.
Ante-	Before; lying adjacent to	Antemortem - before death.
Anti-	Against; opposite	Antilactase - a substance that opposes the action of lactase.
Aut(o)-	Self	Autoanalysis - a patient's own analysis of the mental state underlying his or her mental disorder.
Bi-	Two	Biarticular - pertaining to two joints.
Bio-	Life	Biology - the study of life and living organisms.
Brachy-	Short	Brachycardia - slowness of the heart heartbeat.
Cata-	Down	Catatonic - a syndrome of psychomotor disturbances characterized by periods of physical rigidity, negativism, or stupor.
Circum-	Around	Circumduction - movement of a part or extremity in a circular direction.
Con-	Together	Condensation - making more solid or dense.
Contra-	Against	Contralateral - relating to the opposite side.
De-	Away from	Depression - reduction of the level of functioning.
Di-	Two	Diamelia - absence of two limbs.
Diplo-	Double	Diplocoria - a double pupil in the eye.
Dur-	Hard, firm	Durable - able to withstand abuse or time with little change.

© 2011 Contexo Media

Prefixes and Suffixes

Word Component	Meaning	Example
Dys-	Bad, abnormal	Dyscephalia - malformation of the head and face.
End(o)-	Inward	Endoaneurysmorrhaphy - surgical opening of an aneurismal sac and suturing of its oriface.
Ent-	Within	Entoptic - within the eyeball.
Epi-	On	Epididymotomy - incision into the epididymis.
Eso-	Carry	Esophagus - the portion of the digestive canal between the pharynx and stomach.
Eu-	Normal; health	Eubiotics - the science of healthy and hygenic living.
Eury-	Broad	Eurycephalic - having an abnormally broad head.
Ex-	Outside	Extracranial - outside the skull.
Extra-	Beyond	Extracystic - outside of, or unrelated to, the gallbladder or urinary bladder or any cystic tumor.
Hapto-	Feeling; touch	Haptometer - instrument for measuring sensitivity to touch.
Hemi-	Half	Hemiacardius -one of two fetuses, in which only a part of the circulation is effected by its own heart.
Hept-	Seven	Heptapeptide - a peptide containing seven amino acids.
Hetero-	Different	Heterogenous - of unlike natures.
Homo-	Same	Homomorphic - denoting two or more structures of similar size and shape.
Hyper-	Greater than normal; excessive	Hyperplasia - an increase in number of normal cells in a tissue or organ.
Hypo-	Less than normal	Hypodontia - diminished development, or absence of teeth.
Im- or In-	Not	Imbalance - lack of equality between opposing forces.
Infra-	Beneath	Infracostal - below the rib.
Inter-	Among; between	Interaction - the reciprocal action between two entities in a common event.
Intra-	Within; into	Intrabronchial - within a bronchus.
Intro-	Inwardly; into	Introflection - a bending inward.
Iso-	Equal	Isometric - of equal dimensions.
Juxta-	Adjacent	Juxtaepiphysial - close to or adjoining an epiphysis.
Macr(o)-	Large	Macronychia - abnormally large fingernails or toenails.
Mal-	Bad; abnormal	Malacosteon - softening of the bones.
Medi- or Meso-	Middle	Mediolateral - relating to the median plane and a side.
Mega-	Large; great	Megaesophagus - great enlargement of the lower portion of the esophagus.
Meta-	Change	Metachrosis - the ability to change color in some animals, as in the chameleon.
Micr(o)-	Small	Microrhinia - abnormal smallness of the nose.
Mono-	One	Monoplegia - paralysis of a single limb or a single group of muscles.
Morph(o)-	Shape	Morphography - the classification of organisms by form and structure.
Multi-	Many	Multiparity - the condition of having carried two or more fetuses to viability, regardless of whether the infants were alive at birth.
Neo-	New	Neoplasm - an abnormal tissue that grows by cellular proliferation more rapidly than normal and continues to grow after the stimuli that initiated the new growth cease.
Non-	Not	Nonproteogenic - not leading to the production of proteins.
Nulli-	Non	Nulligravida - a woman who has never conceived a child.
Ob-	Before; obstruct	Obturator - any structure that occludes an opening.
Oct(o)(a)-	Eight	Octapeptide - a peptide made up of eight amino acid residues.
Olig(o)-	Few; little	Oligodactylia - subnormal number of fingers or toes.

Prefixes and Suffixes

Word Component	Meaning	Example
Pachy-	Thick	Pachyderma - abnormally thick skin.
Para-	Beside	Parabiosis - fusion of whole eggs or embryos, as occurs in some forms of conjoined twins.
Pent-	Five	Pentadactyl - having five fingers or toes on each hand or foot.
Per-	By; through	Peranum - by or through the anus.
Peri-	Around	Perimastitis - inflammation of the fibrous tissue around the breast.
Poly-	Many	Polyneuralgia - neuralgia in several nerves.
Post-	Behind; after	Postfebrile - occuring after a fever.
Pre-	Before; in front	Preoral - in front of the mouth.
Pro-	In favor of; for; supporting; in front of	Proal - concerning foward movement.
Pros- or Prox-	Beside	Proximal - nearest the trunk or the point of origin.
Pseudo-	False	Pseudopod - a false foot.
Quar-	Four	Quartan - recurring every fourth day.
Re-	Back; contrary	Reabsorb - to absorb again.
Retr(o)-	Backward	Retrocedent - going backward, returning.
Semi-	Half	Semiflexion - halfway between flexion and extension of a limb.
Sept-	Seven	Septivalent - having a combining power of seven.
Sex-	Six	Sexdigitate - having six digits on one or both hands or feet.
Sub-	Under	Subapical - below the apex.
Super-	Above	Superolateral - above and to one side.
Syn- or Sys-	Together	Synadelphus - conjoined twins with a single head, partially united trunk, and four upper and four lower limbs.
Tachy-	Rapid, accelerated	Tachymeter- a surveying instrument used for the rapid determination of distances, elevations, and bearings.
Tetra- or Quadri-	Four	Tetrabrachius - a deformed fetus with four arms.
Trans-	Across; through	Transaxial - across the long axis of a structure or part.
Tri-	Three	Tribasilar - having three bases.
Ultra-	Excess; beyond	Ultraligation - ligation of a blood vessel beyond the point where a branch is given off.
Uni-	One	Unicellular - having only one cell.

Table of Common Suffixes

Word Component	Meaning	Example
-algia	Pain	Arthralgia - pain in a joint.
-ase	Enzyme	Lipase - any fat-splitting or lipolytic enzyme.
-centesis	Puncture	Arthrocentesis - puncture of a joint space with a needle to remove accumulated fluid from the joint.
-cide	Killer	Suicide - the act of taking one's own life.
-desis	Binding	Arthrodesis - surgical immobilization of a joint.
-ectomy	Excision; Surgical removal	Cystectomy - surgical removal of a cyst.

Prefixes and Suffixes

Word Component	Meaning	Example
-form	Shaped	Aciniform - resembling an acinus or grape like structure.
-iasis	Condition; state	Taeniasis - infection with cestodes of the genus Taenia.
-ism	Condition; practice	Narcissism - a state in which one interprets and regards everything in relation to oneself and not to other persons or things.
-itis	Inflammation	Gastritis - acute or chronic inflammation of the stomach.
-logy	Study of	Gastroenterology - the medical speciality concerned with the function and disorders of the gastrointestinal tract.
-lys(i)(o)	Destruction; breakdown	Hydrolysis - breakdown of a compound by adding water.
-megaly	Large	Cardiomegaly - large heart.
-oma	Tumor	Carcinoma - a new growth or malignant tumor.
-osis	Condition	Stenosis - the constriction or narrowing of a passage or oriface.
-pathy	Disease of	Gastropathy - any disease of the stomach.
-penia	Lack of	Phosphopenia - low serum phosphate levels.
-pexy	Fix	Arthropexy - surgical fixation of a joint.
-phob	Abnormal fear	Agoraphobia - overwhelming symptoms of anxiety that occur on leaving home or venturing into the open; a form of social phobia.
-plasia	Growth	Hyperplasia - excessive proliferation of normal cells in the normal tissue arrangement of an organ.
-plasty	Repair (surgical)	Blepharoplasty - plastic surgery upon the eyelid.
-plegia	Paralysis	Paraplegia - paralysis of both lower extremities and, generally, the lower trunk.
-plexis	Stroke	Cataplexy - a transient attack of extreme generalized weakness, often precipitated by an emotional response.
-pnea	Breathing	Sleep Apnea - failure of the respiratory center to stimulate adequate respiration during sleep.
-poiesis	Production	Hematopoiesis - formation of blood or blood cells.
-praxia	Movement	Atapraxia - defective muscular coordination.
-rrhaphy	Suture	Neurorrhaphy - suturing of ends of severed nerves.
-rrhea	Fluid discharge	Diarrhea - the passage of fluid or unformed stools.
-scope	Observe	Microscope - optical instrument that greatly magnifies minute objects.
-scopy	Visually examining	Endoscopy - inspection of body organs or cavities by use of an endoscope.
-(o)stomy	Opening; forming artificial opening	Colostomy - the opening of a portion of the colon through the abdominal wall to its skin surface.
-taxis	Movement	Ataxis - without movement.
-tome	Cutting instrument	Curettome - a spoon-shaped scraping instrument for removing foreign tissue matter from a cavity.
-tomy	Incision	Hysterectomy - surgical removal of the uterus.
-tripsy	Crushing	Lithotripsy - the application of the physical force of sound waves to crush a stone in the bladder or urethra.
-trophy	Growth	Atrophy - a decrease in size of an organ or tissue.

Practice Quiz: Prefixes and Suffixes

Determine the meaning of the following prefixes:

1. Hyp(o)- _____
2. Mal- _____
3. Anti- _____
4. Mega- _____
5. Poly- _____
6. Semi- _____
7. Trans- _____
8. Meta- _____
9. Hyper- _____
10. End(o)- _____

Add prefixes to the following:

11. _____-duction   process of drawing away from.
12. _____-natal   before birth.
13. _____-cision   cutting out.
14. _____-cision   cutting into.
15. _____-lateral   pertaining to one side.
16. _____-cardia   fast heart beat.
17. _____-drome   a symptom occurring before the onset of disease.

Determine the meaning of the following suffixes:

18. -algia _____
19. -tripsy _____
20. -osis _____
21. -pnea _____
22. -itis _____
23. -stomy _____
24. -desis _____
25. -oma _____
26. -plasia _____
27. -plasty _____
28. -pexy _____
29. -scopy _____
30. -penia _____
31. -rrhaphy _____
32. -ectomy _____
33. -megaly _____
34. -rrhea _____

Chapter 15

ABBREVIATIONS

Abbreviations

Abbreviations are used throughout medical coding. It is imperative that the correct abbreviations are used since the incorrect recording of an abbreviation could mean something entirely different than the original meaning. This could prove to be disastrous for the patient.

Abbreviations with Measurements

When English and metric measurements are used with numeric values (1, 2, 3, etc.), the measurement is ALWAYS abbreviated.

7 mm (NOT 7 millimeters)

When English and metric measurements are used with numeric values (1, 2, 3, etc.), the abbreviation is for the singular and plural forms. An 's' is NEVER added to the abbreviation to make it plural.

7 mm (NOT 7 mms or 7 millimeters)

2 lb (NOT 2 lbs)

When English and metric measurements are used without a number, the measurement is NOT abbreviated.

Please use centimeters instead of millimeters. (NOT Please use cm instead of mm.)

Abbreviations with Latin and Chemical Abbreviations

When using a lowercase Latin abbreviation, use periods.

e.g. (example given)

When Latin and chemical abbreviations are used that contain uppercase and lowercase letters, do NOT use periods.

pH (hydrogen ration)

Na (sodium)

Fe (iron)

General Abbreviations

When using abbreviations to describe general medical terms that are all-capital, do NOT use periods.

EKG (electrocardiogram)

ENT (ear, nose, and throat)

© 2011 Contexo Media

Abbreviations

Abbreviations Commonly Used in Medical Practices

Abbreviation	Definition
A	without, lack of; apathy (lack of feeling); apnea (without breath); aphasia (without speech); anemia (lack of blood)
AA	aortic aneurysm; ascending aorta
AAA	abdominal aortic aneurysm
AAR	active avoidance reaction
AAT	aachen aphasia test, alanine aminotransferase
Ab	antibody
A & P	anterior and posterior; auscultation and percussion
Abd	abdomen
ABE	acute bacterial endocarditis
ABG	arterial blood gases
ABP	arterial blood pressure
ABPA	allergic bronchopulmonary aspergillosis
Ac	before meals
ACBG	aortocoronary bypass graft
ACD	absolute cardiac dullness
ACE	angiotensin converting enzyme
ACG	angiocardiography
Ad	to, toward, near to, adductor, (leading toward); adhesion, (sticking to); adnexa (structures joined to); adrenal (near the kidney)
ACI	acute coronary insufficiency
ACL	anterior cruciate ligament
ACT	anticoagulant therapy; active motion
ACTH	adrenocorticotropic hormone
ADG	atrial diastolic gallop
ADH	antidiuretic hormone
ADL	activities of daily living
Ad lib	as desired, at liberty
AED	automatic external defibrillator
AEI	atrial escape interval
AEP	average evoked potential
AER	average evoked response
AF	aortic flow; atrial fibrillation
AFB	acid-fast bacilli
AFIB	atrial fibrillation
AFP	alpha-fetoprotein
AGA	appropriate for gestational age
AI	aortic insufficiency
AICD	automated implantable cardio-defibrillator
AIDS	acquired immune deficiency syndrome

114

© 2011 Contexo Media

Abbreviations

Abbreviation	Definition
AIP	acute interstitial pneumonia (aka hamman-rich syndrome)
AKA	above knee amputation
ALMI	anterior lateral myocardial infarction
ALP	alkaline phosphatase
ALT	alanine transaminase, alanine aminotransferase
AMA	against medical advice
AMB	ambulatory
Ambi	both, ambidextrous, (ability to use hands equally); ambilaterally (both sides)
AMI	acute myocardial infarction
Amphi	about, on both sides, both, amphibious, (living on both land and water)
Ampho	both, amphogenic, (producing offspring of both sexes)
Ana	up, back, again, excessive, anatomy, (a cutting up); anagenes (reproduction of tissue); anasarca (excessive serum in cellular tissues of body)
Ant	before, forward, antecubital, (before elbow); anteflexion, (forward bending)
Anti	against, opposed to, reversed antiperistalsis (reversed peristalsis); antisepsis (against infection)
AMI	acute myocardial infarction
AO	angle of; aorta
AOD	arteriosclerotic occlusive disease
AP	apical pulse
APE	acute pulmonary edema
Apo	from, away from aponeurosis (away from tendon); apochromatic (abnormal color)
APSGN	acute poststreptococcal glomerulonephritis
ARDS	acute or adult respiratory distress syndrome
ARF	acute renal failure
AS	aortic stenosis
ASCVD	arteriosclerotic cardiovascular disease
ASD	atrial septal defect
ASHD	arteriosclerotic heart disease
AST	aspartate aminotransferase
ATN	acute tubular necrosis
ATRA	all trans-retinoic acid
AU	both ears
AV	aortic valve
AVB	atrio-ventricular block
AVR	aortic valve replacement
BAL	bronchoalveolar lavage
BBS	bilateral breath sounds
BE	barium enema
BG	blood glucose

© 2011 Contexo Media

Abbreviations

Abbreviation	Definition
BI	brain injury
Bi	twice, double biarticulate (double joint); bifocal (two foci); bifurcation (two branches)
BID	bis in di'e (twice a day)
Bilat	bilateral
B/K	below knee
BM	bowel movement or breast milk
BMD	bone mineral density
BMR	basal metabolic rate
BO	bronchiolitis obliterans
BOOP	bronchiolitis obliterans organizing pneumonia
BP	blood pressure
BPD	bronchopulmonary dysplasia
BPH	benign prostatic hypertrophy
BRM	biologic response modifiers
BRP	bathroom privileges
BS	bowel sounds
BSA	body surface area
BSE	breast self examination
BT	bowel tones
BUN	blood urea nitrogen
Bx	biopsy
C	celsius(centigrade)
C (C)	with
C&S	culture and sensitivity
C/o	complaint of
Ca	calcium, cancer, carcinoma
CA	cardiac arrest
CABG	coronary artery bypass graft
CAD	coronary artery disease
CAPD	continuous ambulatory peritoneal dialysis
CAT or CT	computerized tomography scan
Cata	down, according to, complete catabolism (breaking down); catalepsia (complete seizure)
CATH LAB	cardiac catheterization lab
CBC	complete blood count
CBD	common bile duct
CBE	clinical breast examination
CBG	capillary blood gas
CBI	continuous bladder irrigation
CBR	complete bed rest

Abbreviations

Abbreviation	Definition
CC	chief complaint
CCK	cholecystokinin
CCPD	continuous cyclic peritoneal dialysis
CCS	corticosteroids
CCU	cardiac care unit
CD	cardiovascular disease
CEA	cultured epithelial autograft
CF	cystic fibrosis
CFT	complement-fixation test
CHD	coronary heart disease
CHF	congestive heart failure
CI	cardiac insufficiency
CICU	cardiac intensive care unit
CIHD	chronic ischemic heart disease
CIN	cervical intraepithelial neoplasm
Circum	around, about circumflex (winding about); circumference (surrounding); circumarticular (around joint)
CMS	circulation, motion, sensation
CO	cardiac output
COAD	chronic obstructive airway disease
Com	with, together, commissure (sending or coming together)
Con	with, together, conductor (leading together); concrescence (growing together); concentric (having a common center)
Contra	against, opposite contralateral (opposite side); contraception (prevention of conception); contraindicated (not indicated)
CO2	carbon dioxide
COLD	chronic obstructive lung disease
COPD	chronic obstructive pulmonary disease
C/P	cardiopulmonary
CP	chest pain, cleft palate
CPAP	continuous positive airway pressure
CPD	cephalo-pelvic disproportion
CPFT	certified pulmonary function technician
CPP	cerebral perfusion pressure
CPR	cardiopulmonary resuscitation
CPPD	chest percussion and post drainage
CPT	chest physical therapy
CRF	chronic renal failure
CRRT	continuous renal replacement therapy
CRT	capillary refill time
CSF	cerebrospinal fluid, colony stimulating factors
CT	chest tube, computed tomography

© 2011 Contexo Media

Abbreviations

Abbreviation	Definition
CTD	close to death
CVA	cerebral vascular accident, costovertebral angle
CVEA	complex ventricular ectopy
CVP	central venous pressure
CX	circumflex
Cx'd	cancelled
CXR	chest x-ray
DAD	diffuse alveolar damage
DAT	diet as tolerated
DBP	diastolic blood pressure
DC (dc)	discontinue
DCCT	diabetes control and complication trials
DEX (DXT)	blood sugar
De	away from, dehydrate (remove water from); dedentition (removal of teeth); decompensation (failure of compensation)
D5W	dextose 5% in water
D5LR	dextrose 5% with lactated ringers
Di	twice, double, diplopia (double vision); dichromatic (two colors); digastric (double stomach)
Dia	through, apart, across, completely diaphragm (wall across); diapedesis (ooze through); diagnosis (complete knowledge)
DIC	disseminated intravascular coagulation
DIP	desquamative interstitial pneumonitis
Dis	reversal, apart from, separation disinfection (apart from infection); disparity (apart from equality); dissect (cut apart)
DKA	diabetic ketoacidosis
DLCO	diffusing capacity of carbon monoxide
DM	diabetes mellitus
DNA	deoxyribonucleic acid
DNI	do not intubate
DNR	do not resuscitate
DOE	dyspnea on exertion
DPAP	demand positive airway pressure
DPI	dry powder inhaler
DTR	deep tendon reflex
DVT	deep vein thrombosis
Dx	diagnosis
Dys	bad, difficult, disordered, dyspepsia (bad digestion); dyspnea (difficult breathing); dystopia (disordered position)
E, ex	out, away from, enucleate (remove from); eviscerate (take out viscera or bowels); exostosis (outgrowth of bone)
EBV	epstein-barr virus
Ec	out from, ectopic (out of place); eccentric (away from center); ectasia (stretching out or dilation)
ECF	extracellular fluid, extended care facility
ECG (EKG)	electrocardiogram/electrocardiograph

Abbreviations

Abbreviation	Definition
ECHO	echocardiogram
Ecto	on outer side, situated on ectoderm (outer skin); ectoretina (outer layer of retina)
EEG	electroencephalogram
EENT	eye, ear, nose, and throat
Em, en.	empyema (pus in); encephalon (in the head)
EMC	ensephalomyocarditis
EMG	electromyogram
EMO	extracorporeal membrane oxygenator
EMT	emergency medical technician
Endo	within, endocardium (within heart); endometrium (within uterus)
ENT	ear, nose, and throat
Epi	upon, on, epidural (upon dura); epidermis (on skin)
ERCP	endoscopic retrograde cholangiopancreatography
ERV	expiratory reserve volume
ESRD	end stage renal disease
ET	endotracheal tube
Exo	outside, on outer side, outer layer, exogenous (produce outside); exocolitis (inflammation of outer coat of colon)
Extra	outside, extracellular (outside cell); extrapleural (outside pleura)
F & R	force and rhythm
FA	fatty acid
FBS	fasting blood sugar
FD	fatal dose, focal distance
FDA	Food & Drug Administration
FEF	forced expiratory flow
FPF	familial pulmolary fibrosis
FRC	functional residual capacity
Fx	fracture
FUO	fever of unknown origin
FVC	forced vital capacity
FVD	fluid volume deficit
GB	gallbladder
GERD	gastroesophageal reflux disease
GFR	glomerular filtration rate
GGT	gamma-glutamyl transferase
GI	gastrointestinal
GOT	glutamic oxalic transaminase
GU	genitourinary
GVHD	graft-versus-host-disease
HA	headache

© 2011 Contexo Media

Abbreviations

Abbreviation	Definition
Hb	hemoglobin
HCG	human chorionic gonadotropin
HCVD	hypertensive cardiovascular disease
HCO3	bicarbonate
HCT	hematocrit
HD	heart disease, hemodiaysis
HDL	high density lipoprotein
HEENT	head, eye, ear, nose, and throat
Hemi	half, hemiplegia (partial paralysis); hemianesthesia (loss of feeling on one side of body)
HEPA	high efficiency particulate air (filter or mask)
Hgb	hemoglobin
HIV	human immunodeficiency virus
HM	heart murmur
HMO	health maintenance organization
H/o	history of
HPI	history of present illness
HR	heart rate
HRCT	high resolution CT scan
HRT	hormone replacement therapy
HS	hour of sleep
HSP	hypersensitivity pneumonitis
HTN (BP)	hypertension
Hx	history
Hyper	over, above, excessive hyperemia (excessive blood); hypertrophy (overgrowth); hyperplasia (excessive formation)
Hypo	under, below, deficient hypotension (low blood pressure); hypothyroidism (deficiency or underfunction of thyroid)
IBC	iron binding capacity
IBD	inflammatory bowel disease
IBS	irritable bowel syndrome
IBW	ideal body weight
IC	inspiratory capacity
ICCE	intracapsular cataract extraction
ICF	intermediate care facility
ICP	intracranial pressure
ICS	intercostal space
ICT	inflammation of connective tissue
ICU	intensive care unit
IDM	infant of diabetic mother
IDDM	insulin dependent diabetes mellitus
IE	inspiratory exerciser

Abbreviations

Abbreviation	Definition
IH	infectious hepatitis
IHD	ischemic heart disease
IHR	intrinsic heart rate
IIP	implantable insulin pump
ILD	interstitial lung disease
IM	intramuscular
Im, in	in, into, immersion (act of dipping in); infiltration (act of filtering in); injection (act of forcing liquid into)
Im, in	not, immature (not mature); involuntary (not voluntary); inability (not able)
Imp	impression
IMT	inspiratory muscle trainer
IMV	intermittent mandatory ventilation
Infra	below, infraorbital (below eye); infraclavicular (below clavicle or collarbone)
INR	international normalization ratio
Inter	between, intercostal (between ribs); intervene (come between)
Intra	within, intracerebral (within cerebrum); intraocular (within eyes); intraventricular (within ventricles)
Intro	into, within, introversion (turning inward); introduce (lead into)
I&O	intake and output
IPD	intermittent peritoneal dialysis
IPF	idiopathic pulmonary fibrosis
IPPB	intermittent positive pressure breathing
IRV	inspiratory reserve volume
ITP	immune thrombocytopenic purpura
IV	intravenous
IVF	in vitro fertilization
IVP	intravenous pyelography
JAMA	journal of the american medical association
JVP	jugular venous pressure
K	potassium
Kcl	potassium chloride
KI	potassium iodide
KS	kartagener's syndrome
KUB	kidney, ureter, bladder
KVO	keep vein open
L & A	light and accommodation
LAM	lymphangioleiomyomatosis
LB	large bowel
LDL	low density lipoprotein
LE	lupus erythematosus
LFT	lipid/liver function tests

Abbreviations

Abbreviation	Definition
LIP	lymphocytic interstitial pneumonia
LLQ	left lower quadrant
LMP	last menstrual period
LOX	liquid oxygen
LP	lumbar puncture
LPM	litres per minute (02 flow rate)
LRCP	licensed respiratory care practitioner
LRI	lower respiratory tract infection
LUQ	left upper quadrant
LVRS	lung volume reduction surgery
Lytes	electrolytes
MAP	mean arterial pressure
MAR	medication administration record
MCS	multiple chemical sensitivity
MDI	multiple daily vitamin
MET	metabolic equivalents
Meta	beyond, after, change; metamorphosis (change of form); metastasis change (beyond original position); metacarpal (beyond wrist)
MI	myocardial infarction
MLC	midline catheter
MM	mucous membrane
Moabs	monoclonal antibodies
MOM	milk of magnesia
MRDD	mental retarded/developmentally disabled
MRI	magnetic resonance imaging
MRM	modified radical mastectomy
MS	multiple sclerosis, morphine sulfate
MV	mitral valve
MVP	mitral valve prolapse
MVV	maximal voluntary ventilation
Na	sodium
Nacl	sodium chloride
NAD	no apparent distress
NC	nasal cannula
NED	no evidence of disease
Neg	negative
NETT	national emphysema treatment trial
NICU	neonatal intensive care unit
NIDDM	noninsulin dependent diabetes mellitus
NKA	no known allergies
NKDA	non-ketotic diabetic acidosis

Abbreviations

Abbreviation	Definition
NKMA	no known medication allergies
Noc	night
NPD	nightly peritoneal dialysis
NPO	nothing by mouth
NPPV	noninvasive positive pressure ventilation
NS (NIS)	normal saline
NSAID	nonsteroidal anti-inflammatory drug
NSIP	non-specific interstitial pneumonitis
NSR	normal sinus rhythm
NT	nasotracheal
NTD	neural tube defect
NV	nausea & vomiting
NYD	not yet diagnosed
O2	oxygen
OA	occupational asthma
ODTS	organic dust toxic syndrome
OLB	open lung biopsy
OLD	occupational lung disease
OOB	out of bed
Opistho	behind, backward, opisthotic (behind ears); opisthognathous (beyond jaws)
ORIF	open reduction internal fixation
OS	left eye
OSA	obstructive sleep apnea
OT	occupational therapy
OTC	over-the-counter
OU	both eyes
P	after
P	pulse
PA	pulmonary artery
PABA	para-aminobenzoic acid
Para	beside, beyond, near to paracardiac (beside the heart); paraurethral (near the urethra)
PCA	patient controlled analgesia, posterior communicating artery
PCN	penicillin, primary care nurse
PCV	packed cell volume
PD	peritoneal dialysis
PDA	patent ductus arteriosus
PDD	pervasive development disorder
PDR	physician's desk reference
PE	physical examination
PEFR	peak expiratory flow rate

© 2011 Contexo Media

Abbreviations

Abbreviation	Definition
PEG	percutaneous endoscopic gastrostomy
PEJ	percutaneous endoscopic jejunostomy
PEP	positive expiratory pressure
Peri	around, periosteum (around bone); periatrial (around atrium), peribronchial (around bronchus)
PERL	pupils equal, react to light
Permeate	(pass through); perforate (bore through); peracute (excessively acute)
PERRLA	pupils equal, round, react to light, accommodation
PET	positron emission tomography
PF	pulmonary fibrosis
PFM	peak flow meter
PFT	pulmonary function test
PG	prostaglandin
PH	past history
PI	present illness
PICC	peripherally inserted central venous catheter
PID	pelvic inflammatory disease
PIDS	primary immunodeficiencies
PLB	pursed lip breathing
PMI	point of maximal impulse
PMH	past medical history
PND	post nasal drip (or discharge)
PNH	paroxysmal nocturnal hemoglobinuria
PO	by mouth
PO2	oxygen tension in arterial blood
Post	after,behind,postoperative (after operation); postpartum (after childbirth); postocular (behind eye)
Post op	post-operative
PPH	primary pulmonary hypertension
PPV	positive pressure ventilation
PR	pulmonary rehabilitation
PRBC	packed red blood cells
Pre	before, in front of, premaxillary (in front of maxilla); preoral (in front of mouth)
Pre op	pre-operative
Prep	preparation
PRN	as needed
Pro	before, in front of, prognosis (foreknowledge); prophase (appear before)
PS	pyloric stenosis
PSA	prostate specific antigen
PT	prothrombin time
P.T.	physical therapy
PTT	partial thromboplastin time

Abbreviations

Abbreviation	Definition
PTX	pneumothorax
PUD	peptic ulcer disease
PVD	peripheral vascular disease
Px	pneumothorax
Q	every
QD	everyday
QH	every hour
Q2H	every 2 hours
QID	four times a day
Qns	quantity not sufficient
QOD	every other day
QOL	quality of life
Qs	quantity sufficient, quantity required
R	respirations
RAD	reactive airway disease
RAI	radioactive iodine
RAIU	radioactive iodine uptake
RBC	red blood cells
RDS	respiratory distress syndrome
RDW	red cell distribution width
REEDA	redness, edema, ecchymosis, drainage, approximation
Re	back, again, contrary, reflex (bend back); revert (turn again to); regurgitation (backward flowing, contrary to normal)
Retro	backward, located behind retrocervical (located behind cervix); retrograde (going backward); retrolingual (behind tongue)
RHD	rheumatic heart disease, relative hepatic dullness
RLQ	right lower quadrant
RM	respiratory movement
RO or R/O	rule out
ROM	range of motion
ROS	review of systems
RPE	rating of perceived exertion
RPFT	registered pulmonary function technician
RRT	registered respiratory therapist
RT or R	right
RUQ	right upper quadrant
RV	residual volume
Rx	prescription, pharmacy
S/S	signs & symptoms
SAB	spontaneous abortion
SAST	serum aspartate aminotransferase
SB	spina bifida

Abbreviations

Abbreviation	Definition
SBO	small bowel obstruction
Semi	half, semi cartilaginous (half cartilage); semi lunar(half-moon); semiconscious (half conscious)
SGPT	serum glutamic-pyruvic transaminase
SLE	systemic lupus erythematosus
SNF	skilled nursing facility
SOB	shortness of breath
SOBOE	shortness of breath on exertion
SOP	standard operating procedure
SP	spontaneous pneumothorax
SR	sinus rhythm
S (s)	without
SS	social services
STAT	immediately
STD	sexually transmitted disease
STH	somatotropic hormone
STM	short term memory
Sub	under, subcutaneous (under skin); subarachnoid (under arachnoid)
SUI	stress urinary incontinence
Super	above, upper, excessive, supercilia (upper brows); supernumerary (excessive number); supermedial (above middle)
Supra	above, upper, excessive, suprarenal (above kidney); suprasternal (above sternum); suprascapular (on upper part of scapula)
SVR	systemic vascular resistance
Sym	together, with, symphysis (growing together); synapsis (joining together); synarthrosis (articulation of joints together)
Sx	symptoms
T	temperature
T3	triiodothyronine
T4	thyroxine
TBSA	total body surface area
TCDB	turn, cough, deep breathe
TDM	treadmill
TED	thrombo-embolism deterrent
TEP	transesophageal puncture
THR	total hip replacement
THTM	thallium treadmill
TIA	transient ischemic attack
TIBC	total iron binding capacity
TID	three times a day
TIL	tumor infiltrating lymphocytes
TKR	total knee replacement
TLC	total lung capacity
TNF	tumor necrosis factor

Abbreviations

Abbreviation	Definition
TNM	tumor, node, metastases
TNTC	too numerous to count
TP	tuberculin precipitation
TPN	total parenteral nutrition
TPR	temperature, pulse, respiration
Trans	across, through, beyond, transection (cut across); transduodenal (through duodenum); transmit (send beyond)
TTN	transient tachypnea of the newborn
TTO2	transtracheal oxygen
TTP	thrombotic thrombocytopenia purpura
TUPR	trans-urethral prostatic resection
TUR(P)	trans-urethral resection of the prostate
TV	tidal volume
TWB	touch weight bear
TWE	tap water enema
Tx	treatment, traction
UA	urinalysis
UAO	upper airway obstruction
UBW	usual body weight
UGA	under general anesthesia
UGI	upper gastrointestinal
UIP	usual interstitial pneumonitis
Up ad lib	up as desired
Ultra	beyond, in excess, ultraviolet (beyond violet end of spectrum); ultraligation (ligation of vessel beyond point of origin); ultrasonic (sound waves beyond the upper frequency of hearing by human ear)
UPJ	ureteropelvic junction
URI	upper respiratory infection
US	ultrasonic, ultrasound
USA	unstable angina
UTI	urinary tract infection
UVJ	ureterovesical junction
VA	visual acuity
VATS	video assisted thoracic surgery
VBP	venous blood pressure
VBAC	vaginal birth after caesarean
VC	ventricular contraction
VENT	ventral
VF/Vfib	ventricular fibrillation
VLDL	very low density lipoprotein
VMA	vanillylmandelic acid
VP	venous pressure, venipuncture

Abbreviations

Abbreviation	Definition
VPB	ventricular premature beats
VPC	ventricular premature contractions
VS	vital signs
VSD	ventricular septal defect
VT/Vtach	ventricular tachycardia
W	vessel wall
W/C	wheelchair
WBC	white blood cell
WD	well developed
WHO	World Health Organization
WN	well nourished
WNL	within normal limits
WOB	work of breathing
WPW	Wolff-Parkinson - White Syndrome
X	times

Abbreviations and Symbols

Following are some abbreviations and symbols commonly used by health practitioners when writing progress notes by hand in the medical record. If a physician is audited by a payer, a list similar to the following should accompany the records.

Activities

AMB	ambulatory
BRP	bathroom privileges
CBR	complete bed rest
OOB	out of bed
up ad lib	up as desired

Assessment Data

abd	abdomen
BP	blood pressure
bx	biopsy
C	celsius (centigrade)
cc	chief complaint
c/o	complains of
dx	diagnosis
F	fahrenheit
GI	gastrointestinal
GU	genitourinary
h/o	history of
HPI	history of present illness
Imp	impressions
lt or L	left
NAD	no apparent distress
neg	negative
P	pulse
PE	physical examination
PMH	past medical history
R	respirations
R/O	rule out
ROS	review of systems
rt or R	right
RX	treatment
Sx	symptoms
T	temperature
WNL	within normal limits

+	positive
-	negative

Diseases

ASHD	arteriosclerotic heart disease
ASCVD	arteriosclerotic cardio. disease
BPH	benign prostatic hypertrophy
CA	cancer
CAD	coronary artery disease
CHF	congestive heart failure
COPD	chronic obstruct. pul. disease
CVA	cerebrovascular accident
DM	diabetes mellitus
HTN ($\neq$BP)	hypertension
MI	myocardial infarction
PVD	peripheral vascular disease
STD	sexually transmitted disease

Diagnostic Studies

ABG	arterial blood gases
BE	barium enema
CBC	complete blood count
CO_2	carbon dioxide
C&S	culture and sensitivity
CXR	chest x-ray
ECG (EKG)	cardiogram
lytes	electrolytes
RBC	red blood cells
UA	urinalysis
UGI	upper GI
WBC	white blood cells

Symbols

>	greater than
<	less than
/	increasing
\	decreasing
$2°$	secondary to
=	equal to
$\neq$	unequal
°	degree

© 2011 Contexo Media

Abbreviations

Orders

a	before
ad lib	as desired
AMA	against medical orders
BM	bowel movement
BP	blood pressure

Chemical Symbols

Al	Aluminum
Ar	Argon
As	Arsenic
Ba	Barium
B	Boron
Br	Bromine
Ca	Calcium (Ca_2+ ion)
Cd	Cadmium
C	Carbon
CO_2	Carbon Dioxide
pCO_2	Partial Pressure Carbon Dioxide
Cl	Chlorine
Cr	Chromium
Co	Cobalt
Cu	Copper
F	Fluorine
He	Helium
H	Hydrogen
H_2O	Water
I	Iodine
Fe	Iron
K	Potassium
Kr	Krypton
Pb	Lead
Li	Lithium
Mg	Magnesium
Mn	Manganese
Hg	Mercury
Ne	Neon
N	Nitrogen
O	Oxygen
P	Phosphorus

Abbreviation Confusion

Some abbreviations may look similar, but have different meanings. Here are some examples:

AAL

Acute lymphoblastic leukemia

Anterior axillary line

AB

Ace bandage

Active bilaterally

Abd.

Abdomen

Abduction

Abductor

ABE

Activity before exercise

Acute bacterial endocarditis

ABN

Abnormal

Active bulimia nervosa

Acute bacterial nephritis

ACT

Active motion

Anesthesia care team

AD

Advance directive

Alzheimer's disease

Auris dexter right ear (right ear)

AI

Adequate intake

Aortic insufficiency

Articulation index

AO

Abdominal aorta

Acid output

Ankle orthosis

Anterior oblique

AP

Acid phosphatase

Active pepsin

Ante partum

Abbreviations

AR
Active-resistance
Aortic regurgitation

ARF
Acute respiratory failure
Acute rheumatic fever

AROM
Active range of motion
Artificial rupture of membranes

Art
Arterial
Articulation

AS
Aortic stenosis
Auris sinistra (left ear)

AU
Ad usum (according to custom)
Auris unitas (both ears)

AV
Aortic valve
Atrioventricula

AW
Able to work
Above waist

Ax.
Axial
Axilla
Axillary

B.U.O.
Bleeding of undetermined origin
Bruising of undetermined origin

BA
Brachial artery
Bronchial asthma

BAO
Basal acid output
Brachial artery output

BAP
Behavior activity profile
Brachial artery pressure

BAR
Bariatrics
Barometer
Barometric
Beta-adrenergic receptor

BAT
Basic aid training
Blunt abdominal trauma
Brown adipose tissue

BB
Beta-blocker
Blow bottle
Both bones
Breast biopsy
Buffer base oxidase
Breakthrough bleeding

BBS
Bashful bladder syndrome
Bilateral breath sounds

BC
Basal cell
Birth control
Board certified
Breast cancer
Bronchial carcinoma
Buffy coat

BCA
Balloon catheter angioplasty
Basal cell atypia
Breast cancer antigen

BCC
Basal cell carcinoma
Benign cellular changes
Birth control clinic

© 2011 Contexo Media

Abbreviations

BCG
Bacillus Calmette-Guerin (tuberculosis vaccine)

Ballistocardiogram

Ballistocardiography

Bromcresol green (dye)

BD
Band

Barbital-dependent

Behavioral disorder

Bile duct

Blood donor

Brain damage

Brain dead

Brain death

BI
Basilar impression

Biological indicator

Bodily injury

Bone impaction

Burn index

BM
Basal metabolism

Black male

Bone marrow

Bowel movement

BS
Blood sugar

Bowel sounds

Breath sounds

Bronchial secretion

BSR
Basal skin resistance

Blood sedimentation rate

Bowel sounds regular

BT
Bladder tumor

Blood type

Body temperature

Brain tumor

Breast tumor

BTx
Blood transfusion

Brevetoxin

BU
Bethesda unit

Blood urea

Burn unit

Buruli ulcer

BW
Bed wetting

Below waist

Birth weight

C
Caucasian

Cervical

C.
Celsius complement

Centigrade

Gallon

Ca
Calcium

Carcinoma

CA
Cancer

Cardiac arrest

Caucasian adult

CAF
Caucasian adult female

Cell adhesion factor

CBV
Catheter balloon valvuloplasty

Cerebral blood volume

CC
Caucasian child

Chief complaint

CD
Cadaver donor

Cardiac disease

Contagious disease

Abbreviations

CE

Cardiac enlargement

Cardioesophageal

Cataract extraction

Central episiotomy

Chloroform ether

CF

Cardiac failure

Caucasian female

Cystic fibrosis

CHD

Congenital heart disease

Coronary heart disease

CI

Cardiac index

Cardiac insufficiency

Cerebral infarction

CM

Cardiac murmur

Cardiac muscle

Caucasian male

CO

Carbon monoxide

Cardiac output

CP

Cerebral palsy

Chest pain

CRF

Case report form

Chronic renal failure

CRT

Capillary refill time

Cardiac resuscitation team

CV

Cardiac volume

Cardiovascular

Curriculum vitae

CVA

Cerebrovascular accident (stroke)

Costovertebral angle

DC

Discharges

Discontinue

DI

Diabetes insipidus

Diagnostic imaging

DIC

Disseminated coagulopathy

Disseminated intravascular coagulation

DM

Diabetes mellitus

Diastolic murmur

ECF

Extended care facility

Extracellular fluid

ECHO

Echocardiogram

Enterocytopathogenic human orphan virus

GBS

Gallbladder series

Gastric bypass surgery

Group B Streptococcus

Guillain-Barre syndrome

GO

Gonorrhea

Glucose

ICS

Immotile cilia syndrome

Intercostals space

MT

Mammary tumor

Membrana tympani

Malignant teratoma

MDI

Metered dose inhaler

Multiple daily vitamin

© 2011 Contexo Media

Abbreviations

NBM
No bowel movement

Normal bowel movement

Normal bone marrow

Nothing by mouth

NVD
Nausea, vomiting, diarrhea

Neck vein distention

Neovascularization of the disc

Neurovesicle dysfunction

Number of vessels diseased

PAP
Positive airway pressure

Pulmonary alveolar proteinosis

PE
Physical examination

Pulmonary edema

Pulmonary embolism (or embolus)

PI
Pulmonary insufficiency

Past history

RT
Respiratory therapy (or therapist)

Right

TCA
Tricyclic antidepressant

Total cholic acid

Total circulating albumin

Total circulatory arrest

Trichloroacetic acid

VC
Vital capacity

Ventricular contraction

VD
Vascular disease

V&D
Vomiting and diarrhea

Practice Quiz: Abbreviations

Match the following abbreviations with their meanings:

1. ALL _____
2. CHF _____
3. DEXA _____
4. EEG _____
5. FTT _____
6. HX _____
7. IV _____
8. MRI _____
9. OU _____
10. UTI _____

a. history

b. magnetic resonance imaging

c. urinary tract infection

d. acute lymphocyte leukemia

e. dual energy x-ray absorptiometry

f. failure to thrive

g. intravenous

h. both eyes

i. congestive heart failure

j. electroencephalogram

Chapter 16

TERMS TO KNOW

The following definitions are some of the common medical terms found when coding medical procedures.

Abdominal Aorta
The portion of the aorta (main blood vessel of the body) in the abdomen.

Ablation
In radio-frequency or catheter ablation, the term signifies destruction of selected portions of heart's conduction (electrical) system.

Abscess
A localized collection of pus in any part of the body, usually surrounded by inflamed tissue.

ACE (angiotensin-converting enzyme) Inhibitor
A drug that lowers blood pressure by interfering with the breakdown of a substance involved in blood pressure regulation.

Acute
Severe, for a short time.

Acute Sinusitis
Symptoms of sinusitis that begin suddenly, often about one week after a typical "cold".

Adhesion
Fibrous scars caused when body tissues that are normally separate are joined. Abdominal adhesions may be painful when stretched, because fibrous tissue is not elastic.

Allergen
A substance, such as food, fur, pollen, or dust, that is normally harmless but causes an allergic reaction in susceptible persons.

Allergy
Inappropriate or exaggerated reaction of the immune system to substances that, in the majority of people, cause no symptoms.

Alveoli
Air sacs in the lungs where oxygen and carbon dioxide are exchanged to and from the bloodstream.

Amblyopia
Commonly known as lazy eye. A loss of vision in a young child due to the eye not being used. The eye is normal but the brain tends to suppress or ignore the image received by the amblyopic eye. The most common causes include a muscle imbalance, a focusing problem, or a problem such as a cataract or corneal scar. Sometimes both eyes can be affected.

Amniocentesis
The suction of fluid from the amniotic sac through the use of a needle inserted through the abdomen.

Analgesia
Loss of sensibility to pain, loss of response to a painful stimulus.

Analgesic
A medication that reduces or eliminates pain.

Anaphylaxis
A severe and life-threatening allergic reaction to a substance, for example, penicillin or an insect sting.

Anesthesia
Loss of sensation of a body part; or of the body when induced by the administration of a drug.

Anesthetic
An agent that causes loss of sensation with or without the loss of consciousness.

Aneurysm
A sac-like protrusion from a blood vessel or the heart, resulting from a weakening of the vessel wall or heart muscle.

Angina (or angina pectoris)
Pain or discomfort, pressure or squeezing, usually centered in the chest that results from diseased blood vessels restricting blood and oxygen flow to the heart. Tightness or heaviness in the arms, neck or jaw, shortness of breath, nausea, sweating, weakness, or palpitations may also be present. This is usually due to a cholesterol clogged artery to the heart. Angina may be precipitated by exertion and relieved by rest, and may be an early sign of a heart attack, especially if persistent and progressive.

Angiography
An x-ray technique that makes use of contrast ("dye") injected into the coronary arteries to study blood circulation through the vessels. The test allows physicians to measure the degrees of obstruction to blood flow. Circulation through an artery is not

© 2011 Contexo Media

137

seriously reduced until the inside diameter of the vessel is more than 50 to 70% obstructed.

Angioplasty
A non-surgical technique for treating diseased arteries by temporarily inflating a tiny balloon inside an artery, to push aside plaque build-up.

Anterior
Front of the body or situated near the front of the body.

Anterolateral
Situated or occurring in front of and to the side.

Antibiotic
A substance that combats bacterial infection. Antibiotics are usually derived from living organisms.

Antibody
A protein (also called immunoglobulin) manufactured by lymphocytes (a type of white blood cell) to neutralize an antigen or foreign protein.

Anticoagulants
Any drugs that keep blood from clotting ("blood thinners"). These drugs do not actually dilute the blood.

Anticonvulsant
A medication that prevents or relieves seizures.

Antidepressant
A medication that prevents or treats depression.

Antiemetic
A medication that prevents or alleviates nausea or vomiting.

Antifungal
A medication that combats fungal infections.

Antihistamine
A category of drugs that block the effects of histamine, a chemical released in body fluids during an allergic reaction. Antihistamines reduce itching, sneezing, and runny nose.

Antihypertensives
Any drugs or other therapy that lowers blood pressure.

Anti-inflammatory Drugs
Drugs that reduce symptoms and signs of inflammation.

Antiseptic
Any substance that kills infectious agents. Antiseptics are too strong to be swallowed or injected into the body.

Aorta
The largest artery in the body and the initial blood-supply vessel from the heart to the rest of the body.

Aortic Valve
The valve that prevents blood flowing backwards from the aorta into the heart.

Apex
A general term used in anatomical nomenclature to designate the superior aspect of a body, organ, or the pointed extremity of a conical structure such as the heart or lung.

Aphakia
The loss or absence of the lens of an eye.

Aphasia
The inability to speak, write, or understand spoken or written language because of brain injury or disease.

Apnea
Cessation of respiration; inability to get one's breath.

Apoplexy
A sudden event. Often used as equivalent to stroke.

Arrhythmia (or dysrhythmia)
An abnormal rhythm of the heart. It may feel simply like a skipped beat, or feel like a prolonged fluttering or pounding in the chest. Serious arrhythmias can make one light headed, make one pass out or cause a heart attack.

Arterioles
Small, muscular branches of arteries. When they contract, they increase resistance to blood flow, and blood pressure in the arteries increases.

Arteries
Vessels that carry oxygen-rich blood to the body.

Arteritis
Inflammation of the arteries.

Arteriosclerosis
A disease process, commonly called hardening of the arteries, which includes a variety of conditions that cause artery walls to thicken and lose elasticity.

Arthralgia
Joint pain.

Arthritis
Inflammation of a joint or a state characterized by inflammation of joints.

Arthrocentesis
Surgical puncture of the joint space with a needle where synovial fluid is removed for analysis.

Arthrodesis
The fusion of bones across a joint space, thereby limiting or eliminating movement. It may occur spontaneously or as a result of a surgical procedure, such as fusion of the spine.

Arthropathy
Any disease or disorder involving a joint.

Arthroplasty
The surgical remodeling of a diseased or damaged joint.

Arthroscope
An instrument inserted into it's joint cavity to view the interior of a joint and correct certain abnormalities. An arthroscope is an endoscope for use in a joint.

Arthroscopy
The procedure of visualizing the inside of a joint by means of an arthroscope.

Articular
Pertaining to a joint.

Ascending Aorta
The first portion of the aorta, emerging from the heart's left ventricle.

Aspirate, Aspiration
Withdrawal of a fluid from the body by suction, usually through a needle or syringe.

Asthma
A chronic inflammatory lung disease characterized by recurrent breathing problems.

Astigmatism
An irregular curvature of either the cornea (front of the eye) or the lens. If either structure is shaped more like a football rather than a basketball, light is not sharply focused on the retina. This results in blurry vision for both distance and near.

Ataxia
A loss of muscular coordination, abnormal clumsiness.

Atherosclerosis
A disease process that leads to the accumulation of a waxy substance (plaque) inside blood vessels.

Atria
The two (right and left) upper collecting chambers of the heart.

Atrial Fibrillation
The heart contracts and relaxes at an irregular and sometimes rapid rate.

Atrophy
A wasting of tissues, organs, or the entire body.

Atrium
Either of the heart's two upper chambers.

Autoimmune
A condition in which the body makes antibodies against its own tissues, and damages itself.

Autonomic Nervous System
Involuntary nervous system, also termed the vegetative nervous system. A system of nerve cells whose activities are beyond voluntary control.

Avascular
Non-vascular, not provided with blood vessels.

Axillary Lymph Nodes
Numerous nodes around the axillary (below the shoulder joint) veins which receive the lymphatic drainage from the upper limb, scapular region and pectoral region (including mammary gland); they drain into the subclavian trunk.

Benign
Describing an abnormal growth that will neither spread nor recur after removal.

Beta Blocker
An antihypertensive drug that limits the activity of epinephrine, a hormone that increases blood pressure.

Binocular Vision
The blending of the separate images seen by each eye into a single image; allows images to be seen with depth.

Biopsy
The process by which a small sample of tissue is taken for examination.

Blepharitis
An inflammation of the eyelids or lid margins. It is often caused by an infection. A chronic form produces a crusting or flaking of the lid margins. This is treatable by an eye doctor.

Blindness
Legal blindness is defined as: 1) visual acuity of 20/200 (only being able to see the big E on the eye chart) or less in the best eye even with the eyes corrected by glasses or contact lenses; or, 2) The peripheral visual field is reduced to 20 degrees of visual angle or less. Twenty degrees of visual angle is about the size of a one foot ruler held at arms length.

Blood Clot
A jelly-like mass of blood tissue formed by clotting factors in the blood. Clots stop the flow of blood from an injury; they

Terms To Know

can also form inside an artery whose walls are damaged by atherosclerotic build-up and can cause a heart attack or stroke.

Blood Pressure
The force or pressure exerted by the heart in pumping blood; the pressure of blood in the arteries.

Bradycardia
An abnormally slow heartbeat (usually less than 50 beats per minute).

Bradykinesia
Slowness in movement.

Bronchitis
An inflammation of the bronchi (lung airways) resulting in a persistent cough that produces considerable quantities of sputum (phlegm).

Bronchodilator Drugs
A group of drugs that widen the airways in the lungs.

Bundle Branch Block
A condition in which portions of the heart's conduction system are defective and unable to conduct the electrical signals normally.

Bursa
A bursa (bursae, plural for bursa) is a closed fluid-filled sac that functions as a gliding surface to reduce friction between tissues of the body.

Bursectomy
Surgical drainage and removal of the infected bursa sac.

Calcium Channel Blockers (or calcium blockers)
Drugs that lower blood pressure by regulating calcium-related electrical activity in the heart.

Candida
A group of yeast-like fungi that may produce infection.

Capillaries
Microscopically small blood vessels between arteries and veins that distribute oxygenated blood to the body's tissues.

Carcinogen
Any substance that can cause cancer.

Carcinoma
A malignant growth composed of abnormally multiplying surface tissues. Carcinomas, the most common type of cancer, can often be treated successfully if discovered early.

Cardiac
Means pertaining to the heart.

Cardiac Arrest
The stopping of the heartbeat, usually because of interference with the electrical signal (often associated with coronary heart disease).

Cardiac Catheterization
A procedure that involves inserting a fine, flexible, hollow tube (catheter) into an artery, usually in the groin or wrist area and passing the tube into the heart. Often used in conjunction with angiography and other procedures, cardiac catheterization has become a prime tool for visualizing the heart and blood vessels and diagnosing and treating heart disease.

Cardiac Enzymes
Complex substances capable of speeding up certain biochemical processes, found in cardiac muscle. Abnormal blood levels of these enzymes may signal heart attack.

Cardiac Output
The amount of blood the heart pumps through the circulatory system in one minute.

Cardiology
The study of the heart and its function in health and disease.

Cardiomyopathy
A disease of the heart muscle that leads to deteriorization of the muscle and its pumping ability.

Cardiovascular (CV)
Means pertaining to the heart and blood vessels. The circulatory system of the body consists of the heart and blood vessels and is called the cardiovascular system.

Cardioversion
A technique of applying an electrical shock to the chest in order to convert an abnormal heartbeat to a normal rhythm.

Carotid Artery
A major artery (right and left) in the neck that supplies blood to the brain.

Carpal Tunnel
Space under a ligament in wrist through which the median nerve enters the palm of the hand.

Cartilage
The hard, thin layer of white glossy tissue that covers the end of bone at a joint. This tissue allows motion to take place with a minimum amount of friction.

Cataract
An opacity or haziness of the lens of the eye. A cataract is noticed particularly at night when oncoming headlights produce glare disability and/or discomfort. It may or may not reduce the vision depending on size, density, and location. If a cataract reduces

visual acuity significantly, an Ophthalmologist can replace the defective lens with an artificial lens.

Catheter
A small tube used to inject a dye to see the blood vessels, similar to that used for looking at vessels in the heart.

Cauterization
Destruction of tissue by burning it away with a caustic chemical, a red-hot instrument, or electricity. Cauterization can be used to remove growths on the skin or mucous membrane (such as warts).

Central Nervous System
Part of the nervous system which consists of the brain and spinal cord, to which sensory impulses are transmitted and from which motor impulses pass out, and which supervises and coordinates the activity of the entire nervous system.

Cerebral Embolism
A blood clot or small plaque formed in one part of the body and then carried by the bloodstream to the brain, where it blocks an artery.

Cerebral Hemorrhage
Bleeding within the brain resulting from a ruptured blood vessel, aneurysm or a head injury.

Cerebral Thrombosis
The formation of a blood clot in an artery that supplies part of the brain.

Cerebrospinal Fluid (CSF)
Water-like fluid produced in the brain that circulates around and protects the brain and spinal cord. Shrinking or expanding of the cranial contents is usually quickly balanced by increase or decrease of this fluid.

Cerebrovascular
Means pertaining to the blood vessels of the brain.

Cerebrovascular Accident (also called CVA, cerebral vascular accident, stroke or apoplexy)
An impeded blood supply to some part of the brain, resulting in injury to brain tissue.

Cerebrovascular Occlusion
The obstruction or closing of a blood vessel in the brain.

Cervical
Of or relating to the neck.

Cholesterol
An oily substance that occurs naturally in the body, in animal fats and in dairy products, and that is transported in the blood. Limited quantities are required for the normal development of cell membranes.

Chronic Sinusitis
Patients are diagnosed with chronic sinusitis when their sinusitis symptoms persist for greater than 12 weeks despite medical treatment. Chronic sinus disease may be caused by anatomic sinus ostial narrowing, mucociliary disturbances or immune deficiency.

Circulatory System
Pertains to the heart, blood vessels and the circulation of blood.

Claudication
A tiredness or pain in the arms and legs caused by an inadequate supply of oxygen to the muscles, usually due to narrowed arteries.

Coagulation
The process of clotting.

Coccyx
The small bone at the end of the spinal column in humans which is formed by the fusion of four rudimentary vertebrae. The "tail bone".

Collagen
A fibrous protein which is a major constituent of connective tissue. Such as skin, tendons, ligaments, cartilage, and bones.

Collateral Circulation
Blood flow through small, nearby vessels in response to blockage of a main blood vessel ("natural bypass").

Colon
The large intestine.

Coma
A state of deep, often prolonged unconsciousness, usually the result of injury, disease, or poison, in which an individual is incapable of sensing or responding to external stimuli and internal needs.

Computed Tomography (CT or CAT scan)
A non-invasive procedure that takes many x-ray images with the aid of a computer to generate cross-sectional images of the brain or other internal organs to detect any abnormalities that may not show up on an ordinary x-ray.

Concussion
A disruption, usually temporary, of neurological function resulting from a blow or violent shaking.

Congenital
Existing at, and usually before birth referring to conditions that are present at birth, regardless of their causation.

Terms To Know

Congestive Heart Failure (CHF)
A common ailment affecting more than two million Americans. Heart failure means the heart cannot pump all the blood returning to it efficiently, leading to a back-up of blood in vessels, and accumulation of fluid in body tissues, lungs, and abdominal organs. There are several symptoms of heart failure, the most common being shortness of breath and swelling.

Conjunctiva
The membrane that lines the exposed eyeball and the inside of the eyelid.

Conjunctivitis
Inflammation of the membrane covering the surface of the eyeball. It can be a result of infection, irritation, or related to systemic diseases, such as Reiter's syndrome.

Conscious Sedation
Intravenous medication used to help a patient relax during a procedure, without putting the patient to sleep. Usually associated with procedures which are anxiety-producing for the patient.

Contact Dermatitis
Inflammation of the skin or a rash caused by various substances. The more common causes include reaction to detergents left on washed clothes, nickel (in watch straps, bracelets and necklaces), chemicals in rubbery gloves and condoms, certain cosmetics, plants, and topical medications.

Contagious
A term applied to diseases that can spread from person to person.

Contrast Medium
Any material (usually opaque to x-rays) employed to delineate or define a structure during a radiologic procedure.

Contusion
An injury of a part without a break in the skin and with a subcutaneous hemorrhage (e.g. brain contusion – contusion with loss of consciousness as a result of direct trauma to the head, usually associated with fracture of the skull).

Cornea
The cornea is the clear front window of the eye that transmits and focuses light into the eye.

Coronary Artery Bypass Grafting (CABG)
A surgical rerouting ("bypassing") of blood around a diseased vessel that supplies the heart by grafting either a piece of vein from the leg or the artery from under the breastbone or other location. Almost 500,000 bypasses are performed each year.

Coronary Artery Disease (CAD), or Coronary Atherosclerosis
Occurs when there is a buildup of cholesterol rich plaque along the lining of the coronary arteries, greatly increasing a person's risk of having a heart attack.

Coronary Heart Disease
Caused by the atherosclerotic narrowing of the coronary arteries, and likely to produce angina pectoris or heart attack.

Coronary Occlusion
An obstruction of one of the coronary arteries that hinders blood flow to some part of the heart muscle.

Coronary Thrombosis
The formation of a clot in one of the arteries that carry blood to the heart muscle. Also called coronary occlusion.

Cortex
The surface of the brain. The word cortex is derived from the Greek name meaning "bark" (like tree bark). The visual cortex contains 32 or more areas devoted to visual information processing. Two major cortical pathways are the "What" and the "Where" visual pathways, that are devoted to what an object is and where an object is.

Corticosteroid Drugs
A group of anti-inflammatory drugs similar to the natural corticosteroid hormones produced by the cortex of the adrenal glands.

Cyanosis
Blueness of skin caused by insufficient oxygen in the blood.

Cyst
A sac or vesicle in the body.

Death Rate
The ratio of total deaths to total population in a specified community or area over a specified period of time. The death rate is often expressed as the number of deaths per 1,000 of the population per year. Also called fatality rate.

Deep Vein Thrombosis
A blood clot in a deep vein in the calf, thigh, arm, or pelvis.

Defibrillation
Delivery of a large electrical current to the heart when it is beating erratically. The purpose is to restore a regular heartbeat.

Defibrillator (implantable defibrillator or ICD)
Is a surgically implantable electronic device designed to provide an electric shock at the appropriate time to regularize abnormal heart rhythms in a malfunctioning heart.

Degenerative Myopia
Pathologic progressive myopia. Causes retinal pigment epithelium (RPE), choriocapillaris atrophy, and photoreceptor degeneration. Leads to reduced visual acuity, night blindness, and retinal detachment, the latter requires retinal surgery.

Dehydration
Excessive loss of water from the body, often due to severe vomiting or diarrhea.

Depth Perception
The ability to distinguish objects in a visual field.

Dermoid Cyst
A congenital (born with) tumor present in infancy as a yellowish swelling on the surface of the eye. It may enlarge during puberty. The dermoid cyst can be surgically removed by an ophthalmologist.

Detached Retina
A condition in which the retina separates from another layer of cells in the back of the eye, resulting in a decrease in nutrition and visual function. It may be due to a hemorrhage, trauma, tumor, vascular malformation, or from traction of the vitreous to which it is attached. Sometimes, people with high myopia will develop a retinal detachment, which requires emergency surgery.

Diabetes (diabetes mellitus)
A disease in which the body doesn't produce or properly use insulin. Insulin is needed to convert sugar and starch into the energy needed in daily life.

Diabetic Retinopathy
Pathologic changes in the back of the eye, retina, caused by diabetes. Background type is characterized by ongoing microaneurysms, retinal hemorrhages, and swelling of the central part of the eye, known as the macula. The proliferate type involves the growth of abnormal blood vessels in the retina and optic disk, blood leaking into the jelly part of the eye, known as the vitreous, and detachment of the retina.

Diastolic Blood Pressure
The lowest blood pressure measured in the arteries, occurring when the heart muscle is relaxed, between beats.

Dilation
A process by which the pupil is temporarily enlarged with special eye drops (mydriatic); allows the eye care specialist to better view the inside of the eye.

Diplopia
Commonly known as double vision. In children, diplopia is often associated with a muscle imbalance such as esotropia. A refractive error may also cause enough blurring that a person sees two objects.

Distal
Situated away from the center of the body.

Diuretics
Drugs that lower blood pressure by stimulating fluid loss, promoting urine production.

Doppler Ultrasound
A technology that uses sound waves to assess blood flow within the heart and blood vessels and to identify leaking valves.

Drip
The common name for an intravenous infusion (IV). A hollow tube is inserted into a vein, through which the liquid runs from an elevated sterile container.

Dye (contrast)
A radiopaque substance used during an x-ray exam to provide contrast in the different tissues and organs. "Dye" usually refers to the contrast media given intravenously.

Dysarthria
The imperfect articulation of speech resulting from muscular problems caused by damage to the brain or nervous system.

Dyslexia
A learning problem in which a person has difficulty with letter or word recognition. Children often are of normal or above normal intelligence; however, they have difficulty reading and sometimes naming pictures of objects. This is a higher cortical processing problem and NOT a vision or eye problem.

Dyspnea
Shortness of breath.

Echocardiogram (ECHO)
A method of studying the heart's structure and function by analyzing sound waves (similar to those used to visualize a baby in the womb) bounced off the heart and recorded by an electronic sensor placed on the chest. A computer processes the information to produce a one-, two- or three-dimensional moving picture that shows how the heart and valves are functioning.

Edema
Swelling caused by fluid accumulation in body tissues.

Electrocardiogram (ECG/EKG)
A test that measures the electrical output of the heart. It is a simple procedure that will allow a physician to make decisions regarding the health of the heart's muscle, arteries and electrical system.

Electroencephalogram (EEG)
A graphic record of the electrical impulses produced by the brain.

Terms To Know

Electromyography (EMG)
A method of recording the electrical currents generated in a muscle during its contraction.

Electrophysiology Studies (EPS)
Use cardiac catheterization to study patients who have arrhythmias (abnormal heartbeats). An electrical current stimulates the heart in an effort to provoke an arrhythmia. EPS is used primarily to identify the origin of arrhythmias and to test the effectiveness of treatment.

Embolization
The insertion of a substance through a catheter into a blood vessel to stop hemorrhaging, or excessive bleeding.

Embolus (also called Embolism)
A blood clot or plaque that forms in the blood vessel in one part of the body and travels to another part.

Endocarditis
A bacterial infection of the heart's inner lining (endothelium) or heart valves.

Endoscope
A medical device for viewing internal portions of the body. It is usually comprised of fiber optic tubes and video display instruments.

Endoscopy
Inspection of internal body structures or cavities using an endoscope.

Endothelium
The smooth inner lining of many body structures, including the heart (endocardium) and blood vessels.

Enlarged Heart
Enlarged heart is an increase in the size of the heart caused by a thickening of the heart muscle because of increased workload. This increased workload can be due to heart valve disease or high blood pressure. Enlarged heart may also be a dilation (expansion) of the heart due to damage that weakens the heart muscle.

Enucleation
An operation in which the whole eye and the front part of the optic nerve are removed. It is usually performed when the eye contains a tumor or is blind and very painful.

Enzymes
Complex chemicals capable of speeding up specific biochemical processes in the body.

Eosinophil
A type of white blood cell that usually comprises <5% of all white blood cells in the blood. Eosinophils are found in increased numbers in chronic sinusitis, nasal polyps and asthma. They contribute to inflammation by production of inflammatory mediators, such as leukotriene C4.

Epinephrine
A naturally occurring hormone, also called adrenaline. It dilates the airways to improve breathing and narrows blood vessels in the skin and intestines so that an increased flow of blood reaches the muscles and allows them to cope with the demands of exercise.

Eponym
Medical terms that have been named as a result of the person who discovered the body part or disease.

Esotropia
Cross-eyed or, in medical terms, convergent or internal strabismus.

Estrogen
A female hormone, produced by the ovaries, that may protect women against heart disease. Estrogen is not produced after menopause.

Etiology
Cause of a disease.

Excision
Removal by cutting away material.

Exercise Stress Test (exercise test, stress test, or treadmill test)
Is a common test for diagnosing coronary artery disease, especially in patients who have symptoms of heart disease. The test helps physicians assess blood flow through coronary arteries in response to exercise, usually walking, at varied speeds and for various lengths of time on a treadmill. A stress test may include use of electrocardiography, echocardiography, and injection of radioactive substances.

Exogenous
Originating outside of the body.

Exophthalmos
An abnormal protrusion of the eyeball often caused by thyroid disease or a tumor behind the eye. Medical treatment is necessary.

Eye
The organ of sight. The word "eye" come from the Teutonic "auge." The eye has a number of components. These include the cornea, iris, pupil, lens, retina, macula, optic nerve, and vitreous.

Familial Hypercholesterolemia
A genetic predisposition to dangerously high cholesterol levels.

Terms To Know

Fatty Acids (fats)
Are substances that occur in several forms in foods; different fatty acids have different effects on lipid profiles.

Fenestration (of cyst)
Surgical creation of window-like opening.

Fibrillation
Rapid, uncoordinated contractions of individual heart muscle fibers. The heart chamber involved can't contract all at once and pumps blood ineffectively, if at all.

Fibrinolysis
This is what happens when enzymes in the blood dissolve blood clots.

Flutter
The rapid, ineffective contraction of any heart chamber. A flutter is considered to be more coordinated than fibrillation.

Foramen
A natural opening or passage in bone.

Fracture
A disruption of the normal continuity of bone.

Gallbladder Series
A series of x-rays of the gallbladder, taken after the gallbladder has been outlined with a special x-ray dye. The dye is taken by mouth the night prior to the study.

Gastrostomy Tubes
A gastrostomy tube (feeding tube) is inserted into the stomach if the patient is unable to take food by mouth.

Glaucoma
An eye condition in which the fluid pressure inside the eyes rises because of slowed fluid drainage from the eye. Untreated, it may damage the optic nerve and other parts of the eye, leading to vision loss or even blindness.

Heart Attack
Occurs when one of the arteries which supplies blood to the heart muscle becomes suddenly blocked. Symptoms are usually severe and sudden in onset. They may include fullness, discomfort or squeezing in the chest area radiating to the arms, throat, neck or jaw, with nausea and sweating.

Heart Block
A general term for conditions in which the electrical impulse that activates the heart muscle cells is delayed or interrupted somewhere along its path.

Heart Failure
(see Congestive Heart Failure or CHF).

Heart-Lung Machine
An apparatus that oxygenates and pumps blood to the body during open heart surgery.

Hemangioma
A benign tumor consisting of a mass of blood vessels.

Hematoma
A blood clot.

Hemiplegia
Paralysis of one side of the body.

Hemorrhage
Bleeding due to the escape of blood from a blood vessel.

Heredity
The genetic transmission of a particular quality or trait from parent to offspring.

High Blood Pressure
A chronic increase in blood pressure above its normal range.

High Density Lipoprotein (HDL)
A component of cholesterol that helps protect against heart disease by promoting cholesterol breakdown and removal from the blood; hence, its nickname "good cholesterol."

Histamine
A chemical present in cells throughout the body that is released during an allergic reaction.

Histologic
Pertaining to the study of microscopic structures of tissue.

Holter Monitor
A portable device for recording heartbeats over a period of 24 hours or more.

Hyperopia
Commonly known as farsightedness. Most children are hyperopic and see things in the distance better than very close things.

Hypertension
High blood pressure.

Hypoglycemia
Means low levels of glucose in the blood.

Hypotension
Abnormally low blood pressure.

Hypoxia
Less than the normal content of oxygen in the organs and tissues of the body.

Terms To Know

Iliac Bone
A part of the pelvic bone that is above the hip joint and from which autogenous bone grafts are frequently obtained.

Iliac Crest
The large, prominent portion of the pelvic bone at the belt line of the body.

Immobilization
Limitation of motion or fixation of a body part usually to promote healing.

Immunosuppressive Medications
Any drugs that suppress the body's immune system. These medications are used to minimize the chances that the body will reject a newly transplanted organ such as a heart.

Immunotherapy
Allergy shots. Gradually increased doses of an allergen cause the immune system to become less sensitive to the substance, which reduces the symptoms of the allergy when the substance is encountered in the future.

Implantable Defibrillator
An implantable defibrillator is a surgically implantable electronic device designed to provide an electric shock at the appropriate time to regularize abnormal heart rhythms.

Incubation Period
The time lag between infection and appearance of symptoms. During this time, infectious agents are multiplying but are insufficient in number to cause symptoms or infect other people. Incubation periods range from a few days (influenza) to months (hepatitis).

Infarct
The area of heart tissue permanently damaged by an inadequate supply of blood and oxygen.

Inferior
Situated below or directed downward.

Inferior Vena Cava
The large vein returning blood from the legs and abdomen to the heart.

Infuse
To introduce a solution into the body through a vein.

Inotropic Medications
Drugs that increase the strength of the heart's contraction.

Intra-aortic Balloon Pump (IABP)
A balloon on a catheter is inserted into the aorta and inflated intermittently to improve the delivery of blood to the heart.

Intraocular Pressure (IOP)
The pressure that the fluid (vitreous) contained within the eye, exerts on the globe (lining of the eyeball). Increased intraocular pressure is a feature of glaucoma.

Intravascular Echocardiography
A marriage of echocardiography and cardiac catheterization. A miniature echo device on the tip of a catheter is used to generate images inside the heart and blood vessels.

Intrinsic
Situated entirely within or pertaining exclusively to a part.

Iris
The iris is the colored part of the eye that helps regulate the amount of light that enters the eye.

Ischemia
Decreased blood flow to an organ, usually due to constriction or obstruction of an artery.

I.V.
Intravenous. Literally, means through a vein. "An IV" often refers to a particular kind of injection apparatus: a bottle of fluid is held up on a small pole, and gravity causes the fluid to flow down through a flexible tube, through a needle, and into the patient's vein.

Joint
The junction or articulation of two or more bones that permits varying degrees of motion between the bones.

Jugular Veins
The veins that carry blood back from the head to the heart.

Kyphosis
An abnormal increase in the normal kyphotic curvature of the thoracic spine.

Lacrimal Gland
The tear gland located under the upper eyelid at the outer corner of the eye. The fluid it secretes cleans and provides moisture for the cornea. It is responsible for tearing during emotional stimulation or following corneal irritation by a foreign body or chemical.

Lamina
The flattened or arched part of the vertebral arch, forming the roof of the spinal canal.

Lateral
Situated away from the midline of the body.

Laser
Light Amplification by Stimulated Emission of Radiation. The device that produces a focused beam of light at a defined wavelength that can vaporize tissue. In surgery, lasers can be

used to operate on small areas without damaging delicate surrounding tissue.

LASIK

LASIK (Laser in-Situ Keratomileusis) combines the precision of the excimer laser delivery system with the benefits of Lamellar Keratoplasty (LK) which has been proven to treat a wide range of refractive errors. Using the accuracy and precision of the excimer laser, LASIK changes the shape of the cornea to improve the way light is focused or "refracted" by the eye. First, a thin corneal flap is created, as an instrument called a microkeratome glides across the cornea. Then, in just seconds, ultraviolet light and high energy pulses from the excimer laser reshape the internal cornea with accuracy up to 0.25 microns. By adjusting the pattern of the laser beam, it is possible to treat high levels of nearsightedness and moderate amounts of farsightedness and astigmatism.

Lazy Eye

A term often used instead of amblyopia. A loss of visual function, usually measured by visual acuity, in one or both eyes that cannot be explained by identifiable causes(s) such as a cataract or retinal disease. An eye that turns in (esotropia) or out (exotropia) may have a certain degree of central visual loss (amblyopia). A lazy eye is often treated by placing a patch over the stronger eye and forcing use of the lazy eye. The earlier the detection of the lazy eye the better for recovery of central vision with patching. If left untreated, after the age of about 8 or 9 years, patching therapy is no longer effective and the child will have a permanent loss of vision and loss of binocular vision and depth perception.

Lens

The lens is the transparent structure inside the eye that focuses light rays onto the retina.

Lesion

An injury or a wound. An atherosclerotic lesion is an injury to an artery due to hardening of the arteries.

Ligament

A band of flexible, fibrous connective tissue that is attached at the end of a bone near a joint. The main function of a ligament is to attach bones to one another to provide stability of a joint, and to prevent or limit some joint motion.

Lipids

Fatty substances insoluble in blood.

Lipoproteins

Lipids surrounded by a protein; the protein makes the lipid soluble in blood.

Lordosis

Curvature of the spine with the convexity forward.

Lumbar

The lower part of the spine between the thoracic region and the sacrum. The lumbar spine consists of five vertebrae known as (L1-L5).

Lumen

The hollow area within a tube, such as a blood vessel.

Macular Degeneration

A degeneration or loss of the macula of the eye, usually hereditary. The most common form of macular degeneration is Age-Related Macular Degeneration (ARMD). It is believed that one contributing factor for ARMD is excessive light exposure over a person's lifetime. Limiting excessive light exposure (e.g., wearing sunglasses and a hat outside) and a diet rich in antioxidants as well as zinc may prevent the development of ARMD. In general, the lighter a person's complexion the greater the risk of ARMD.

Magnetic Resonance Angiography (MRA)

A technique that produces images of the heart and other body structures by measuring the response of certain elements (such as hydrogen) in the body to a magnetic field. When stimulated by radio waves, the elements emit distinctive signals in a magnetic field.

Magnetic Resonance Imaging (MRI)

A non-invasive study which is conducted in a Magnetic Resonance Imager. The magnetic images are assembled by a computer to provide an image of the arteries in the head and neck. No contrast material is needed, but some patients may experience claustrophobia in the imager.

Malignant

Designating an abnormal growth that tends to spread (metastasize), and eventually cause death. Malignant tumors sometimes recur after apparent removal (see benign).

Mammography, Mammogram

A mammogram is an X-ray of the breast. It is used to detect breast cancer and other abnormalities of the breast.

Medial

Toward the inside or center of the body (i.e., the big toe is medial to the small toe).

Miosis

Constriction of the pupil.

Mitral Valve

The structure that controls blood flow between the heart's left atrium (upper chamber) and left ventricle (lower chamber).

Mitral Valve Prolapse

A condition that occurs when the leaflets of the mitral valve between the left atrium (upper chamber) and left ventricle (lower chamber) are longer than needed, thereby allowing bulging into the ventricle, which may allow some backflow of blood into the atrium (called mitral regurgitation).

Monounsaturated Fats

Types of fat found in many foods, but predominantly in avocados and canola, olive and peanut oils. Monounsaturated fats tend to lower LDL cholesterol levels, and some studies suggest that it may do so without also lowering HDL cholesterol levels.

Mortality Rate

The total number of deaths from a given disease in a population during an interval of time, usually a year.

Murmur

The noises superimposed on normal heart sounds. They are caused by congenital defects or damaged heart valves that do not close properly and allow blood to leak back into the chamber from which it has come.

Mydriasis

Dilation of the pupil.

Mydriatic

A drug that dilates the pupil. Sometimes used to treat amblyopia, particularly if the child will not wear an eye patch over the stronger eye.

Myocardial Infarction (MI)

The damage or death of an area of the heart muscle (myocardium) resulting from a blocked blood supply to the area. The affected tissue dies, injuring the heart. Symptoms include prolonged, intensive chest pain and a decrease in blood pressure that often causes shock.

Myocardium

The muscular wall of the heart. It contracts to pump blood out of the heart and then relaxes as the heart refills with returning blood.

Myopia

Commonly known as nearsightedness. A refractive error in which the light rays focus in front of the retina producing blurry distance vision. External optical correction (glasses or contact lenses) are required for clear distance vision. It is now believed that myopia is partly hereditary; one is more likely to become myopic if one's parents are myopic. Also, near work can lead to a further worsening of the myopia. If the myopia is greater than 6 diopters, a condition known as high myopia, the possibility of retinal detachment is increased.

Necrosis

Refers to the death of tissue within a certain area.

Needle Biopsy

A small needle is inserted into the abnormal area in almost any part of the body, guided by imaging techniques, to obtain a tissue biopsy. This type of biopsy can provide a diagnosis without surgical intervention.

Neoplasm

Any new or abnormal growth, specifically a new growth of tissue in which the growth is uncontrolled.

Neuralgia

A paroxysmal pain extending along the course of one or more nerves.

Nitroglycerin (NTG)

A drug that helps relax and dilate arteries, often used to treat cardiac chest pain (angina).

Non-Invasive Procedures

Any diagnostic or treatment procedures in which no instrument enters the body.

Nystagmus

Rapid rhythmic repetitious involuntary (unwilled) eye movements. Nystagmus can be horizontal, vertical or rotary.

Obesity

The condition of being significantly overweight. It is usually applied to a condition of 30% or more over ideal body weight. Obesity puts a strain on the heart and can increase the chance of developing high blood pressure, diabetes, and heart disease.

Occluded Artery

An artery in which the blood flow has been impaired by a blockage.

Ocular Dexter (OD)

Right eye.

Open Heart Surgery

An operation in which the chest and heart are opened surgically while the bloodstream is diverted through a heart-lung (cardiopulmonary perfusion) machine.

Ophthalmoscope

A lighted instrument used to examine the inside of the eye, including the retina and the optic nerve.

Optician

A technician who fits a person for glasses. He/she does not test for glasses. Some opticians also fit contact lenses.

Optometrist (OD)

A licensed non-physician educated to detect eye problems with special emphasis on correcting refractive errors. Depending on training, an Optometrist may use diagnostic and therapeutic medicines. An Optometrist does not perform surgery.

Orthopedics
The medical specialty involved in the preservation and restoration of function of the musculoskeletal system that includes treatment of spinal disorders and peripheral nerve lesions.

Oculus Sinister (OS)
Left eye.

Osteoma
A benign tumor of bone.

Osteoporosis
A disorder in which bone is abnormally brittle, less dense, and is the result of a number of different diseases and abnormalities.

Ossification
The process of forming bone in the body.

Oculus Uterque (OU)
Both eyes.

Pacemakers
Small, surgically implantable devices, which can control the heart's rhythm when it has a tendency to beat too slowly. Pacemakers can usually be implanted in 1 to 2 hours and require only a small incision to place the generator under the skin. Most pacemakers will last 5 to 10 years before generator replacement is necessary.

Palpate
To touch, or feel.

Palpitations
Uncomfortable sensations within the chest caused by an irregular heartbeat.

Paraplegia
Paralysis of the lower part of the body including the legs.

Pathology
The study of disease states.

Patent Ductus Arteriosus
A congenital defect in which the opening between the aorta and the pulmonary artery does not close after birth.

Percuss
To tap firmly on the body with the fingers, used to map out the area of an organ and detect possible changes in the consistency of its tissues.

Percutaneous Transluminal Coronary Angioplasty (PTCA)
Opens arteries blocked by atherosclerosis and allows blood to flow freely to the heart muscle. Angioplasty is not surgery. It opens a clogged artery by inflating a tiny balloon in the vessel, pushing the plaque aside.

Pericarditis
The inflammation of the outer membrane surrounding the heart. Rheumatic fever, heart surgery, viral, and bacterial infections are some of its possible causes.

Pericardiocentesis
A diagnostic procedure using a needle to withdraw fluid from the sac or membrane surrounding the heart (pericardium).

Pericardium
The outer fibrous sac that surrounds the heart.

Peripheral Vision
Side vision; the ability to see objects and movement outside of the direct line of vision.

Photophobia
Severe discomfort to bright lights. Usually a symptom of eye disease, such as glaucoma, in an infant or retinal disease in a child or adult. Sometimes treated with dark sunglasses.

Physical Therapy
The treatment consisting of exercising specific parts of the body such as the legs, arms, hands or neck, in an effort to strengthen, regain range of motion, relearn movement and/or rehabilitate the musculoskeletal system to improve function.

Physiology
The science of the functioning of living organisms, and of their component systems or parts.

Plaque
A deposit of fatty (and other) substances in the inner lining of the artery wall; it is characteristic of atherosclerosis.

Platelets
One of three types of cells found in blood; they aid in the clotting of the blood.

Polyunsaturated Fat
The major fat constituent in most vegetable oils including corn, sunflower and soybean. These oils are liquid at room temperature. Polyunsaturated fat actually tends to lower LDL cholesterol levels but may also reduce HDL cholesterol levels as well.

Positron Emission Tomography (PET SCAN)
A test that uses positron emitting substances to assess information about the metabolism of elements that can be used to indicate whether heart muscle is alive and functioning. A ring of radiosensitive detectors positioned around the chest reconstructs a two-or three-dimensional image of the heart.

Terms To Know

Posterior
The back of the body or situated nearer the back of the body.

Post-Ictal
State following a seizure, often characterized by altered function of the limbs and/or mentation.

Presbyopia
The normal decrease in focusing power (accommodation) of the eye which occurs with aging. It begins about age twelve but becomes most noticeable to the average farsighted person after age forty. Bifocals or reading glasses are required for clear near vision.

Prevalence
The total number of cases of a given disease that exist in a population at a specific time.

Prosthesis
An artificial body part such as an artificial leg or arm. The term prosthesis is also used to describe some of the implants used in the body such as a hip or knee replacement device.

Prosthetic Valve
An artificial heart valve.

Proximal
Nearest the center of the body.

Pulmonary
Refers to the lungs and respiratory system.

Pulmonary Valve
The heart valve between the right ventricle and the pulmonary artery. It prevents blood flowing from the lungs into the heart.

Pulmonary Vein
The blood vessel that carries newly oxygenated blood from the lungs back to the left atrium of the heart.

Pupil
The pupil is the dark aperture in the iris that determines how much light is let into the eye.

Pupillary Response
The constriction or dilation of the pupil as stimulated by light.

Pyelogram, IV Urogram, IVP
An X-ray of the pelvis, showing the kidney and associated structures, after injection of a radiopaque dye.

Quadriplegia
Complete paralysis of the body from the neck down. Quadriplegia is most likely to occur when a spinal cord injury is in the area of the 5th to 7th cervical vertebrae (bones in the neck that make up part of the structure surrounding the spinal cord).

Refraction
The bending of light that takes place within the human eye. Refractive errors include nearsightedness (myopia), farsightedness (hyperopia), and astigmatism. Lenses can be used to control the amount of refraction, correcting those errors.

Renal
Pertains to the kidneys.

Retina
The retina is the nerve layer that lines the back of the eye, senses light and creates impulses that travel through the optic nerve to the brain.

Retinal Detachment
A retina that separates from its connection at the back of the eye. The process of retinal detachment is usually due to a tear (a rip) in the retina, often when the vitreous gel pulls loose or separates from its attachment to the retina, most commonly along the outside edge of the eye. This rip is sometimes accompanied by bleeding if a blood vessel is also torn. After the retina has torn, liquid from the vitreous gel passes through the tear and accumulates behind the retina. The buildup of fluid behind the retina is what separates (detaches) the retina from the back of the eye. As more of the liquid vitreous collects behind the retina, the extent of the retinal detachment can progress and involve the entire retina, leading to a total retinal detachment. A retinal detachment almost always affects only one eye. The second eye, however, must be checked thoroughly for any signs of the problem.

Rheumatic Fever
A disease, usually occurring in childhood, that may follow a streptococcal infection. Symptoms may include fever, sore or swollen joints, skin rash, involuntary muscle twitching, and development of nodules under the skin. If the infection involves the heart, scars may form on heart valves and the heart's outer lining may be damaged.

Risk Factor
An element or condition involving a certain hazard or danger. When referring to heart and blood vessels, a risk factor is associated with an increased chance of developing cardiovascular disease, including stroke.

Rods
The rods are the visual cells of the retina that are important for night vision and peripheral vision. The rods are the first affected in rod-cone degenerations such as retinitis pigmentosa (RP).

Rubella
A mild contagious eruptive disease caused by a virus and capable of producing congenital defects in infants born to mothers infected during the first three months of pregnancy. Rubella is also called German measles.

Sacrum
A part of the spine that is also part of the pelvis. It articulates with the ilia at the sacroiliac joints and articulates with the lumbar spine at the lumbosacral joint. The sacrum consists of five fused vertebrae that have no intervertebral discs.

Sagittal
Longitudinal.

Saturated Fat
The type of fat found in foods of animal origin and a few of vegetable origin; they are usually solid at room temperature. Abundant in meat and dairy products, saturated fats tend to increase LDL cholesterol levels and it may raise the risk of certain types of cancer.

Sciatica
A lay term indicating pain along the course of a sciatic nerve, especially noted in the back of the thigh and below the knee.

Scintigraphy
The use of radioactive substances to record images of their distribution in body tissues.

Sclera
The tough white outer coat of the eyeball.

Scoliosis
Lateral (sideways) curvature of the spine.

Sepsis
A state of infection of tissue due to disease-producing bacteria or toxins.

Skeleton
The rigid framework of bones that gives form to the body, protects and supports the soft organs and tissues, and provides attachments for muscles.

Septal Defect
A hole in the wall of the heart separating the atria or in the wall of the heart separating the ventricles.

Septum
The muscular wall dividing a chamber on the left side of the heart from the chamber on the right.

Shock
A condition in which the body function is impaired because the volume of fluid circulating through the body is insufficient to maintain normal metabolism. This may be caused by blood loss or by a disturbance in the function of the circulatory system.

Shunt
A connector that allows blood to flow between two locations.

Sick Sinus Syndrome
The failure of the sinus node to regulate the heart's rhythm.

Silent Ischemia
An episode of cardiac ischemia not accompanied by chest pain.

Sinus (SA) Node
The "natural" pacemaker of the heart. The node is a group of specialized cells in the top of the right atrium which produces the electrical impulses that travel down to eventually reach the ventricular muscle, causing the heart to contract.

Sinusitis
An inflammation of the membrane lining the facial sinuses, often caused by bacterial or viral infections.

Sodium
A mineral essential to life found in nearly all plant and animal tissue. Table salt (sodium chloride) is nearly half sodium.

Snellen Chart
The familiar eye chart with larger letters at the top and smaller ones at the bottom. It is used for measuring central vision.

Sphygmomanometer or Sphygmometer
An instrument for measuring blood pressure in the arteries; especially one consisting of a pressure gauge and a rubber cuff that wraps around the upper arm and inflates to constrict the arteries.

Spinal Canal
The bony channel that is formed by the intravertebral foramen of the vertebrae and in which contains the spinal cord and nerve roots.

Spinal Cord
The longitudinal cord of nerve tissue that is enclosed in the spinal canal. It serves not only as a pathway for nervous impulses to and from the brain, but as a center for carrying out and coordinating many reflex actions independently of the brain.

Spine
The flexible bone column extending from the base of the skull to the tailbone. It is made up of 33 bones, known as vertebrae. The first 24 vertebrae are separated by discs known as intervertebral discs, and bound together by ligaments and muscles. Five vertebrae are fused together to form the sacrum and four vertebrae are fused together to form the coccyx. The spine is also referred to as the vertebral column, spinal column, or backbone.

Stenosis
The narrowing or constriction of an opening, such as a blood vessel or heart valve.

Terms To Know

Stent
A device made of expandable, metal mesh that is placed (by using a balloon catheter) at the site of a narrowing artery. The stent is then expanded and left in place to keep the artery open. They are effective in preventing recurrent obstruction of the blood vessel following the procedure.

Sterile
Free from living organisms.

Stethoscope
An instrument for listening to sounds within the body.

Strabismus
A condition in which the visual axes of the eyes are not parallel and the eyes appear to be looking in different directions.

Streptococcal Infection ("strep" infection)
An infection, usually in the throat, resulting from the presence of streptococcus bacteria.

Streptokinase
A clot-dissolving drug used to treat heart attack patients.

Sternum
The breastbone.

Steroid
A group of chemicals, many normally found in the body. Most steroids are hormones and affect body processes such as the overcoming of inflammation. Steroids medication decreases inflammation and inhibits immune reactions.

Stress
Bodily or mental tension resulting from physical, chemical or emotional factors. Stress can refer to physical exertion as well as mental anxiety.

Stroke
A sudden disruption of blood flow to the brain (e.g., by a clot or a leak in a blood vessel).

Subarachnoid Hemorrhage
Bleeding from a blood vessel on the surface of the brain into the space between the brain and the skull.

Sudden Death
Death that occurs unexpectedly and instantaneously or shortly after the onset of symptoms. The most common underlying reason for patients dying suddenly is cardiovascular disease, in particular, coronary heart disease.

Superior
Situated above or directed upward toward the head of an individual.

Superior Vena Cava
The large vein that returns blood from the head and arms to the heart.

Syncope
A temporary, insufficient blood supply to the brain which causes a loss of consciousness. Usually caused by a significant arrhythmia.

Systolic Blood Pressure
The highest blood pressure measured in the arteries. It occurs when the heart contracts with each heartbeat.

Tachycardia
Rapid beating of the heart.

Tendon
The fibrous band of tissue that connects muscle to bone. It is mainly composed of collagen.

Tetany
Muscle twitching and cramps caused by a lack of calcium in the blood.

Thallium Stress Test
An x-ray study that follows the path of radioactive potassium carried by the blood into heart muscle. Damaged or dead muscles can be defined, as can the extent of narrowing in an artery.

Thoracic
The chest level region of the spine that is located between the cervical and lumbar vertebrae. It consists of 12 vertebrae which serve as attachment points for ribs.

Throat culture
A mucus sample taken from the throat to detect the possible presence of infection.

Thrombolysis
The breaking up of a blood clot.

Thrombosis
A blood clot that forms inside the blood vessel or cavity of the heart.

Thrombolytic Therapy
A drug that dissolves blood clots.

Thrombus
A blood clot.

Tissue Plasminogen Activator (TPA)
A clot-dissolving drug used to treat heart attack patients.

Titration, Titrate

Adjusting the concentration of a solution (such as an injectable drug) so that the smallest possible amount (or lowest concentration) of the active ingredient is used that will achieve the desired effect.

Tomography

From the Greek words "to cut or section" (tomos) and "to write" (graphein), in nuclear medicine, it is a method of separating interference from the area of interest by imaging a cut section of the object.

Trans Fat

Created when hydrogen is forced through an ordinary vegetable oil (hydrogenation), converting some polyunsaturates to monounsaturates, and some monounsaturates to saturates. Trans fat, like saturated fat, tends to raise LDL cholesterol levels and, unlike saturated fat, trans fat also lowers HDL cholesterol level at the same time.

Transesophageal Echocardiography (TEE)

A diagnostic test that analyzes sound waves bounced off the heart. The sound waves are sent through a tube-like device inserted in the mouth and passed down the esophagus (food pipe), which ends near the heart. This technique is useful in studying patients whose heart and vessels, for various reasons, are difficult to assess with standard echocardiography.

Transient Ischemic Attack (TIA)

A temporary, stroke-like event that lasts for only a short time and is caused by a temporarily blocked blood vessel.

Transplantation

Replacing a defective organ with one from a donor.

Tricuspid Valve

The structure that controls blood flow from the heart's right atrium (upper chamber) into the right ventricle (lower chamber).

Triglycerides

The most common fatty substances found in the blood; normally stored as an energy source in fat tissue. High triglyceride levels tend to accompany high cholesterol levels and other risk factors for heart disease such as obesity.

Tumor

A swelling or an abnormal growth of tissue resulting from uncontrolled, progressive multiplication of cells, and serving no physiological function.

Tunnel Vision

A reduced visual field in which the eyes only see straight ahead (no peripheral vision). It may be due to certain eye diseases, such as glaucoma or retinitis pigmentosa (RP).

Ultrasound

High-frequency sound waves. Ultrasound waves can be bounced off of tissues using special devices. The echoes are then converted into a picture called a sonogram. Ultrasound imaging, referred to as ultrasonography, allows physicians and patients to get an inside view of soft tissues and body cavities, without using invasive techniques.

Unilateral

Having, or relating to, one side.

Upper GI Series

An X-ray exam of the upper part of the digestive tract.

Urokinase

An enzyme derived from human urine that dissolves blood clots.

Urticaria

A skin condition commonly known as hives.

Uvea

The vascular middle layer of the eye constituting the iris, ciliary body, and choroid.

Valvular Regurgitation

Regurgitation of blood (blood moving the wrong way) in the heart. Caused by a heart valve malfunction.

Valvuloplasty

The reshaping of a heart valve with surgical or catheter techniques.

Varicose Vein

Any vein that is abnormally dilated, usually from long-standing pressure within it.

Vascular

Pertaining to the blood vessels.

Vasodilators

Any medications that dilate (widen) the arteries.

Vasopressors

Any medications that elevate blood pressure.

Veins

Any of a series of blood vessels of the vascular system that carry blood from various parts of the body back to the heart. Veins return oxygen-depleted blood to the heart.

Ventricles (right and left)

The two lower chambers of the heart.

Terms To Know

Ventricular Fibrillation
A condition in which the ventricles contract in a rapid, unsynchronized fashion. When fibrillation occurs, the ventricles cannot pump blood throughout the body.

Ventricular Tachycardia
An arrhythmia (abnormal heartbeat) in the ventricle, characterized by a very fast heartbeat.

Vertebra
One of the 33 bones of the spinal column. A cervical, thoracic, or lumbar vertebra has a cylindrically-shaped bony anteriorly and a neural arch posteriorly (composed primarily of the laminae and pedicles as well as the other structures in the posterior aspect of the vertebra) that protects the spinal cord. The plural of vertebra is vertebrae.

Vertigo
A feeling of dizziness or spinning.

Visual Acuity
The clarity or clearness of the vision, a measure of how well a person sees. The ability to distinguish details and shapes of objects; also called central vision.

Vitreous Humor
The vitreous humor is a clear, jelly-like substance that fills the middle of the eye.

Wolff-Parkinson-White Syndrome
A condition in which an extra electrical pathway connects the atria (two upper chambers) and the ventricles (two lower chambers). It may cause a rapid heartbeat.

X-ray
A form of radiation used to create a picture of internal body structures on film.

Practice Quiz: Terms to Know

Please define the following terms:

1. antibody _____

2. arthroscopy _____

3. benign _____

4. contusion _____

5. edema _____

6. necrosis _____

7. plaque _____

8. thrombosis _____

9. occlusion _____

10. vertigo _____

For 11-20, please choose whether the following are:

a. compound words

b. root words

c. suffixes

d. prefixes

e. eponyms

11. cardio _____

12. desis _____

13. bradycardia _____

14. plasia _____

15. Moh's micrographic surgery _____

16. gastro _____

17. ante _____

18. mast(o) _____

19. peri _____

20. Kaposi's Sarcoma _____

Chapter 17

PRACTICE QUIZ ANSWERS

Chapter 1 – Introduction to Anatomy
1. Midsagittal plane
2. Anatomical
3. Median, sagittal, and transverse

Chapter 2 – Integumentary System
1. d
2. a. Epidermis
   b. Dermis
3. Dermal Papillae
4. Keratin
5. Hands and Feet
6. Phagocytes
7. a. Hair
   b. Glands
   c. Nails
8. b
   c
   a
9. Figure 2.1
   1. Free nerve endings
   2. Hair shaft
   3. Pore
   4. Dermal papilla
   5. Cuticle
   6. Internal sheath
   7. External sheath
   8. Glassy membrane
   9. Connective tissue
   10. Vein
   11. Sensory nerve
   12. Artery
   13. Motor nerve
   14. Sebaceous gland
   15. Hair cuticle
   16. Hair matrix
   17. Papilla of hair follicle
   18. Sweat gland
   19. Arrector muscle
   20. Reticular layer
   21. Stratum basale
   22. Stratum spinosum
   23. Stratum granulosum
   24. Stratum lucidum
   25. Stratum corneum
   26. Pacinian corpuscle
   27. Meissner's corpuscle
10. Figure 2.2
    1. Dead hair
    2. New hair
    3. Hair bulb
    4. Dermis
    5. Hair follicle
    6. Epidermis
    7. Hair shaft
11. Figure 2.3
    1. Free edge
    2. Nail body
    3. Lunula
    4. Cuticle
    5. Nail root

Chapter 3 – Musculoskeletal System
1. a. Protection
   b. Muscle attachment sites
   c. Blood cell production
   d. Mineral storage
2. Supportive connective tissue

© 2011 Contexo Media

157

Practice Quiz Answers

3 Bone

4. Ossification

5. a. Cuboidal
   b. Flat
   c. Sesamoid
   d. Tubular
   e. Irregular

6. Joint

7. Appendicular, Axial

8. Sinuses

9. Spine

10 a. Cervical
   b. Thoracic
   c. Lumbar

11. a. Smooth
    b. Cardiac
    c. Skeletal

12. Voluntarily muscles require conscious will to make them contract

    Involuntary muscles do not require conscious will to make them contract

13. Muscles become rigid

14. b

15. a

16. b

17. b

18. a

19. a

20. b

21. b

22. a

23. a

24. a

25. b

26. a

27. a

28. b

29. d

30. c

31. b

32. a

33. d

34. Figure 3.1
   1. Flat (Parietal)
   2. Short (Talus)
   3. Long (Femur)
   4. Sesamoid (Patella)
   5. Irregular (Sphenoid)

35. Figure 3.2
   1. Parietal bone
   2. Orbit
   3. Zygomatic bone
   4. Nasal Septum
   5. Mandible
   6. Hyoid bone
   7. Clavicle
   8. Coracoclavicular ligament
   9. Articular capsule
   10. Subscapularis tendon
   11. Body of sternum
   12. Xiphoid process
   13. Costal cartilages
   14. Anterior longitudinal ligament
   15. Ulnar collateral ligament
   16. Radial collateral ligament
   17. Annular ligament
   18. Iliac crest
   19. Anterior sacroiliac ligament
   20. Interosseous membrane
   21. Inguinal ligament
   22. Iliofemoral ligament
   23. Coccyx
   24. Pubic symphis
   25. Femur
   26. Quadriceps femoris tendon
   27. Tibial collateral ligament
   28. Fibular collateral ligament
   29. Patellar ligament
   30. Tibia
   31. Fibula

Practice Quiz Answers

32. Interosseous membrane
33. Medial malleolus
34. Lateral malleolus
35. Tibial tuberosity
36. Head of fibula
37. Patella
38. Lateral epicondyle
39. Medial epicondyle
40. Head of femur
41. Greater trochanter
42. Sacrum
43. Anterior superior iliac spine
44. Ulna
45. Radius
46. Lateral epicondyle
47. Medial epicondyle
48. False ribs (8-12)
49. True ribs (1-7)
50. Humerus
51. Scapula
52. Head of humerus
53. Greater tubercle
54. Acromion
55. Coracoid process
56. Manubrium of sternum
57. Maxilla
58. Nasal conchae
59. Temporal bone
60. Frontal bone
A. Scaphoid
B. Trapezium
C. Trapezoid
D. Capitate
E. Lunate
F. Pisiform
G. Triquetrum
H. Hamate
J. Intermediate cuneiform
K. Lateral cuneiform
L. Cuboid

M. Talus
N. Navicular
O. Calcaneous
P. Medial cuneiform

36. Figure 3.3
1. Mastoid process
2. Mandible
3. Clavicle
4. Scapular notch
5. Spine of scapula
6. Greater tubercle
7. Head of humerus
8. Infraspinous fossa
9. Humerus
10. Medial epicondyle
11. Lateral epiondyle
12. Head of radius
13. Olecranon of ulna
14. Posterior superior iliac spine
15. Sacrum
16. Greater sciatic notch
17. Head of femur
18. Greater trochanter
19. Medial epicondyle
20. Lateral epicondyle
21. Lateral condyles
22. Head of fibula
23. Medial condyles
24. Tibia
25. Fibula
26. Medial malleolus
27. Lateral malleolus
28. Metatarsals
29. Talus
30. Calcaneus
31. Calcaneal (Achilles) tendon
32. Posterior talofibular ligament
33. Posterior tibiofibular ligament
34. Interosseos membrane
35. Posterior cruciate ligament

Practice Quiz Answers

36. Lateral meniscus
37. Fibular collateral ligament
38. Anterior cruciate ligament
39. Medial meniscus
40. Tibial colateral ligament
41. Phalanges
42. Metacarpals
43. Sacrotuberous ligament
44. Ischiofemoral ligament
45. Iiliofemoral ligament
46. Posterior sacroiliac ligament
47. Ilium
48. Ulna
49. Radius
50. Annular ligament
51. Radial collateral ligament
52. Ulnar collateral ligament
53. Scapula
54. Teres minor tendon
55. Infraspinatus tendon
56. Acromion
57. Supraspinous fossa
58. Axis
59. Atlas
60. Temporal bone
61. Occipital bone
62. Parietal bone
A. Lunate
B. Triquetrum
C. Hamate
D. Capitate
E. Scaphoid
F. Trapezium
G. Trapezoid

37. Figure 3.4
1. Coracoclavicular ligament
2. Acromioclavicular ligament
3. Coracoacromial ligament
4. Coracohumural ligament
5. Transverse humeral ligament

6. Long tendon of biceps
7. Subscapularis tendon
8. Articular capsule
9. Articular capsule
10. Radial collateral ligament
11. Annular ligament
12. Biceps tendon
13. Interosseous membrane
14. Radius
15. Ulna
16. Anterior ligament
17. Ulnar collateral ligament
18. Supraspinous fossa
19. Clavicle
20. Scapular notch
21. Acromion
22. Spine of scapula
23. Greater tubercle
24. Head of humerus
25. Infraspinous fossa
26. Lateral epicondyle
27. Olecranon fossa
28. Olecranon process
29. Ulna
30. Radius
31. Medial epicondyle
32. Humerus
33. Olecranon of ulna
34. Interosseous membrane
35. Ulna
36. Radius
37. Annular ligament
38. Radial collateral ligament
39. Ulnar collateral ligament
40. Humerus
41. Scapula
42. Teres minor tendon
43. Infraspinatus tendon
44. Acromioclavicular ligament
45. Humerus

Practice Quiz Answers

46. Medial epicondyle
47. Trochlea
48. Coronoid process
49. Ulnar tuberosity
50. Ulna
51. Radius
52. Radial tuberosity
53. Head of radius
54. Capitulum
55. Lateral epicondyle
56. Coronoid fossa
57. Humerus
58. Scapula
59. Subscapular fossa
60. Lesser tubercle
61. Greater tubercle
62. Head of humerus
63. Acromion
64. Coracoid process
65. Scapular notch
66. Clavicle

38. Figure 3.5

1. Anterior longitudinal ligament
2. Iiliolumbar ligament
3. Anterior sacroiliac ligament
4. Coccyx
5. Sacrotuberous ligament
6. Sacrospinous ligament
7. Iliofemoral ligament
8. Pubofemoral ligament
9. Inguinal ligament
10. Obturator membrane
11. Pubic symphysis
12. Femur
13. Quadriceps femoris tendon
14. Medial patellar retinaculum
15. Fibular collateral ligament
16. Tibial collateral ligament
17. Lateral patellar retinaculum
18. Patellar ligament
19. Interosseous membrane
20. Fibula
21. Tibia
22. Medial condyles
23. Tibial tuberosity
24. Head of fibula
25. Lateral condyles
26. Patella
27. Lateral epicondyle
28. Medial epicondyle
29. Pubis
30. Obturator foramen
31. Spine of ischium
32. Lesser trochanter
33. Head of femur
34. Greater   trochanter
35. Anterior inferior iliac spine
36. Ilium
37. Anterior superior iliac spine
38. Iliac crest
39. Sacrum
40. Sacral promontory
41. Femur
42. Tibia
43. Fibula
44. Posterior cruciate ligament
45. Lateral meniscus
46. Fibular collateral ligament
47. Anterior cruciate ligament
48. Medial meniscus
49. Tibial collateral ligament
50. Posterior superior iliac spine
51. Sacrum
52. Greater sciatic notch
53. Ischium
54. Femur
55. Ischiofemoral ligament
56. Iliofemoral ligament
57. Sacrotuberous ligament
58. Ilium

© 2011 Contexo Media

Practice Quiz Answers

59. Posterior sacroiliac ligament

39. Figure 3.6
    1. Sphenoid bone
    2. Frontal lobe
    3. Frontal bone
    4. Nasal bone
    5. Zygomatic arch
    6. Maxilla
    7. Mandible
    8. Coronoid process
    9. Mastoid process
    10. Right cerebral hemisphere

40. Figure 3.7
    1. Cervical vertebrae
    2. Thoracic vertebrae
    3. Lumbar vertebrae
    4. Sacrum
    5. Coccyx
    6. Pelvic curve
    7. L5
    8. Intervertebral foramina
    9. Lumbar curve
    10. L1
    11. T12
    12. Foveae for ribs
    13. Thoracic curve
    14. Intervertebral discs
    15. T1
    16. C7
    17. Cervical curve
    18. Axis (C2)
    19. Atlas (C1)

41. Figure 3.8
    1. Fronatalis m.
    2. Zygomaticus minor m.
    3. Zygomaticus major m.
    4. Orbicularis oris m.
    5. Depressor anguli oris m.
    6. Levator scapulae m.
    7. Pectoralis minor m.

8. Internal intercostal m.
9. Coracobrachialis m.
10. Brachialis m.
11. Rectus sheath
12. Rectus abdominus m.
13. Linea alba
14. Internal abdominal oblique m.
15. Transversus abdominus m.
16. Palmaris longus m.
17. Flexor pollicis longus m.
18. Flexor digitorum superficialis m.
19. Abductor pollicis brevis m.
20. Flexor pollicis brevis m.
21. Abductor digiti minimi m..
22. Iliopsoas m.
23. Pectineus m.
24. Adductor brevis m.
25. Adductor magnus m.
26. Vastus lateralis m.
27. Vastus medialis m.
28. Patella
29. Patellar ligament
30. Medial patellar retinaculum
31. Tibia
32. Flexor digitorum longus m.
33. Abductor hallucis m.
34. Extensor hallucis brevis m.
35. Extensor hallucis longus m.
36. Extensor digitorum longus m.
37. Soleus m.
38. Peronius brevis m.
39. Peronius longus m.
40. Gastrocnemius m.
41. Tibialis anterior m.
42. Lateral patellar retinaculum
43. Gracilis m.
44. Vastus medialis m.
45. Iliotibial tract
46. Vastus lateralis m.
47. Rectus femoris m.

Practice Quiz Answers

48. Adductor longus m.
49. Sartorius m.
50. Tensor fasciae latae m.
51. Superficial inguinal ring
52. Flexor carpi radialis m.
53. Palmaris longus m.
54. Extensor carpi radialis longus m.
55. Brachioradialis m.
56. External abdominal oblique m.
57. Brachialis m.
58. Biceps brachii m.
59. Serratus anterior m.
60. Pectoralis major m.
61. Deltoid m.
62. Trapezius m.
63. Sternocleidomastoid m.
64. Buccinator m.
65. Masseter m.
66. Orbicularis oculi m.
67. Temporalis m.

42. Figure 3.9
    1. Galea aponeurotica
    2. Occipitalis m.
    3. Splenius capitis m.
    4. Splenius cervicis m.
    5. Levator scapulae m.
    6. Supraspinatus m.
    7. Rhomboid minor
    8. Rhomboid major
    9. Spinalis thoracis m.
    10. Iliocostalis thoracis m.
    11. Longissimus thoracis m.
    12. Serratus posterior inferior m.
    13. External abdominal oblique m.
    14. Anconius m.
    15. Supinator m.
    16. Gluteus minimus m.
    17. Piriformis m.
    18. Superior gemellus m.
    19. Obturator internus m.

20. Inferior gemellus m.
21. Quadratus femoris m.
22. Adductor magnus m.
23. Gracilis m.
24. Biceps femoris
25. Semimembranous m.
26. Gastrocnemius m.
27. Plantaris m.
28. Popliteus m.
29. Soleus m.
30. Tibialis posterior m.
31. Flexor digitorum longus m.
32. Flexor hallucis longus m.
33. Peroneus longus m.
34. Peroneus brevis m.
35. Calcaneal t. (Achilles)
36. Peroneus longus m.
37. Soleus m.
38. Gastrocnemius m.
39. Semimembranosis m.
40. Semitendinosis m.
41. Iliotibial tract
42. Biceps femoris m.
43. Adductor magnus m.
44. Gluteus maximus m.
45. Gluteus medius m.
46. Extensor pollicis longus t.
47. Extensor pollicis brevis m.
48. Abductor pollicis longus m.
49. Extensor carpi ulnaris m.
50. Extensor carpi radialis brevis m.
51. Extensor digitorum m.
52. Flexor carpi ulnaris m.
53. Extensor carpi radialis longus m.
54. Brachioradialis m.
55. Latissimus dorsi m.
56. Triceps
57. Teres major m.
58. Teres minor m.
59. Infraspinatus m.

© 2011 Contexo Media

Practice Quiz Answers

60. Deltoid m
61. Trapezius m.
62. Sternocleidomastoid m.
63. Occipitotemporalis m.
64. Temporalis m.

43. Figure 3.10
1. Extensor digitorum tt.
2. Extensor digiti minimi m.
3. Extensor carpi ulnaris m.
4. Extensor retinaculum
5. Extensor digiti minimi t.
6. Extensor digitorum tt.
7. 2nd, 3rd, 4th Dorsal interosseous mm.
8. 1st Dorsal interosseous m.
9. Extensor carpi radialis longus t.
10. Extensor pollicis longus t.
11. Extensor pollicis brevis t.
12. Extensor carpi radialis brevis t.
13. Extensor pollicis brevis m.
14. Abductor pollicis longus m.
15. Ulna
16. Lunate
17. Triquetrum
18. Hamate
19. Capitate
20. Metacarpals
21. Trapezoid
22. Trapezium
23. Scaphoid
24. Radius
25. Abductor pollicis longus m.
26. Radius
27. Extensor pollicis brevis t.
28. Opponens pollicis m.
29. Abductor pollicis brevis m.
30. Flexsor pollicis brevis m.
31. Flexor pollicis longus t.
32. Adductor pollicis m.
33. Flexor digitorum profundus t.
34. Flexor digitorum superficialis tt.

35. Deep transverse metacarpal II.
36. Lumbrical mm.
37. Opponens digiti minimi m.
38. Flexor digiti minimi brevis m.
39. Abductor digiti minimi m.
40. Flexor retinaculum
41. Antebrachial fascia
42. Ulna
43. Flexor carpi ulnaris m.
44. Flexor digitorum superficialis m.
45. Flexor pollicis longus m.

Chapter 4 – Respiratory System

1. a. inhaling
   b. exhaling
2. CO_2
3. Breathing
4. Digestive
5. Lungs
6. Windpipe
7. Cilia
8. Figure 4.1
   1. Sphenoid sinus
   2. Frontal sinus
   3. Superior concha
   4. Middle concha
   5. Middle meatus
   6. Inferior concha
   7. Hard palate
   8. Soft palate
   9. Uvula
   10. Tongue
   11. Epiglottis
   12. Thyroid cartilage
   13. Trachea
   14. Rib
   15. Intercostal muscle
   16. Heart
   17. Left lung
   18. Diaphragm

19. Right lung

20. Pulmonary vessels

21. Bronchioles

22. Secondary bronchus

23. Primary brochus

24. Esophagus

25. Larynx

26. Vocal cords

27. Laryngopharynx

28. Oropharynx

29. Nasopharynx

30. Opening of Eustachian tube

31. Brain stem

9. Figure 4.2

1. Nasal Bone

2. Orbicularis oculi m.

3. Lateral cartilage

4. Greater alar cartilage

5. Septal cartilage

10. Figure 4.3

1. Epiglottis

2. Thyrohoid membrane

3. Superior horn of thyroid cartilage

4. Thyroid cartilage

5. Corniculate cartilage

6. Arytenoid cartilage

7. Cricoid cartilage

8. Tracheal cartilage

9. Trachea

10. Cricothyroid ligament

11. Vocal fold

12. Vestibular fold

13. Thyrohyoid ligament

14. Hyoid bone

11. Figure 4.4

1. Deoxygenated blood from the heart

2. Bronchiole

3. Oxygenated blood to the heart

4. Alveolus

5. Capillary network

6. Oxygen diffuses from alveolus

7. Carbon-dioxide diffuses from blood to alveolus

12. Figure 4.5

1. Trachea

2. Superior lobe of left lung

3. Lobar bronchus

4. Inferior lobe

5. Main bronchi

6. Inferior lobe

7. Middle lobe

8. Superior lobe of right lung

Chapter 5 – Cardiovascular System

1. d

2. c

3. a

4. b

5. Valves

6. Arterioles

7. Venules

8. Aorta

9. Systemic arteries

10. Superior and inferior vena cavae

11. Systemic veins

12. Capillaries

13. Coronary arteries

14. Figure 5.1

1. Left subclavian artery

2. Left brachiocephalic vein

3. Aortic arch

4. Ligamentum arteriosum

5. Pulmonary trunk

6. Left pulmonary artery

7. Left pulmonary vein

8. Left auricle

9. Circumflex artery

10. Great cardiac vein

11. Left anterior descending artery

12. Left ventricle

13. Apex

Practice Quiz Answers

14. Descending aorta
15. Inferior vena cava
16. Right marginal artery
17. Small cardiac vein
18. Right ventricle
19. Anterior cardiac vein
20. Right artium
21. Right pulmonary vein
22. Right coronary artery
23. Right pulmonary artery
24. Ascending aorta
25. Superior vena cava
26. Right brachiocephalic vein
27. Brachiocephalic artery
28. Left common carotid artery
29. Aorta
30. Left pulmonary artery
31. Left pulmonary vein
32. Left atrium
33. Aortic semilunar valve
34. Bicuspid (left AV) valve
35. Left ventricle
36. Interventricular septum
37. Myocardium
38. Trabeculae carneae
39. Inferior vena cava
40. Papillary muscle
41. Right ventricle
42. Chordae tendineae
43. Tricuspid (right AV) valve
44. Right atrium
45. Right pulmonary vein
46. Right pulmonary artery
47. Pulmonary semilunar valve
48. Superior vena cava

15. Figure 5.2

1. Internal jugular v.
2. Superior vena cava
3. Subclavian a. & v.
4. Aortic arch
5. Pulmonary a.
6. Pulmonary v.
7. Cardiac a.
8. Hepatic v.
9. Celiac trunk
10. Superior mesenteric a.
11. Left renal a. & v.
12. Gonadal a. & v.
13. Inferior mesenteric a.
14. Common iliac a. & v.
15. Internal iliac a. & v.
16. External iliac a. & v.
17. Femoral a. & v.
18. Deep femoral a. & v.
19. Saphenous v.
20. Popliteal a.
21. Popliteal v.
22. Medial genicular aa.
23. Anterior tibial a.
24. Anterior tibial v.
25. Peroneal a.
26. Posterior tibial a.
27. Posterior tibial v.
28. Dorsalis pedis a.
29. Dorsal venous arch
30. Arcuate a.
31. Lateral tarsal a.
32. Small saphenous v.
33. Lateral genicular aa.
34. Descending genicular a.
35. Superficial venous palmar arch
36. Superficial palmar arch
37. Deep palmar arch
38. Medial antebrachial v.
39. Ulnar a.
40. Radial a.
41. Median cubital v.
42. Right renal a. & v.
43. Abdominal aorta
44. Inferior vena cava

45. Basilic v.

46. Cephalic v.

47. Brachial a.

48. Axillary a. & v.

49. Brachiocephalic v.

50. Brachiocephalic trunk

51. Common carotid a.

52. External jugular v.

53. Internal carotid a.

54. Vertebral a.

Chapter 6 – Digestive System

1. Alimentary canal

2. Peristalsis

3. Mouth

4. Chyme

5. a. Duodenum

   b. Jejunum

   c. Ileum

6. Bile

7. Stores bile until needed

8. Appendix

9. Colon

10. Figure 5.1

    1. Mouth

    2. Tongue

    3. Esophagus

    4. Left liver lobe

    5. Stomach

    6. Transverse colon

    7. Jejunum

    8. Descending colon

    9. Ileum

    10. Sigmoid colon

    11. Rectum

    12. Appendix

    13. Cecum

    14. Iliocecal valve

    15. Ascending colon

    16. Pancreas

17. Duodenum

18. Gall bladder

19. Right liver lobe

20. Pharynx

Chapter 7 – Urinary System

1. Urination

2. Renal capsule

3. a. Renal cortex

   b. Renal medulla

   c. Renal pelvis

4. Bladder

5. The female urethra is shorter

6. Figure 7.1

   1. Superior mesenteric a.

   2. Celiac trunk

   3. Adrenal gland

   4. Left kidney

   5. Renal a.

   6. Fibrous capsule

   7. Papilla

   8. Minor calyx

   9. Major calyx

   10. Cortex

   11. Renal pyramid

   12. Renal column

   13. Renal pelvis

   14. Left ureter

   15. Left common iliac a.

   16. Left common iliac v.

   17. Urethra

   18. Trigone

   19. Opening of ureter

   20. Urinary bladder

   21. Right common iliac a.

   22. Right common iliac v.

   23. Abdominal aorta

   24. Inferior mesenteric a.

   25. Right gonadal a. & v.

   26. Renal pelvis

Practice Quiz Answers

27. Right renal aa.

28. Right renal v.

29. Right kidney

30. Adrenal gland

31. Inferior vena cava

7. Figure 7.2

1. Renal capsule

2. Cortex

3. Medulla

4. Renal pyramid

5. Renal column

6. Minor calyx

7. Major calyx

8. Ureter

9. Renal pelvis

10. Papilla

8. Figure 7.3

1. Interlobar arteries

2. Cortical radiate (interlobular) arteries

3. Arcuate arteries

4. Inferior segmental artery

5. Uteric branch

6. Posterior branch of renal artery

7. Renal artery

8. Anterior branch of renal artery

9. Inferior suprarenal artery

10. Anterior superior segmental artery

11. Superior (apical) segmental artery

Chapter 8 – Male Genital System

1. Testosterone

2. Muscular tube through which sperm travels

3. b

4. Peristalsis

5. Scrotum

6. Figure 8.1

1. Bladder

2. Trigone

3. Prostate

4. Prostatatic utricle

5. Bulbourethral gland

6. Bulb of penis

7. Crus of penis

8. Opening of bulbourethral gland

9. Corpus cavernosum

10. Deep artery of penis

11. Corpus spongiosum

12. Corona

13. Glans of penis

14. Urethral opening

15. Penile urethra

16. Membranous urethra

17. Prostatic urethra

7. Figure 8.2

1. Ductus deferens

2. Epididymis

3. Efferent ductules

4. Rete testes

5. Seminiferous tubule

6. Tunica albuginea

7. Septum

8. Lobule

8. Figure 8.3

1. Sigmoid colon

2. Sacrum

3. Rectum

4. Anal sphincter

5. Anus

6. Epididymis

7. Testis

8. Scrotum

9. Prepuce

10. Urethral opening

11. Navicular fossa

12. Glans of penis

13. Ductus deferens

14. Urethra

15. Corpus spongiosum

16. Corpus cavernosum

17. Urogenital diapragm

18. Prostate gland

19. Ejaculatory duct

20. Pubic symphysis

21. Suspensory ligament

22. Seminal vesicle

23. Urinary bladder

24. Ampulla of ductus deferens

25. Peritoneum

Chapter 9 – Female Genital System

1. Corpus luteum

2. Infundibulum

3. Fimbrae

4. Uterus

5. The vulva

6. a. Estrogen

   b. Progesterone

7. Figure 9.1

   1. Fundus of uterus

   2. Isthmus of fallopian tube

   3. Ampulla of fallopian tube

   4. Mesposalpinx

   5. Infundibulum of falopian tube

   6. Oocyte

   7. Fimbriae of fallopian tube

   8. Corpus luteum

   9. Uterine cavity

   10. Broad ligament

   11. Body of uterus

   12. Cervical canal

   13. Cervix

   14. Vagina

   15. Uterosacral ligament

   16. Endometrium

   17. Myometrium

   18. Perimetrium

   19. Ovary

   20. Fimbriae

   21. Suspensory ligament

   22. Ovarian ligament

8. Figure 9.2

   1. Sigmoid colon

   2. Sacrum

   3. Rectouterine pouch

   4. Cervix

   5. Rectum

   6. Anal sphincter

   7. Anus

   8. Vaginal orifice

   9. Labium minus

   10. Labium majus

   11. Clitoris

   12. Vagina

   13. Urethra

   14. Urinary bladder

   15. Pubic symphysis

   16. Uterus

   17. Peritoneum

   18. Round ligament of uterus

   19. Ovary

   20. Fallopian tube

   21. Suspensory ligament

Chapter 10 – Endocrine System

1. e

2. b

3. g

4. h

5. c

6. d

7. f

8. a

Chapter 11 – Nervous System

1. a. CNS

   b. PNS

2. a. Forebrain

   b. Brainstem

   c. Hindbrain

3. c

4. a

Practice Quiz Answers

5. b

6. Spinal cord

7. a. Sensory

   b. Mixed

8. b

9. b

   a

   c

10. Figure 11.1

    1. Lateral cord
    2. Medial cord
    3. Posterior cord
    4. Musculocutaneous n.
    5. Ulnar n.
    6. Median n.
    7. Radial n.
    8. Subcostal n.
    9. Iliohypogastric n.
    10. Ilioinguinal n.
    11. Genitofemoral n.
    12. Lateral femoral cutaneous n.
    13. Femoral n.
    14. Muscular branch of Femoral n.
    15. Sciatic n.
    16. Common peroneal n.
    17. Deep peroneal n.
    18. Superficial peroneal n.
    19. Tibial n.
    20. Saphenous n.
    21. Pudendal n.
    22. Obturator n.
    23. Sacral plexus
    24. Lumbar plexus
    25. Intercostal nn.
    26. Spinal cord
    27. Brachial plexus
    28. Cervical plexus
    29. Brain Stem
    30. Cerebellum
    31. Cerebrum

    32. Brain

11. Figure 11.2

    1. Olfactory bulb
    2. Olfactory tract (I)
    3. Optic chiasm
    4. Optic n. (II)
    5. Pituitary gland
    6. Oculomotor n. (III)
    7. Trochlear n. (IV)
    8. Trigeminal n. (V)
    9. Abducens n. (VI)
    10. Facial n. (VII)
    11. Vestibulocochlear n. (VIII)
    12. Glossopharyngeal n. (IX)
    13. Vagus n. (X)
    14. Hypoglossal n. (XII)
    15. Accessory n. (XI)
    16. Cervical n. (I)
    17. Medulla oblongata
    18. Cervical n.(II)
    19. Spinal cord
    20. Posterior inferior cerebellar a.
    21. Cerebellum
    22. Anterior spinal a.
    23. Anterior inferior cerebellar a.
    24. Vertebral a.
    25. Pons
    26. Basilar a.
    27. Pontine aa.
    28. Superior cerebellar a.
    29. Posterior cerebral a.
    30. Posterior communicating a.
    31. Middle cerebral a.
    32. Internal carotid a.
    33. Anterior cerebral a.
    34. Anterior communicating a.
    35. Cerebrum

Practice Quiz Answers

Chapter 12 – Immune System

1. Fever
2. IgG
3. IgE
4. Mechanical

Chapter 13 – Root Words

1. angi(o)
2. cardi(o)
3. cyan(o)
4. derm
5. hepat(o)
6. lymph(o)
7. ot
8. psych(o)
9. rhin
10. thromb(o)
11. A
12. C
13. B
14. C
15. A

Chapter 14 – Prefixes and Suffixes

1. less than normal
2. bad; abnormal
3. against; opposite
4. large; great
5. many
6. half
7. across; through
8. change
9. excessive; greater than normal
10. inward
11. de-
12. pre-
13. ex-
14. in-
15. uni-
16. tachy-
17. syn-
18. pain
19. crushing
20. condition
21. breathing
22. inflammation
23. opening; forming artificial opening
24. binding
25. tumor
26. growth
27. repair (surgical)
28. surgical fixation
29. visually examining
30. lack of
31. suture
32. excision; surgical removal
34. large
35. fluid discharge

Chapter 15 – Abbreviations

1. D
2. I
3. E
4. J
5. F
6. A
7. G
8. B
9. H
10. C

Chapter 16 – Terms to Know

1. A protein manufactured by lymphocytes to neutralize an antigen or foreign protein
2. The procedure of visualizing the inside of a joint by means of an arthroscope
3. Describing an abnormal growth that will neither spread nor recur after removal
4. An injury of a part without a break in the skin and with a subcutaneous hemorrhage
5. Swelling caused by fluid accumulation in body tissues
6. Refers to the death of tissue within a certain area

Practice Quiz Answers

7. A deposit of fatty substances in the inner lining of the artery wall

8. A blood clot that forms inside the blood vessel or cavity of the heart

9. Blood flow impaired by a blockage

10. A feeling of dizziness or spinning

11. B

12. C

13. A

14. C

15. E

16. B

17. D

18. B

19. D

20. E

Introduction to FALL PROTECTION

J. Nigel Ellis, Ph.D., CSP, P.E.

Second Edition

 American Society of Safety Engineers

1800 East Oakton Street, Des Plaines, IL 60018-2187

American Society of Safety Engineers
1800 East Oakton Street
Des Plaines IL 60018-2187
708-692-4121
708-296-9221 fax

© 1988, 1993 by
J. Nigel Ellis, Ph.D., CSP, PE
Dynamic Scientific Controls
3101 N. Market
Wilmington DE 19802
302-762-4304
302-762-4305 fax

All rights reserved. No part of this book may be reproduced or transmitted in any form or by any means, electronic or mechanical, including photocopying, recording, or by any information storage and retrieval system, without permission in writing from the Publisher.

American Society of Safety Engineers
1800 East Oakton Street
Des Plaines, Illinois 60018
708-692-4121
Michael F. Burditt, Manager Technical Publications

Library of Congress Cataloging-in-Publication Data

Ellis, J. Nigel, 1942-
    Introduction to fall protection / J. Nigel Ellis — 2nd ed.
     p. cm.
    Includes bibliographical references and index.
    ISBN 0-939874-97-0 : $54.95
    1. Industrial safety—Standards—United States. 2. Industrial
safety—Standards—Europe. 3. Falls (Accidents)—United States.
4. Falls (Accidents)—Europe. I. Title.
T55.E35 1994
620.8'6—dc20   93-47067
                                              CIP

Editor: Barbara Behof Jaron
Design, Composition and Typesetting: Lois Stanfield, LightSource Images
    The text of this book is composed in Baskerville, with display type
    set in Eurostile Condensed.
Cover Design: Lois Stanfield, LightSource Images
Copy Editor: Nancy E. Kaminski

Printed in the United States on recycled paper.
Second Edition

Dedication

This book is dedicated to Hope, my wife, for all of her constructive critiques and support over the many years I've strived to make fall protection a reality in the workplace.

Fond reminiscence lingers in North America of American Indian skilled labor at heights. This centers around the Navajo in the West, and the Mohawk of the Iroquois Nation in the East, whose employment during the great railroad building boom of the 1880s led to bridge building experience and later to the highrise construction skills of today. Nerves of steel are associated with these and other ironworkers who are willing and able to work at heights and get things done. Like many construction managers, the author deeply respects the efforts of these and the many other skilled workers who perform at heights or depths. We must all work to minimize the hazards and risks for these workers. To them this book also is dedicated.

TABLE OF CONTENTS

Dedication	*iii*
Foreword to the Second Edition	*xi*
Preface	*xiii*
Acknowledgements	*xv*
Introduction	*xvii*
Special Author's Note	*xxi*

1 Is America Working Safely at Elevation?   1

- Is There a Difference Between Slips, Trips and Falls from Elevation?   2
- What Do Available Statistics Reveal?   2
- Is Every Industry Affected by Falls?   2
- Has Fall Protection Been Available To and Used By Elevated Fall Victims?   5
- When Do Falls Occur?   5
- Economics of a Fall   6
- What is the Status of North American Fall Protection
  and Emergency Escape Standards and Regulations?   8
  - ANSI   9
  - OSHA   11
  - Foreign Standards   12
- Are Company Fall Protection Policies and Rules Effective?   12

2 Who Needs Fall Protection?   15

- Who Has the Responsibility to Protect Workers from Elevated Falls?   16
- How Should Responsibility Flow?   17
- When to Plan Anchorage Points   17
- Guidelines for Architects/Engineers   18
- Guidelines for Building Managers/Owners   18
- Guidelines for Consulting Engineers   19
- Guidelines for Steel Fabrication Suppliers   19
- Guidelines for Corporate Counsel   20
- Guidelines for General Contractors   20

- Guidelines for Subcontractors   20
- Guidelines for Employers   20
- Guidelines for Owners   20
- Guidelines for Equipment Manufacturers   21
- What is the Function of Insurance?   22
- What Level of Fall Protection is Adequate?   22
- What's Wrong with Present Methods?   24
- Exploding the Myths and Mysteries of Fall Protection   26
- Should Existing Work Practices Set the Standards?   28

3 What Are the Principles of Fall Protection?   33

- Slips: Falls on the Same Level   34
- Trips: Falls on the Same Level   34
- Stair Falls: Falls on One or More Levels   35
- More on Slips and Trips   36
- Slip/Trips and Fall Signage   36
- Elevated Falls: Falls from One Level to Another   37
- Elements of a Fall Hazard   37
- Prevention or Fall Arrest as a Means of Fall Protection?   39
- Setting Fall Arrest Equipment Objectives   39
- The Personal Fall Arrest Equipment Triangle   40
- Personal Lifelines (Backup) vs. Positioning Lines
  (Primary)   48
- Manual vs. Automatic Equipment   48
- Confined Space Retrieval Planning:
  Avoiding Multiple Fatalities   49

4 Where is Fall Protection Needed?   51

- Are There Fall Hazards in Every Industry?   52
- Fall Protection Needs   52
- Can One Fall Protection System Meet the Needs of a Work Task?   53
- What Does Fall Protection Protect Against?   53
- Fall Protection by Worker Activity   53
- Risk: Should Every Fall Hazard Be Controlled?   54
- A Role for the Unions   55

5 How to Organize a 100% Fall Protection Program   57

- Should Fall Protection Always Be Provided?   58
- What Is 100% Fall Protection?   58
- Can 100% Fall Protection Be Achieved?   58
- Developing an Effective Fall Protection Program   59
  - Establishing Policy and Developing Rules   59
  - Conducting a Fall Hazard Analysis   67
  - Determining Appropriate Hazard Control Measures   68
  - Orientation, Personnel Selection and Training   69

- Inspection and Maintenance	71
- Program Audit and Feedback	71
• Additional Considerations for Confined Entry Operations	71
• Return on Investment	72

6 Fall Hazard Analysis — **75**

• How Are Fall Hazards Analyzed?	76
• Identifying Hazardous Exposures	76
• Appraising Risk	76
- Qualitative Risk Appraisal	76
- Quantitative Risk Appraisal	77
• Classifying Related Tasks	79
• Prioritizing Control Measures	79
• Providing Needed Personal Protection	80
• The Engineering of Anchorage Points	80
• Interpretation of Dynamic Peak Loads in Fall Arrest Systems	82

7 Which Fall Protection System Should Be Used? — **85**

Part I - Hierarchy of Fall Protection Solutions	*86*
Part II - Fall Arrest Equipment Capability	*86*
• Summary of ANSI Z359.1 Key Requirements	87
• Selecting Fall Arrest Equipment	89
• Nets	90
- Personnel Nets	90
- Debris Nets	90
• Body Supports	91
- Body Belts	91
- Work-positioning Belts and Harnesses	93
- Full Body Harnesses	93
• Lanyards	94
• Connecting Snaphooks	95
• Knots: A Traditional Method of Connection	96
• Climbing Protection Systems	97
- Cables	98
- Rails	98
- Self-retracting Lanyards/Lifeline Devices	99
- Climbing Assists	100
• First-Worker-Up Devices	100
• Lifeline Systems	100
- Vertical Rope Grab Lifeline Systems	101
- Self-retracting Lanyards/Lifeline Devices (Locking)	105
- Self-retracting Lanyards/Lifeline Devices (Lowering)	107
- Horizontal Lifelines (Permanent, Semi-Permanent, Temporary)	107
• Confined Space Entry and Retrieval	111
• Emergency Descent and Lowering Systems	115
- Vertical Descent	116

- Angled Descent	118
- Emergency Escape Training	118
• Personal Rescue Systems	118
- Rescue from Above-Ground Level	119
- Load Arresting Systems	120

Part III - Residual Hazards Associated with the Use of Fall Arrest Equipment   *120*

• Body Belt Use for Significant Fall Arrest	121
• Swing Falls	122
• Roll-out	122
• Mixing and Matching Equipment	125
• Equipment Misuse	125
• Electrical	126
• Heat	126
• Cutting Edges	126
• Intense Cold	126
• Corrosion and Dirt	126

Part IV - Equipment Inspection and Maintenance   *127*

• Maintenance and Inspection Guide	127
• Cleaning	128
- Synthetic Ropes, Belts and Harnesses	128
- Fall Arrester Devices	128
• Storage	128

8 Anchorage Points   **131**

• Anchorage Planning: The Key to Fall Protection	132
• Elevated Falls Kill Workers	137
• Tools for Safety	138
• Elimination of Hazards	138
• Employing Competent Persons	138
• Tying It All Together	139

9 Applications   **141**

• Roofing Work	142
• Swinging/Suspended Scaffolds	147
• Scaffolds	151
• Aerial Lifts and Platforms	152
• Ladders	153
• Confined Spaces	155

10 Safety Rules and Maintenance   **165**

• Aerial Lifts	166

- Fall Arrest Equipment 166
- Guardrails 166
- Safety Nets 166
- Scaffolds 166
- Steel Erection 167
- Stockpickers 167
- Design and Construction Fall Protection Planning 167
- General Industry Fall Protection Planning 167

11 Training 169

- Training to Meet OSHA Safety Regulations 170
- Supervisor Training 170
- Employee Training 170

Postscript 173

Glossary of Terms 175

Answers to Review Questions 181

Appendices 183

- A-1 Fall Protection, Escape and Rescue Standards 184
- A-2 Calculation of Vertical Fall Arrest Forces 188
- A-3 Calculation of Horizontal Lifeline Forces 193
- A-4 Equipment Installation and Use Engineering Guide 200
- A-5 Outdated Fall Protection Methods 204
- A-6 OSHA Guidance on Fall Planning 208

Bibliography 211

Index 221

About the Author 227

FOREWORD TO THE SECOND EDITION

During the past several years, evolving OSHA standards have affected many industries. In addition, new ANSI fall protection standards have emerged. These major changes have been noted in this book.

New sections have been added to this book, as well, including material on fall clearance distance, in order to educate the industry on the hazards associated with shock absorption deceleration distance. Other sections address anchorage points, inspection, maintenance and training. Fall protection issues in specific industries are addressed in new chapters. In addition, the author's views on many issues have been offered for such areas as steel erection, scaffolding, piperacks and roofing. And the new chapters offer a greater number of review questions, in order to provide practice for the CSP and P.E. (Safety) examinations. The Appendices have been updated to reflect easier-to-understand engineering calculations for fall arrest systems, including horizontal lifelines.

☞ SPECIAL NOTE: Many key points of information, especially new areas of discussion, are highlighted in this new edition with the icon: (☞).

PREFACE

The recommendations in this book may or may not meet specific local jurisdiction requirements. In addition, some states, provinces, or countries have more advanced requirements than those promulgated by U.S. Federal OSHA standards at this time. However, I believe that the limits and criteria proposed in this text are reasonable, feasible, and practical where no stricter requirements apply. Be sure to study applicable equipment standards and proposed testing requirements, drafts of proposed standards, and local legal requirements in your area before making final decisions on a course of protective action.

—J. Nigel Ellis

Who can use this book?

- Employer Safety Directors
- Corporate Managers, Supervisors, Foremen
- Structural, Industrial, Civil, and Mechanical Engineers
- Inspectors Exposed to Fall Hazards
- Architects
- Consulting Engineers
- Building Managers
- Contractors
- Owner Contract Administrators
- Equipment and Prefab Manufacturers
- Plaintiff Lawyers
- Defense Lawyers
- OSHA Officials
- Standards Writers and Construction Specifiers
- Justice and Court Officials
- Insurance Company Loss Control Engineers
- Union Officials and Workers
- Students in Safety Engineering and Systems Safety

The basic purpose of this book is to introduce the reader to a planning guide for thinking out personal security at heights before the fall hazard exposure occurs. Its intention also is to develop understanding and perspective on acrometry — the geometry of heights — and acrotechnology, meaning the use of the knowledge of heights to prevent severe injury from falls.

This book does not claim to interpret OSHA regulations, or ANSI standards, or court decisions in the USA. But the author believes that many opinions can be supported by existing regulations in the USA, and that these opinions may help to cut through the fog of court decisions, jurisdictional interpretations, and the towering wall of outdated industry work practices, to help provide protection to those who need it most.

This edition addresses elevated fall hazards primarily, and does not address to the same extent the vast data available for researching slip or trip hazards. This edition does, however, reference some important factors relating to surface slip control, floor coverings, stairs, and awareness of slip/trip hazards.

Review questions found at the end of each chapter are intended to be suitable in aiding preparation for the CSP core and specialty examinations of the Board of Certified Safety Professionals, Savoy, Illinois. The author periodically submits questions to the BCSP for possible use in its examinations.

ACKNOWLEDGEMENTS

The first edition of this book took five years to organize. This second edition has taken just as long to update.

Many changes in standards have occurred in the USA, Canada and Europe during this time, and their impact is just beginning to be felt, thereby justifying this updated edition.

I want to thank the hundreds of participants in my Fall Protection classes who have contributed to my knowledge of the real world and who have offered me their constructive comments on the first edition of this book.

Thank you to Edie Hazeldine, my assistant, without whose tireless efforts this edition would not have been finished.

And thanks to Pat Macht, whose fall protection sketches over the past 16 years have educated us far better than can words alone.

This second edition would not have been possible without the first, which was the work of many dedicated and talented people. Reviewers of that first edition included many recognized on both sides of the Atlantic for their fall protection knowledge. My thanks again go to all those who took the time to broaden my knowledge and experience of fall protection methods over more than 23 years in the industrial safety business, and who continue to do so.

Howard B. Lewis provided enormous support for organizing and assembling the early draft of the first edition. His background in safety education helped him develop the step-by-step, how-to guide of the Fall Protection Program section of the book.

The untiring help, determination and conviction of Bob Sisterson of Vallen Corporation is again noted for disseminating this information throughout the Southwest through seminars and education.

The basis of published test data and test methods, undertaken and developed by Andrew Sulowski of Ontario Hydro, provided a foundation for the fall protection equipment standards developed in North America. He has made invaluable contributions to my knowledge.

I continue to have high regard for the people I have met from the OSHA Office of Standards and from the Regional Field Offices, in particular, Tom Seymour and Chappel Pierce. Their dedicated, patient and reasonable approach to doing what is right for worker safety is not fully appreciated.

And I again note the invaluable guidance Vince Pollina has provided to me.

J. Nigel Ellis, Ph.D., CSP, P.E.
Wilmington, Delaware
February 1994

INTRODUCTION

More and more safety professionals realize that fall protection *can* be provided economically, can be practical, is being planned and implemented, and must be planned in the future. They also know that fall protection can be profitable.

This book is for all those who have heard "It can't be done!", even though they know in their hearts that "It *should* be done!".

Present losses in injury costs and suffering are staggering. The investment cost for protection can be minimal and reasonable. To continue to ignore, or to fight, responsibility for reasonable control of fall hazards at the work site is — just like the ostrich straining to bury its head in the sand — to incur a personal liability few of us can afford. Those individuals who have chosen to ignore these facts in the past must act now . . . or face the consequences.

The cost of fall protection currently is incurred at the legal and compensation end of the economic cycle. American industry has been insuring its way to fall safety, accepting risk and avoiding equipment use planning and worker training. Workers who are given the option of wearing, or even are required to use, belts and lanyards, generally do not receive appropriate tools or adequate planning, and generally cannot be expected to know any more than what their employers tell them. A policy of tying off when stationary is simply not credible to workers who are unprotected 99% of the time. As a result, experts believe industrial falls are costing up to one-half of all occupational injury expenses; and if this is true, the payout is shocking and unconscionable.

The loud, angry response of many foremen and managers — "It can't be done practically!" — remains. Actually, they don't want to even tackle the problem. To the detriment of owners and equipment manufacturers, plaintiff lawyers know that violation of OSHA standards and other rules, and the general lack of common sense when it comes to fall hazards, is rampant in almost every industry in the USA.

Some OSHA Review Commission administrative law judges seem to support the position that unless a method of fall protection has been previously used in exactly the same situation, and in the same part of the country, a fall hazard citation is invalid. So-called "industry practice" then becomes a barrier to progress. The employer becomes emboldened to fight OSHA instead of fighting falls.

Most expert witnesses would agree that many steel erection connectors only become seriously safety-minded after a fall. After a serious injury, they get religion!

Moreover, no jury has yet been convinced that gravity doesn't work. Yet it is often the employer who has permitted the situation to exist, and who traded on the blind ignorance of the worker. Elevated fall hazards are a risk we all, in all good conscience, shouldn't be taking . . . or imposing on others.

Reaction time in an emergency is 0.75 seconds — optimistically — according to the Delaware Motor Vehicle Drivers' Manual.[1] But by then it is too late.

What is Fall Protection?

Fall protection is the backup system planned for a worker who could lose his or her balance at height, in order to control or eliminate injury potential.

Fall protection is a planned response to foreseeable fall hazards. Fall protection can minimally be applied by:

1. Keeping the fall distance to a working surface to a minimum by using a scaffold platform, an aerial platform, or a work basket, for example.
2. Installing personnel nets (this can be done without a fall hazard using fall arrest equipment, if necessary).
3. Use of personal fall protection equipment with pre-designated anchorage points that fit the required work task mobility, including travel to and from the workstation.

Fall hazard distance begins at and is measured from the level of a workstation on which a worker must initially step and where a fall hazard exists. It ends with the greatest distance of possible continuous fall, including steps, openings, projections, roofs, and direction of fall (interior or exterior). Protection is required to keep workers from striking objects and to avoid pendulum swing, crushing, and foreseeable impact with any part of the body to which injury could occur.

The objective of elevated fall protection is to convert the hazard to a slip or minor fall at the very worst — a fall from which, hopefully, no injury occurs. And the purpose of this book is to further that objective.

THE HARD-BOILED OPPOSITION

How Long Does It Take To Fall?

Height (feet)	Time (seconds)
4	0.5
16	1.0
36	1.5
64	2.0
100	2.5
144	3.0
256	4.0
576	6.0
1600	10.0

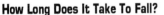

Fall Protection from an Historical Perspective

"When one falls, it is not one's foot that is to blame."
—Chinese proverb

For thousands of years man has used ropes and various knots to help move or secure objects against the forces of gravity. Bend knots were used to gain a reliable hold, and hitch knots were used in moving a load by sliding along another rope and, if necessary, gripping to lock the load in place.

The practice of people climbing ladders and/or being

suspended on ropes and using these same knots for positioning has primarily grown from the rigging trades. Some of the earlier users could be found on sailing ships, in church steeple construction and maintenance, and in tree-trimming trades. A similar development of harness, rope and knot usage originated more recently from cliff and cave rescue as well as from mountaineering.

The use of ropes and some type of body belt for restraint or work positioning support found particular interest during stormy seas and above the decks of ships. In the middle 1800s, another type of arrangement became prevalent in the telegraph industry for pole climbers. Surprisingly, much of the advice on the utility industry lineman's belt care and maintenance offered in a 1928 textbook still is valid today[2].

Safety devices that were designed to be passive until a fall occurred began to develop in the early part of the 20th century. Perhaps due to much publicity of investigations following accidents, high-rise window cleaners were the first to take an interest in independent lifelines. Between World Wars I and II, several manufacturers of body belts and other fall protection equipment came into being.

The first retracting lifelines were introduced in Sweden after World War II. Around the same time, the first climbing protection devices were developed, which required no manipulation for use.

In 1952, the National Safety Council (NSC) and the American Society of Safety Engineers published a report on maximum arrest force based on rapid deceleration tests of cadavers and anesthetized dogs[3]. Later, these findings helped to lay the foundation for Japan's 1800-lb. fall protection equipment force limit.

In 1967, the Boeing Company published a test report demonstrating the superiority of harnesses and shock absorber lanyards over belts and ropes[4].

Ladder safety devices began to be widely recognized in the 1950s and 1960s. And during the 1960s and 1970s, the availability and characteristics of synthetic fibers caused a shift away from the natural fibers used in lifelines and from the leather used in belts. Parachute-type harnesses became popular for emergency retrieval through narrow top openings of confined spaces.

Research in Europe showed the use of a full body harness to be a necessity for fall protection because of superior support both during and after a fall arrest. Equipment standards were developed in the 1970s in many countries based on widespread research into force levels on the body.

Fall hazard acquiescence by employers in the USA had been on a plateau in the 1970s and 1980s. ANSI A10.14-1975 and other A10 standards reflected industry practice: where anchorage points are natural and convenient, then tying off is the answer. Otherwise, no protection becomes a logical conclusion. ANSI A10.14-1975 was retired in 1977 under the ANSI sunset rule.

It was not until the mid-1980s that several companies in North America began to seriously address the objective of continuous fall protection.

Even though use of specific equipment is not the only indicator of fall hazard approaches on different continents, for the purposes of comparison, the following 1980's estimates are useful:

1. Employers invest in approximately 10 times more safety equipment per worker in Scandinavia than in the USA for some types of personal protection equipment[5].
2. Fall protection and respiration protection equipment are approximately equal in purchase volume invested per year by employers in Europe. Yet in the USA, an

estimated 10 times more capital is invested in respiratory protection than in fall protection equipment, despite twice as many losses per year from falls than from respiratory incidents[6].

Fall hazards can be analyzed and the appropriate planning steps can be made toward the goal of performing elevated work with no fall injury potential. OSHA had proposed fall protection standards for a number of industries by 1986.

By 1992, many OSHA standards had been put into effect, with the notable exception of construction fall protection and scaffold fall protection. A former member to the OSHA Review Commission was asked to review the issue of ironworker fall protection; a recommendation for negotiated rule making has been accepted and is in process.

The early 1990s saw the revision of the ANSI A10.14-1991 standard; the introduction of the new ANSI Z359.1-1992 standard; the introduction of the European fall protection standards; the OSHA Region 8 (Denver-based) 100% fall protection policy; and the State of Washington's ban on belts for fall arrest use. In addition, fall protection has become a major force of the proposed OSHA Reform Act (1992 Congress).

Notes

1. Division of Motor Vehicles, Driver's Manual, State of Delaware, Rev. 1989.
2. Kurtz, Edwin B. *The Lineman's Handbook.* McGraw Hill (1928 and 1942).
3. "Final Report on the ASSE Project: Safety Belts, Harnesses, and Accessories." American Society of Safety Engineers, 1952. National Safety Council, Chicago, IL.
4. "Evaluation of Safety Belts, Lanyards, and Shock Absorbers." Boeing Report #2-1886-09. September 15, 1967.
5. Westerdal, Roland. Bilsom International, Inc. Personal communication to the author, July 1987.
6. Texas Employers Insurance Association. NSC Accident Facts 1985; and other sources of the author.

SPECIAL AUTHOR'S NOTE

Since 1970, I have had the opportunity to review hundreds of falls that produced serious injury or death. As a manufacturer of emergency escape and fall arrest equipment, I have always been a strong proponent of correct equipment usage and proper training, with particular emphasis on understanding what the equipment does and does not do for worker protection.

Battle lines have frequently been drawn over the philosophies of fall protection. Original safety dogma was to make the belt and lanyard as strong as possible so that they wouldn't break, and then provide the individual product components to the worker. Of less consideration and importance were the impact forces on the worker and the choice of anchorage.

As safety planning grew through HAZOP and various state requirements in recent years, some engineers threw up their hands at what they perceived as impossible fall protection safety factors. But new methods and perspectives have begun to emerge, and modern systems have begun to gain wider acceptance. Yet fall protection planning is still in its infancy at many corporations where the worker is still expected to know about safety under the convenient term "common sense". While the common sense of the average worker is a factor in fall protection, in my experience it plays far less a role than might at first be apparent. The need to learn, plan and apply alternative measures continues.

My tort case experience as expert witness on both sides of negligence, intentional tort, peculiar risk and OSHA cases has taught me the essence of "standards of care". Common law always has called for a safe workplace, notwithstanding any lack of specific safety standards addressing every particular hazard. Recognition of hazards likely to produce serious injury and death is nowhere more important than in the case of falls from height.

Through my own experience, I understand how each employer owes it to the health of his or her business to search out fall hazards, eradicate them, or protect against falls. This new edition of *Introduction to Fall Protection* is my own personal continued commitment towards providing sufficient practical knowledge on how to recognize the many fall hazards that abound and practical insight on what to do about them.

IS AMERICA WORKING SAFELY AT ELEVATION?

Industrial falls are the number-one cause of on-site, occupational fatalities in the USA today. Yet, personal fall protection is the most underdeveloped safety program resource in the country.

❖ Is there a difference between slips, trips, and falls from elevation?
❖ What do available statistics reveal?
❖ Is every industry affected by falls?
❖ Has fall protection been available to and used by elevated fall victims?
❖ When do falls occur?
❖ Economics of a fall
❖ What is the status of fall protection and emergency escape standards in North America?
  • ANSI
  • OSHA
  • Foreign standards
❖ Are company fall protection policies and rules effective?

Is There a Difference Between Slips, Trips and Falls from Elevation?

There is no doubt that gravity works. When a person loses his balance and his body moves from an erect position to a prone or semi-prone position, a fall has taken place. The sudden energy release and subsequent absorption during impact with one or more body parts often produces an injury.

Unlike other types of incidents, falls rarely have near misses from which to be warned or learn about the consequences. It is reasonable to assume that some disabling injury occurs with nearly every accidental and uncontrolled fall.

Falls are classified into four general categories: Slips, trips, falls on stairs, and falls from elevation. Slips and trips occur on the same level. Stair and elevated falls occur from one level to another. (See Figure 1.1.)

The frequency of slips and trips tends to be very high; however, injuries typically consist of sprains and strains. Conversely, an elevated fall that may only take place every two or three years at a particular site usually results in serious or fatal injury. If falls on the same level can produce severe injury, certainly each foot above grade level increases that likelihood.

What Do Available Statistics Reveal?

Statistics in the National Safety Council's (NSC) annual Accident Facts in 1992[1] indicate that there were 88,000 accidental deaths during 1992[2], of which 12,200 were due to falls. The Council reported that of 9,900 deaths that took place in 1991 in the workplace, 1,247 were due to industrial falls. Based on approximately one million cases involving disability from 14 states, the Bureau of Labor Statistics (BLS), in its Supplementary Data System, 1988, indicates that approximately 180,000 were due to falls. (Note: Accident Facts includes motor vehicle deaths; the BLS study only includes highway motor vehicle injuries.)

Loss of Balance Results In:

Fall	Elevated Fall: fall from one level to another.
Trip	Fall at same level; fall down.
Slip	Fall at same level; fall down.

Stair falls may include slips and trips leading to falls.

Slips and trips may lead to falls when close to exposed or leading edges.

Slips/Trips: high frequency — low severity.

Elevated Falls: low frequency — high severity.

FIGURE 1.1

A June 1984 Bureau of Labor Statistics study showed that 85 percent of surviving workers involved in falls from elevation during 1982 lost time from their jobs. The average lost time for those workers was 31 days, 14 days more than the average for all other work-related injuries that year. In other words, elevated falls resulted in a productivity loss of six work-weeks, nearly twice the average for all other work-related injuries.[2]

Many of the 744 injuries in this BLS study could have been avoided by effective fall prevention or protection measures. Although 47 percent of the fall survivors were working at heights exceeding 10 feet every day, 14 percent stated that fall protection was not required. Twenty percent said they felt fall protection was not needed, and 47 percent did not consider it practical. These findings suggest a low awareness of the potential severity of falls from elevation or of the availability of effective control measures.

Almost half of the companies surveyed in this BLS study had no requirements for the use of fall protection equipment. At the same time, 75 percent conducted no training. Sixteen injured workers were using fall protection equipment, but because the equipment was not selected, installed, or used properly, they sustained injuries. For example, one worker fell 10 feet and hit the ground because his lanyard was too long to arrest his fall in time.

These National Safety Council and Bureau of Labor Statistics findings are not isolated occurrences. A BLS study conducted in California in 1976 determined that 24,179 people were injured that year in accidental falls from one level to another.[3] In New York, a study of Workers' Compensation cases filed between the years 1966 and 1970 found falls represented one-third of the 120,682 work-related injury claims filed during this period.[4]

A number of OSHA regional offices periodically publish a newsletter entitled OSHA Fatal Facts. Each newsletter details the events surrounding a fatal incident (including a technical illustration) and suggests recommendations to prevent another such incident. Approximately 50 percent of the available summaries are about fatalities caused by falls from elevation, many while moving. See Figures 1.2, 1.3, 1.4 and 1.5 for samples of these summaries.

Is Every Industry Affected by Falls?

Although elevated falls occur at any time in nearly every industry, studies show that certain industries are plagued by a higher rate of incidents. The 1984 BLS Elevated Fall Injury Survey found the construction industry to have the highest number of injuries (41%),

IS AMERICA WORKING SAFELY AT ELEVATION?

US Department of Labor
January 1992
Occupational Safety & Health Administration
Washington DC

ACCIDENT SUMMARY

Employee was suspended to the work site in a harness made of lightweight chain on the end of a crane load line. During the operation the load line separated from a revolving drum due to improper crane operation. The victim was dropped into approximately 40 feet of water and was drowned. The supervisor in charge at the time of the accident was the designated competent person at the site.

ACCIDENT PREVENTION RECOMMENDATIONS

1. The contractor should provide conventional means such as ladders, personnel hoists, aerial lifts, elevated work platforms or scaffolds for employees to reach the work site [29 CFR 1926.550(g)(2)].
2. The contractor should perform a trial lift on the equipment to determine that all systems, controls and safety devices are functioning properly immediately prior to hoisting employee to work site [29 CFR 1926.550(g)(5)].
3. The contractor should not permit inadequately trained employees to operate equipment or machinery [29 CFR 1926.20(b)(4)].

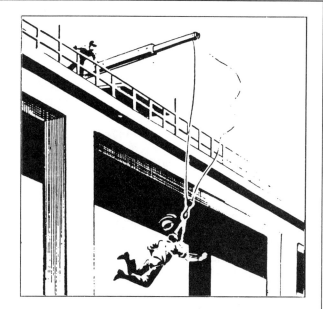

4. Contractor should provide appropriate personal protective equipment such as safety belts and lanyards for employees in operations where there is exposure to hazardous conditions [29 CFR 1926.28(a)].
5. Employer should comply with manufacturer's specifications applicable to operation of cranes or derricks [29 CFR 1926.550(a)(1)].

FIGURE 1.2
Figures 1.2 through 1.5 illustrate examples of the fatal incidents detailed in OSHA *Fatal Facts* newsletters.

USA Department of Labor
February 1984
Occupational Safety & Health Administration
Kansas City Region - Wichita Area Office - Region VII

ACCIDENT SUMMARY
Kansas
Employee Killed by Suspension Scaffold Failure

A 35-year-old man was killed when he fell approximately 40 feet from a two-point suspension scaffold on which he was standing while caulking windows on a construction site. The scaffold gave way without any warning. One of the workers was not wearing any safety devices. A co-worker was also working on the scaffold, but he escaped serious injury because he was attached to a safety harness.

RECOMMENDATIONS:
1. Ensure that each employee is instructed in the work practices applicable to the proper erection of two-point suspension scaffolds in accordance with the training require-

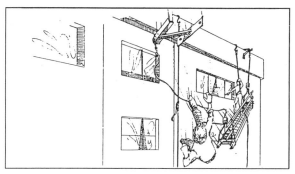

anchored and tiebacks of 3/4-inch manila rope, or equivalent, are secured to a structurally sound portion of the building installed as a secondary means of anchorage in accordance with [29 CFR 1926.451(i)(4)].
3. Ensure each employee working on a two-point suspension scaffold(s) is protected by an approved safety life belt attached to a lifeline in accordance with [29 CFR 1926.451(i)(g)].
For safety and health information in Kansas, contact the Wichita Area Office at the following toll free number: 1-800-362-2896

FIGURE 1.3

ACCIDENT SUMMARY 84-38

!!!! OSHA/GEORGIA FATALFAX !!!!
OCCUPATION: Apprentice Electrician
ESTABLISHMENT: Electrical Contractor
AGE: 26
SEX: Female
TIME: 11:20 a.m.
FATAL ACCIDENT: FALL from elevation
DESCRIPTION OF ACCIDENT

An employee was assigned the task of tying electrical cables in a cable tray located 18 feet above the concrete floor of a manufacturing plant under construction. The employee used a scissor-type vertical lift platform in order to reach the work level. The employee climbed out of the platform onto a ladder-type cable tray. She stood up on the cable tray and a short time later fell to the concrete floor and suffered fatal head injuries.

ACCIDENT PREVENTION RECOMMENDATION
1. Employee shall be instructed in the recognition and avoidance of unsafe conditions in accordance with [29 CFR 1926.21(b)(2)].
2. Employees should stand firmly on the floor of the platform, and should not sit or climb on the edge of the platform or use planks, ladders, or other devices for a work position.

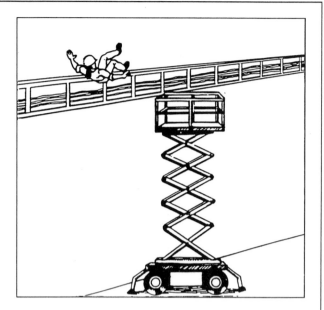

FIGURE 1.4
Figures 1.2 through 1.5 illustrate examples of the fatal incidents detailed in OSHA *Fatal Facts* newsletters.

ACCIDENT SUMMARY 84-36

LOUISIANA

OCCUPATION: Boilermaker Helper
ESTABLISHMENT: Power Plant Construction
AGE: 21
CAUSE: Fall from elevation - Failure to wear personal protective equipment

The victim, who had about two months' experience, was assisting in the rig-up of a hoist. This was atop structural steel members of a boiler building some 220 feet above an air pre-heater below. He was not making use of the static line, safety belt and lanyard provided. As he walked the beams, he lost his balance and fell to the level of the pre-heater.

Recommendation:
Supervisors should visit work areas to ensure employees are using the personal protective equipment provided.
For further information, contact the OSHA Baton Rouge Area Office at 2156 Wooddale Blvd., Hoover Annex, Suite 200, Baton Rouge, LA 70806; (504) 389-0474

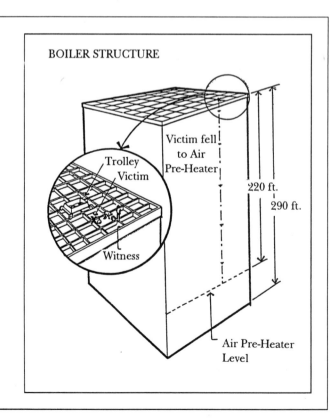

FIGURE 1.5

followed by manufacturing (23%).[5] (See Figure 1.6. Also see Figures 1.7, 1.8, 1.9, and 1.10 for additional data on construction industry accidents and fatalities.)

Of the 3,700 injuries to construction laborers in March of 1983, 11 percent can be directly attributed to falls from elevation, according to a March 1986 BLS report entitled "Injuries to Construction Laborers."[6] Fractures, cuts and bruises were most often caused by the impact of falling. Falls occurred from scaffolds, ladders, piled materials and vehicles, and into shafts. More construction fall statistics were provided by OSHA in its publication of proposed standards (Federal Register, Volume 51, Number 22, pages 42700-42719, November 25, 1986).

A National Institute of Occupational Safety and Health (NIOSH) study of fatalities and accidents in Texas and California between 1973 and 1978 found the rate in the drilling industry was six times that of general industry. Of 106 fatalities in the study, falls from derricks accounted for 31 percent[7]. Other industry categories in which fall incidents occurred with frequency, according to the BLS, include transportation and public utilities, forestry, mining, agriculture, fishing, wholesale and retail trade and services.[8]

Has Fall Protection Been Available To and Used By Elevated Fall Victims?

According to the 1984 BLS study, 74 of the 744 victims surveyed were provided with safety belts; however, more than 75 percent were not attached to a lifeline or structure. The majority of these workers reported that they were unwilling or unable to connect their safety belts because they were moving around. A few stated that there was no place to connect their equipment. Sixteen workers were using fall protection equipment at the time of their elevated fall. For 10 of these workers, the fall protection consisted of a belt tied off with a lanyard, yet four sustained back injuries from the fall arrest.

This small sample of work-related incidents clearly indicates that too many workers in American industry are injured or killed falling from one level to another. This problem is not isolated within one industry or one work task. Either fall protection is not being provided, or the equipment that is provided does not fit in with the required mobility of the work task, making the system impractical.

When Do Falls Occur?

Industrial falls can take place during a variety of elevated work tasks. Loading and unloading material was

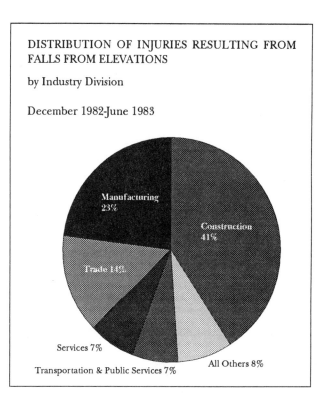

FIGURE 1.6
Source: Elevated Fall Injury Survey, 1984.
US Bureau of Labor Statistics.

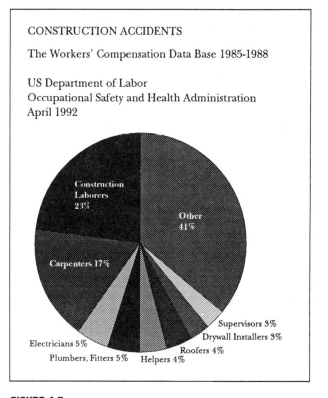

FIGURE 1.7
Source: US Department of Labor, Occupational Safety and Health Administration, April 1992.

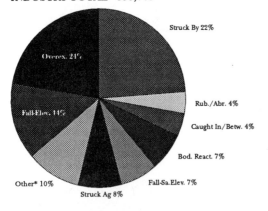
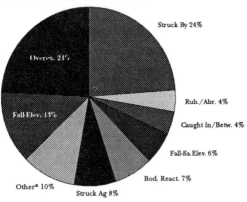
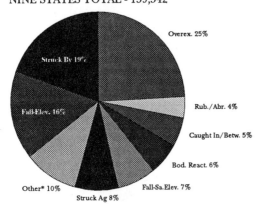

FIGURE 1.8.
Source: Construction Accidents: The Workers' Compensation Data Base, 1985-1988. OSHA, April 1992.

determined by the BLS to be the most common activity – 17 percent – at the time of the fall. Thirteen percent of the studied workers stated that they were involved in operating, repairing, cleaning or installing equipment. Ten percent were performing carpentry tasks. Other activities reported mainly consisted of work tasks associated with construction, including painting, welding, roofing, sheet metal work and masonry or bricklaying.[9]

The BLS survey asked participants to describe their specific movements at the time of the fall. Twenty-eight percent said they were climbing up to or down from an elevated position or location; 13 percent were walking; 11 percent were stepping from one surface to another, and 10 percent were moving backwards.

The structures from which the victims fell consisted primarily of scaffolds (17 percent) and roofs (14 percent). Another 14 percent were standing on objects such as equipment or work materials. Catwalks and walkways were reported by eight percent, as was being on ground or floor level and being close to holes, openings or trenches. To a lesser extent (approximately five percent), loading docks, piled or stacked materials, attic beams or other building structures, and telephone or utility poles were cited as the structure from which the fall took place.

The results of another study, done by OSHA and based upon fatal falls the agency had investigated in 1992, are shown in Figure 1.11.

Economics of a Fall

Falls from elevation are expensive. The cost of a single elevated fall incident usually starts at around $500,000 and easily reaches $1 million or more when third-party suits are involved in severe injury cases (Travellers Insurance and Harry Philo). Minimally, elevated falls result in $10,000-$20,000 cost, according to a study by Stanford University (Tech Report 260, August, 1981).

Medical expenses tend to be high due to the severity of elevated falls. Fractures, brain damage, paraplegia and death are typical results. The 1984 BLS study reported an average hospital stay of 10 nights. For those injuries that are not fatal, foreseeable payout can extend over the remaining course of the worker's employment years, perhaps 30 years or more unless settled earlier. These direct costs, along with the lost-work-time figures cited earlier in this chapter, make up a significant part of the overall financing of fall hazards by industry up until now.

The largest portion of the costs due to elevated falls are incurred through third-party liability suits. The yel-

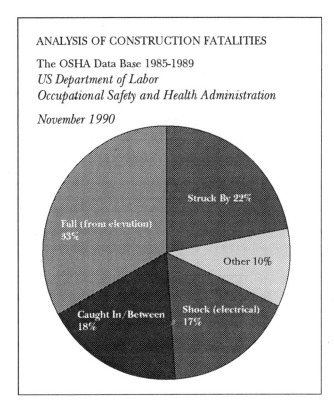

FIGURE 1.9.
Source: US Department of Labor, Occupational Safety and Health Administration, November 1990.

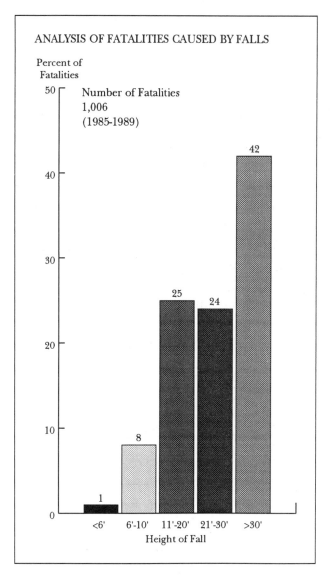

FIGURE 1.10
Source: Analysis of Construction Fatalities. The OSHA Data Base 1985-1989. US Department of Labor, Occupational Safety and Health Administration, November 1990.

low pages ad shown in Figure 1.13 and the newspaper article shown in Figure 1.14 help illustrate this growing trend. An award for $1 million seems small compared with documented decisions of $19 and $24 million. Little has to be said for the drastic increase in the number of cases and size of awards each year. The Yellow Pages ads shown in Figures 1.13 and 1.14 are samples of this growing trend.

More importantly, as the legal emphasis in each state continues to shift from worker contributory negligence and assumption of risk to comparative negligence, principals will become increasingly more responsible for identifying hazards at their sites and ensuring that appropriate precautions are taken and that protection and training provided.[10] No longer may a simple warning in the form of a small clause in the bid document to meet OSHA requirements be enough; owners must reasonably enforce their contracts.

Indirect costs are recognized to be at least equal to benefits paid by insurance administration costs alone. Workers' Compensation (WC) laws are now being challenged. The WC law in the state of Ohio has been breached. Injured employees in that state can now directly sue their company under the "intentional tort" doctrine. Several other states permit such suits.[11]

The Structural Work Act of Illinois, the Scaffold Act of Montana, and the New York State Code all permit liability of an owner for a contractor employee's injury.

The Business Roundtable Report A-3, "Improving Safety Performance" 1982, provides the basis for proving that good owner safety programs are highly profitable. The tragedy of the costs associated with elevated falls is that little is invested in the control of elevated fall hazards and, therefore, tremendous losses can be incurred. Investment consists of pre-job planning and fall protection design, equipment selection, training and maintenance. Currently, most companies in American industry are "insuring" fall safety, and keeping their fingers crossed.

Fatal Falls Investigated by OSHA in 1992

Fall From	
Ladders	16%
Sloped Roof	14%
Scaffold	13%
Flat Roof	12%
Size of Company	
2-10 employees	30%
11-25	16%
20-50	15%
51-100	11.5%
501-1000	17.6%
1000+	—
Age of Victim	
20-29 years	29%
30-39	31%
40-49	20%

FIGURE 1.11

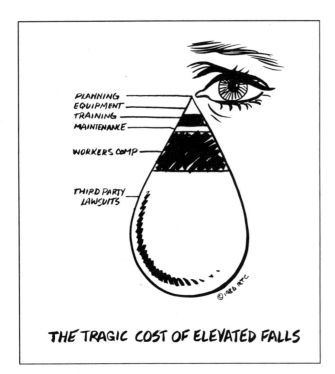

FIGURE 1.12
Copyright 1986, Research and Training Corporation (RTC).

The aim of an effective fall protection program is to increase the investment in planning and shrink the losses through Workers' Compensation payout and third-party liability suits or subrogation.

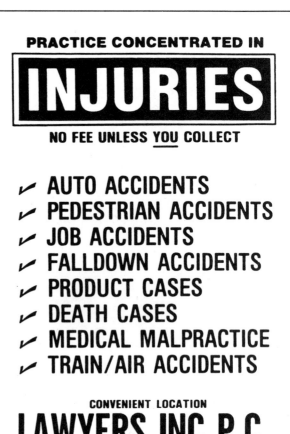

FIGURE 1.13
A typical yellow pages ad. Attorneys' advertisements make up between 2% and 6% of telephone directory yellow pages in the USA.

What Is the Status of North America Fall Protection and Emergency Escape Standards and Regulations?

The purpose of industrial safety standards is to provide design and performance requirements for equipment that can be used for fall protection. The purpose of regulation is to require the use of fall protection generally or by industry. Fall equipment can be one way to meet regulatory requirements. Standards and regulations (see Figure 1.15) provide a basis for enforcement.

IS AMERICA WORKING SAFELY AT ELEVATION?

B4 ··· The News-Journal papers ··· Wednesday, June 24, 1987

Disabled man wins $2.1 million award

By TED CADDELL
Staff reporter

A Superior Court jury on Tuesday ordered a construction company to pay $2.1 million to a Pennsylvania man who was disabled in a fall from a highway bridge project in 1980.

The award was part of a complicated, $5.1 million settlement involving two construction companies and the victim, Robert Mapes.

The jury ruled that Ashland-Warren Inc., which is incorporated in Delaware, was partly at fault for the fall that broke Mapes' neck in November of 1980 in Dallas County, Texas. Ashland-Warren Inc. was ordered to pay $2.1 million to Mapes.

Mapes, 28, of Beech Creek, Pa., sued Ashland-Warren Inc. and Bridge Builders Inc. for unspecified damages. Bridge Builders Inc. settled out of court for $2.3 million before the trial began.

In its decision Tuesday, the jury awarded a total of $5.1 million to Mapes. That figure did not take into account the $2.3 million Mapes already collected from Bridge Builders Inc.

The jury determined that Ashland-Warren and Bridge Builders Inc. each were responsible for 42.5 percent of the accident. They found Mapes 15 percent responsible.

Ashland-Warren's share came to $2,167,000. Mapes' attorney, Stephen Feldman of Philadelphia, said that figure would probably grow to $2.3 million after interest.

Mapes was working for a Claymont-based subcontractor, Bridge & Paving Services Inc., on a raised section of the Carpenter Freeway in Texas on Nov. 11, 1980. That company was not named as a defendant in the suit.

Mapes was carrying construction material when he stepped on a section of bridge decking which slipped. Mapes fell 35 feet and broke his neck, severing part of his spinal column. He has been a quadraplegic since.

In his suit, Mapes argued that Ashland-Warren and Bridge Builders should have had a safety net beneath the raised section of highway while work was in progress. Wilmington attorney Richard Pell, representing Ashland-Warren, contended that the bridge decking satisfied federal Occupational Safety & Health Administration regulations as a safety floor.

Mapes, who has incurred $180,000 in medical expenses since the accident, attended the trial every day in a motorized wheelchair. A heavy-set man who looks shorter than his 6 feet, Mape could be seen many days sitting outside Judge John E. Babiarz Jr.'s courtroom with his parents, reading newspapers and talking about baseball.

He lives with his parents in a specially-constructed ranch house in Beech Creek, about 30 miles from Williamsport, Pa.

FIGURE 1.14

This newspaper article appeared in the Wednesday, June 24, 1987 issue of the Wilmington, Delaware News-Journal. In the same issue, a front-page headline and photo showed an ironworker perilously perched on the top, final steel member of the new Manufacturers Hanover Plaza building in Wilmington.

ANSI

☞ The American National Standards Institute (ANSI) is a standards organization that accredits sponsor associations to develop consensus standards for industry, including safety standards. ANSI represents the interests of the USA internationally through the Technical Advisory Group (TAGS) to the International Standards Organization (ISO). Consensus for safety standards became much more difficult to achieve in the 1980s. Consequently, OSHA moved ahead with its own fall protection standards.

One of the first fall protection equipment standards in the USA was developed by the American National Standards Committee on Safety in Construction and Demolition Operations, A10. The A10.14 Subcommittee stated its belief in 1975 that:

FALL PROTECTION STANDARDS, USA AND CANADA*

PRESENT STANDARDS

ANSI A10.14-1991
Belts and Lanyards

ANSI A14.3-1992
Fixed Ladders

ANSI A39.1-1987
Window Cleaning

ANSI Z117-1989
Confined Spaces

ANSI Z359.1-1992
Fall Arrest Systems

OSHA 1910.23/1926.451
Scaffold Structures

OSHA 1910.36
Emergency Action Plan

OSHA 1910.66 Append.C
900 lbs. Belts
1800 lbs. Harnesses
Fall Arrest Systems

OSHA 1910.146-1993
Tank Vessel &
Confined Space Entry

OSHA 1910.272
Grain Storage & Handling
Facilities

OSHA 1926.1050/3
Stairways & Ladders

OSHA 1926.104
Construction (6 ft. max. free-fall,
5400 lbs. rope strength)

CSA Z259.1-M1976
Belts, Lanyards

CSA Z259.2-M1979
Fall Arrest Devices

CSA Z259.3-M1978
Fall Arrest Devices

CSA Z259.10-M90
Harnesses

CSA Z259.11-M1992
Shock Absorbers for Personal
Fall Arrest Systems

NFPA 101 (1991) A30-2.2
Controlled Descent Devices

OSHA PROPOSED STANDARDS

OSHA 1910.129
1,800lbs/10g Max. Force (Type 1,
General Industry; Fall Arrest)

OSHA 1910.130
(Type II) General Industry;
Work Positioning

OSHA 1910.131
For Climbing Activities

OSHA 1910.270 Oil & Gas Well
Drilling and Servicing

OSHA 1910.269
Electric Power Generation,
Transmission and Distribution;
Electrical Protective Equipment

OSHA 1926 (Sub L)
Scaffolding

OSHA 1926 (Sub M)
1800 lbs. Max. Force
Construction

OSHA 1935.611 and 612
(Type I & II) Test Methods

FIGURE 1.15

A quick summary of present and proposed US and Canadian fall protection standards.

...this standard represents the first nationwide attempt to standardize the construction and use of safety belts and harnesses and their appurtenances. The Standards Committee realizes that this standard will raise many questions that are not at present covered and that the state of the art will advance considerably in the future. This standard, therefore, will be in a continuous state of review by the A10.14 Subcommittee.

It should, perhaps, be explained that the A10 Committee feels that belts and lanyard specifications and structures should be carefully tailored to the use to which they are to be put. In all instances the structure must be designed to interrupt the most severe fall that can occur on the job without doing injury to the person. Additionally, the belt or harness must be designed to provide reasonable comfort and freedom of movement. It seems essential to the Standards Committee to consider each general type of belt or harness together with its associated hardware and lanyard as a system for delivering personal safety. It does not seem possible to achieve a safe system otherwise, and this is the philosophy which the Committee has tried to follow consistently in the writing of this Standard. As a single example, if a D-ring and snap hook are designed to mate, it will not be possible for the ring to bring pressure on the keep in such a way as to be

released. A change in either component may make inadvertent release possible and negate the safety of the system although each component, considered alone, is still perfectly satisfactory. This is why tests of systems as units have been specified.

The A10 Committee solicits comment, experience and injury or accident case histories that may be pertinent to the revision of this standard.

Suggestions for improvement of this Standard will be welcome...[12]

On September 10, 1985, 10 years after publication with no revision or amendments, the withdrawal of the A10.14-1975 standard was initiated following the mandatory ANSI moratorium period. The ANSI A10.14 Standard was revised in 1991 to include rope grabs, shock absorbing lanyards, and to some extent, positioning systems. Additionally, an ANSI A10.32 standard is intended to address fall arrest devices for construction and demolition operations in the future. The ANSI A10.14-1991 standard is similar to the OSHA 1910.66 Appendix C, except that a body belt is made equivalent in safety value to a body harness, a fact which is not recognized by the OSHA standard.

ANSI Z359 Standards

Fall Arrest	Z359.1-1992
Positioning & Restraint	Z359.2- *
Personnel Riding	Z359.3- *
Rescue & Evacuation	Z359.4- *

*Standard is "in process" and has not been finalized as of publication date.

FIGURE 1.16

Safety nets are covered by the ANSI A10.11 Committee. The A10.32 standard has been added to address debris nets.

As a result of a division in thinking, a new free-standing ANSI committee, ANSI Z359, was established in the mid-1980s, with the American Society of Safety Engineers as Secretariat, to address fall protection for all industry areas except construction and demolition. A standards matrix will cover systems, anchorages and testing for the following: 1) fall arrest; 2) climbing; 3) work positioning; 4) man-riding; and 5) rescue and evacuation. (See Figure 1.16.) The first standard, Z359.1-1992, covers fall arrest systems, including components to allow users to connect different manufacturers' parts. Body belts are not permitted for fall arrest.

The ANSI Z117 Committee revised its 1977 standard in 1989. Many current State confined space standards merely require an attendant tending the rope. The revised ANSI Z117.1 standard requires fall arrest equipment be worn before entry if practical and helps define the criteria for fall protection and retrieval through training.

OSHA

☞ The Federal Government administers work safety and health through an agency of the Department of Labor, the Occupation Safety and Health Administration (OSHA). At OSHA's inception in 1971, very limited fall protection rules were promulgated. Some State OSHA plans have developed more detailed and specific requirements. OSHA rules supersede ANSI standards where they overlap or are in conflict.

OSHA has proposed a number of rules and regulations to provide workers with greater protection against industrial falls. OSHA is planning to amend the General Industry Standards Section Subpart I dealing with personal protective equipments. This regulation will establish new standards for fall arrest systems, work positioning systems, travel restricting systems, and fall protection systems for climbing (Proposed OSHA 1910.129-.131).[13] The analogous proposal for the construction series (Proposed OSHA 1926 Subpart M) was proposed in late 1986, along with Subpart L Scaffolds, and Subpart X Stairs and Ladders[14]. Subpart X became a final standard in 1990.[15]

Where 5400-lb. anchorages were previously required, OSHA would round this figure to 5000 lbs. Both general industry and construction fall protection standards include similar testing requirements for equipment and will be cross referenced from future OSHA industry standards.

The US Department of Labor's proposed standard preamble to the 1910.129 Standard states:

> "OSHA believes that such systems, by increasing their usage, can enhance employee protection from injury or death due to falls to different elevations."

These guidelines incorporate new fall protection technology for increased employee safety. In particular, OSHA is recommending a maximum fall arrest force on the body to help control compounding injuries. Additionally, shock absorbing lanyards, retracting lifelines, controlled descent and other systems that can provide protected mobility are addressed.

Although revisions to the general industry standards – including 1910.21-32 Subpart D, Walking and Working Surfaces, and the Oil and Gas Well Drilling and Servicing Industry (1910.270)[16] – have not become final standards as of this printing, the new fall protection requirements are present in two final standards, specifically, the Grain Storage and Handling Industry (1910.272)[17], effective March 31, 1988, and, particularly, the Powered Platform Industry (1910.66), effective 01/24/90[18]. The 1910.146[19] Confined Space Standard was issued January 14, 1993, and requires the use of harnesses and winches for rescue below five-ft. depths.

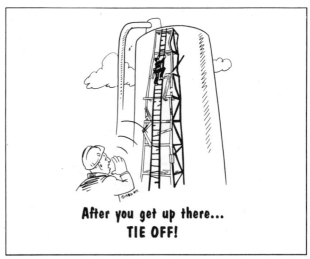

FIGURE 1.17

Copyright 1986, Research and Training Corporation (RTC).

Reasonably detailed safety standards and regulations are needed to provide a basis for equality among contract bidders so that more effective safety planning can be provided.

Foreign Standards: Status Relative to USA

The United States still trails behind many foreign countries relative to the requirements of its standards and the degree of fall protection offered to many workers, perhaps by as much as 20 years.

Canadian fall protection regulations are administered by the Ministry of Labour in each province. Canadian Standard Association (CSA) standards are rapidly advancing by issue of fall arrest equipment component standards.

France, Britain, Sweden, Finland, Germany, Japan and Canada are considerably more advanced in this area of safety standards. For example, in 1978 France banned the use of a body belt to meet its national fall arrest requirements. A year later, Britain followed suit by limiting the use of body belts to where free falls are less than two feet. The ISO Fall Arrest Equipment standard is still pending.

European Community (EC) standards for fall protection are becoming effective 1993-1994. (For a detailed listing of foreign standards, see Appendix A-1).

It is time for the USA to address fall hazards with a wholesale effort and not just in isolated instances within proactive companies.

Are Company Fall Protection Policies and Rules Effective?

While the low frequency of elevated falls has, no doubt, contributed to complacency – "It's not a problem here; we haven't had a fall in ten years"– there are two words in safety terminology that could be responsible for tacitly permitting thousands of deaths and disabling injuries each year. Those two words are "Tie Off!"

For most elevated work tasks, tie-off fall protection is erroneously and unconsciously interpreted to mean climbing up unprotected, tying off, untying, moving unprotected, tying off, and untying to climb back down. (See Figure 1.17.) Is this partial protection any different from asking workers to wear half of a hard hat or one lens in a pair of safety glasses? OSHA Fatal Facts and the Mine Safety and Health Administration's MSHA Fatal Grams both confirm that workers fall when they are moving, rather than when they are stationary at a workstation. And, quite often, moving represents a major portion of the work task.

Tying off, as it appears in standards as well as in company policies and rules, has lulled principals, contractors and employees into feeling comfortable with this

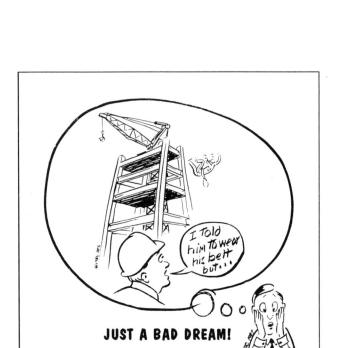

FIGURE 1.18
Copyright 1986, Research and Training Corporation (RTC).

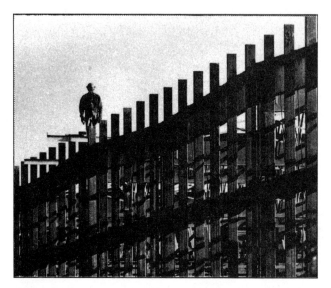

FIGURE 1.19
"Nerves of steel — A construction worker walks atop the shadow-dappled skeleton of part of Federal-Mogul Corp.'s $64 million plant being built at Lititz, Pa." This caption and photo appeared in The News-Journal papers, Wilmington, Delaware, Saturday, November 23, 1985. Photo Credit: Marty Heisey.

partial form of safety. A tie-off fall protection program also gives a company a false sense of security because managers believe fall hazards have been fully addressed and workers simply use what is given to them. In essence, the assertion that fall hazards have been addressed is only a misguided notion. The training so crucial to proper use of personal protective equipment is missing. Can workers reasonably try out a body belt and lanyard so that they know how their safety equipment will perform in an emergency? How can they truly understand the capabilities and limitations of their equipment without first-hand experience? If they could, they would surely see that tying off, as we know it, is a false concept.

As was pointed out earlier in this chapter, the 1984 BLS study on elevated fall injuries found that most workers were "unwilling or unable to connect their safety belts because they were moving around".

If we take this predominant situation and create the scenario of a fall incident, it usually goes like this:

1. Management has established a tie-off rule such as, "If you are more than 10 feet above grade level, you must be tied off."
2. A body belt and 6-ft. lanyard is made available to the worker.
3. Because of the time constraints imposed, and lack of available anchorages, the worker elects to not tie off during the performance of a short-term work task. Management overlooks the hazards.
4. The workers loses his balance, falls from elevation, and is injured.
5. Company management states, "We try to get our people to tie off." And their position remains that the worker did not follow the written company procedure.
6. The worker later states that management either never provided proper equipment or enforced its use, or never trained him effectively.

The irony of this not so infrequent situation is that the employer never really provided or enforced adequate employee protection as required by the Occupational Safety and Health Act of 1970. The "protection" provided was not practical for the work task, nor could it provide complete and continuous protection.

A similar situation exists when a standard or company rule states: "Fall protection equipment must be worn when working more than 10 feet above ground." Without performance guidelines on the proper attachment and use of the equipment, regardless of the type, a worker simply "wears" his fall protection. (See Figure 1.18.) Technically, he is in compliance with the requirements. Again, the practicality of the system is the key to effective protection.

Tying off means that no one is planning or thinking out the job. Statements such as "Fall protection is impossible for roof panel construction or maintenance; you can't tie off to blue sky!" clearly indicate that a work method analysis, including the fall hazards, has not been studied for that work task. Yet equipment and methods are available to protect workers from falling while still allowing necessary mobility.

Public misconception regarding safe work at elevation is frequently fueled by the media and by advertising agencies. For example, newspaper captions such the one shown in Figure 1.19 misrepresent the real danger of the situation and glamorize flagrant violation of federal law. The unsafe situation is seen as "macho" rather than as a deficiency in the company's safety program or its enforcement.

What will bring down the high rate of industrial fall incidents along with their tremendous consequential costs? No OSHA, ANSI or local standard will do it. The diversity of work tasks is too great for generalized standards to be effective. It will be up to individual company policies and rules to bring about the change and provide employees with adequate protection. In the long run, proper enforcement will benefit companies as much as it does the individuals exposed to fall hazards. The objective is to make safety pay, to demonstrate that better, safer work methods dramatically increase profits by lowering operating costs.

Notes

1. Accident Facts, 1984-1992. National Safety Council, 444 N. Michigan Ave., Chicago IL 60611.

2. Injuries Resulting From Fall From Elevations, (Bulletin 2195). June 1984. USA Department of Labor, Bureau of Labor Statistics. USA Government Printing Office, Washington, D.C. 20402.

3. Bureau of Labor Statistics Supplemental Data System, State of California (Excerpt 1976).

4. Summary Tabulations Characteristics and Costs of Work Injuries in New York State–An Industry Report 1966-1970, Vol. II. USA Department of Labor, NY 1966-1970, p.55.

5. Injuries Resulting From Fall From Elevations, (Bulletin 2195). June 1984. USA Department of Labor, Bureau of Labor Statistics. USA Government Printing Office, Washington, D.C. 20402.

6. Injuries to Construction Laborers (Bulletin 2252). March 1986. USA Department of Labor, Bureau of Labor Statistics. USA Government Printing Office, Washington, D.C. 20402.

7. Health and Safety Guide for Oil and Gas Well Drilling and Servicing; National Institute for Occupational Safety and Health, Publication No. 78-190, Cincinnati, OH 45226.

8. Injuries Resulting From Fall From Elevations, (Bulletin 2195). June 1984. USA Department of Labor, Bureau of Labor Statistics. USA Government Printing Office, Washington, D.C. 20402.

9. Ibid.

10. Philo, H. and R.L. Steinberg. "A Partial Revocation of the Legal License to Kill Construction Workers." Trial Magazine. Vol. 15, No. 6. June 1979. pp. 24-28.

11. Industrial Commission of Ohio, Workers' Compensation. Revised Code Section 4121.80 (Intentional) August 22, 1986.

12. ANSI A10.14-1991 Requirements for Safety Belts, Harnesses, Lanyards, Lifelines and Droplines for Construction and Industrial Use. American National Standards Institute, 1430 Broadway, New York, NY 10018.

13. OSHA 1910.129-131. 4/10/90 Proposed Rule for General Industry. Personal Protective Equipment. US Department of Labor, Washington, DC.

14. OSHA. 1926 Subpart L, M, X Safety Standards for Scaffolds Used in the Construction Industry; Notice of Proposed Rulemaking. Federal Register,. Tuesday, November 25, 1986. US Department of Labor, Washington, DC.

15. OSHA 1926.1050-1053. Subpart X, Stairways and Ladders, Federal
Register, November 14, 1990.

16. OSHA 1910.270. Final Rule for Oil and Gas Well Drilling and Servicing. Federal Register, Wednesday, December 28, 1983. US Department of Labor, Washington, DC.

17. OSHA 1910.272. Final Rule for Grain Handling Facilities. Federal Register, December 31, 1987. US Department of Labor, Washington, DC.

18. OSHA 1910.66. Final Rule for Powered Platforms for Building Maintenance. Federal Register, January 24, 1990. US Department of Labor, Washington, DC.

19. OSHA 1910.146. Final Rule for Permit Required Confined Spaces. January 14, 1993. US Department of Labor, Washington, DC.

Review Questions

1. How can falls from elevation be characterized?
   a. High frequency.
   b. High frequency, high severity.
   c. Low severity, high frequency.
   d. Low frequency, high severity.
   e. Low severity.

2. According to the BLS (1984) report on injuries resulting from elevated falls, what was the most frequent response fall survivors reported for not using fall protection equipment?
   a. Not available.
   b. Not practical.
   c. Not required.
   d. Not needed at the height they were working
   e. Too much trouble.

3. At present the costs associated with elevated falls are disproportionate. In order to change or shrink the tear drop shape of the expenditures, where should money be invested?
   a. More effective legal counsel.
   b. Maintenance.
   c. Planning.
   d. Self-insurance.
   e. Training.

4. What does a "tie-off" fall protection program most represent?
   a. No elevated fall hazards.
   b. Partial safety.
   c. Lack of worker compliance.
   d. Low awareness of hazard severity.
   e. Attaching lanyard with a knot.

5. What is one of the more critical developments in OSHA requirements for minimizing the potential for compounding injuries during a fall arrest?
   a. Establishing a maximum fall arrest force.
   b. Banning the use of a body belt.
   c. Preventing exposure.
   d. Limiting the free fall distance to two feet.
   e. Preventing swing falls.

WHO NEEDS FALL PROTECTION?

Who has the responsibility to
protect workers from elevated falls?
How should responsibility flow?

❖ When to plan anchorage points
❖ Guidelines for architects
❖ Guidelines for building managers
❖ Guidelines for consulting engineers
❖ Guidelines for corporate counsel
❖ Guidelines for general contractors
❖ Guidelines for sub-contractors
❖ Guidelines for owners
❖ Guidelines for equipment manufacturers
❖ What is the function of insurance?
❖ What level of fall protection is adequate?
❖ What is wrong with present methods?
❖ Exploding the myths and mysteries of fall protection
❖ Should existing work practices set the standard?

Who Has the Responsibility to Protect Workers from Elevated Falls?

The Owner and the Employee

Ultimately, the owner as principal is responsible for limiting or excluding fall hazards from his or her property. Both reputation and pocketbook are at stake. To the extent that the knowledgeable owner employs architects and engineering consultants to advise about the construction of a building structure, the owner must clearly require state-of-the-art, built-in safety precautions wherever possible, both for contractor employees and his or her own workers. After construction is complete, exterior maintenance contractor employees such as window cleaners must be adequately protected by design of anchorage points, regardless of who owns the access equipment.

It is not reasonable to ignore exposure to fall hazards at any time during the life cycle of the building or structure. Evidence should show that fall protection was a major, upfront consideration in the bid documents and contract awards, and that monitoring, inspection and enforcement efforts were reasonably made.

Many courts are probing the workers' compensation law barriers in the USA and calling for action against employer negligence. The "intentional tort" committed by an employer against an employee is a remedy in a few states. Consequently, some courts are building a record of holding employers accountable for fall injuries to contractor employees, and in some cases to their own employees. State courts limit recovery to contributory negligence by the worker; in a few remaining states, 1% is sufficient to bar recovery by a worker from a product manufacturer or an owner. The majority of states have comparative negligence where damages are reduced up to 50%; over 50% contribution by the worker, as determined by the finder of fact, bars recovery. Federal courts usually follow local state courts in matters of law.

The factual basis of these views might serve as a guide to answer the question, "Who should know that falls can hurt workers, and that falls are a predictable consequence of working at heights without protection?". The courts are increasingly showing that the owner should know about this potential for injury. The owner should be holding contractors responsible and should be willing to invest in their demonstrated adequate performance in this area. Particularly, advisors like architects and engineering consultants, who must be highly and consciously aware of fall hazards on the job, should help educate owners instead of being silent. Fall protection should be a major issue in contract wording for services provided by such advisors. The old shibboleth of existing industry work practice not requiring fall protection is an increasingly redundant, empty defense when cited after the fact, as it is time and time again in the face of poor des)gn and no planning. The employer has notice of the severity of falls through books such as this one and the annual Accident Facts report from the National Safety Council.

The Worker

The worker's responsibility for his or her own safety is a reasonable requirement, provided he or she has been physically trained and mentally prepared, educated in policy, equipped with state-of-the-art equipment, and has been furnished with suitable, identified anchor points based on a credible employer fall protection program.

The questions after an accident are, "Did the worker know of the danger, and thus was negligent?" or, "Did the worker not know of the danger, but still was negligent?" Safety experts increasingly are convinced workers do not necessarily possess an innate sense of safety or common sense, and thus must be trained effectively. Nevertheless, education of foremen and workers in good safety practice is an on-going difficult process that must inch forward, often over the objections and ignorance of the exposed parties. A more frequent observation of work by a competent person, knowledgeable in fall protection methods, may be required. As the chance of death from a fall moves closer to 100%, based on height and impact consequences, so fall hazards may be classified as ultra-hazardous and non-delegable duty to control at the principal level.

The technology and communication required for meeting federal hazard communication and state/provincial "right to know" laws is producing a drive that also should accomplish fall protection through greater worker knowledge and participation concerning what can hurt them. The same applies to OSHA 1910.119 process safety rules. Automobile seat belt laws are also providing excellent precedents for workers.

SAFETY ENGINEERING
FALL PROTECTION PRINCIPLES

Eliminate

Prevent

Arrest

Warn

FIGURE 2.A

WHO NEEDS FALL PROTECTION?

The prime rule is to apply fall protection when the height hazard exceeds a reasonable figure of a few feet, or at any height if continued exposure to the hazard is not preventable. The responsibility of the vendor of the equipment to educate is limited to the extent of whether the customer has a bona-fide "no fall" policy in lieu of a tie-off policy so common to the majority of employers. It also depends on the manufacturer's instructions, labeling, and product literature if the employer and employees were or could have been guided by these items for reasonably foreseeable or permitted uses. Workers should be exposed to, and permitted to read and understand, product instruction and labeling of fall arrest equipment. A book of instruction for safety products should be kept in the same location as the Material Safety Data Sheets (MSDS).

How Should Responsibility Flow?

The owner must set safety policy, which permits the safety department to make reasonable rules on fall protection that must be followed in work practice. Construction managers must be required to enforce the safety rules as part of their job requirements. It is the owner's chief operating officer's job to ensure that this is done in a formal way.

The owner sets the standards and enforces them, based on the procedures for his or her own employees engaged in plant or construction use. If the owner does not set and enforce standards because of unfamiliarity with construction or maintenance practices, then the obligation falls to the architect/engineer, consulting engineer and/or general contractor. But the owner must consciously intend to give the responsibility to the contractor or engineering firm and not supervise anyone. And then the owner must still see that the engineering firm/architect accepts this responsibility.[1]

The unknowledgeable owner must rely on a competent architect for price and completion, and for prevention of accidents and death to anyone on the job.

Both the architect's duty and the general contractor's duty is to formally warn the unknowledgeable owner about elevated fall hazards and the reasonable cost of controlling them. Recent evidence shows that construction projects can benefit from an average of 35% bare labor savings when a 100% fall policy is adopted and applied.

☞ Safety specifications must be spelled out by the owner or the architect, detailing all hazards that might reasonably be expected during construction as well as methods that will reasonably prevent injury resulting from those hazards. The "low bid" without safety will not protect the owner or architect from lawsuits. If the subcontractor employer is negligent in allowing fall hazards, then, following a fall, the owner faces the burden of having hired an incompetent contractor. Contract safety provisions must be effectively enforced.

Ideally, the architect's or consulting engineer's services should be made available for a price under the contract to answer fall protection engineering questions by the general contractor or the subcontractors. Either party also could be required to provide (upon request) anchorage points that meet OSHA requirements and that can be used to install fall arrest equipment according to clear sketches and application requirements submitted in advance. Work method details are critical, and prompt coordination is essential for success.

Anchor strength requirements should equal at least twice the dynamic load or the maximum arrest force the fall system can experience when tested in a worst-case anticipated situation. The equipment manufacturer's installation instructions should serve minimally as a guide for the architect/engineer to follow. For commercial building roof tie-backs, the anchorage points should offer at least the strength anticipated in reasonable foreseeable applications.

When to Plan Anchorage Points

☞ Anchorage points are the key to designing fall protection systems. The strength, location and design must

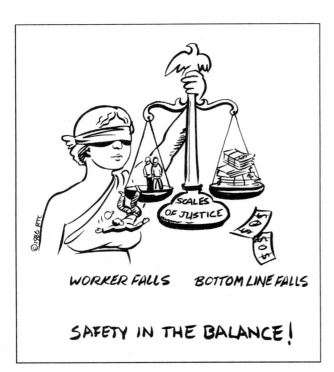

FIGURE 2.1

fit in with the required work task mobility. Quite often, more than one work task is involved. For a building, this means designing the structure for life-cycle fall protection,[2] actually planning:

- prior to construction
- prior to occupancy
- prior to maintenance
- prior to renovation
- prior to demolition

This is the only way fall hazards can be controlled effectively.

The following guidelines indicate more specifically how some roles in industry need to address anchorage points.

Guidelines for Architects/Engineers

☞ The architect must be competent in writing safety specifications for a contract. If no owner's representative is available, then the architect must employ an architect's superintendent to supervise enforcement. Because the architect is the designer, he or she must be knowledgeable of construction methods available to build the design and must understand that all hazards and risks involved must be addressed by him or her in detail. Mere attention to blueprints is not acceptable.

The information learned at or after engineering school regarding 5,400-lb. lifelines and five-times safety factor needs to be modified. Heavy steel beams are very different from radar antennae as sources of anchorage points. At the very least, architects should offer as an addendum in their contract with the owner to design anchorage points for contractors to suit desired work practice upon request. Architects who know workers will be exposed to fall hazards while building the structures they design must be ready to provide the means for safe anchorage feasibilities in those designs, without which fall protection methods become much more difficult.

Guidelines for Building Managers/Owners

☞ Building managers and owners need to address the safety of those who will be responsible for elevated maintenance, inspection, and usage of buildings, including employees and contractor employees. This includes such operations as window cleaning; installation of exterior lighting; inspection and work in shafts, ducts, boiler room pipe systems, pits and sewers; and roof work of all kinds.

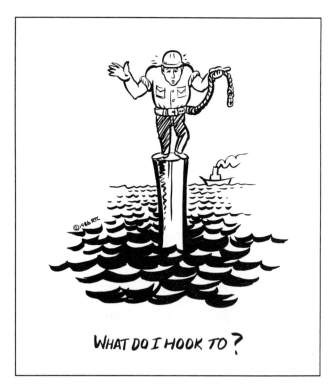

FIGURE 2.2

Long overdue is the need of building managers nationwide to foresee permanent exterior anchorage point requirements for scaffold tie-backs and lifeline anchors at roof level. Pad eyes welded to plates attached to roof deck area structural members, and capable of withstanding 6000 lbs. per person, should be treated and painted a bright yellow or orange. Permanent signs close by should explain their purpose.

Every atrium and sloped side needs special consideration for window cleaning systems and lifeline anchorage points.

Roof edge work within 12 ft. is a protected zone for restraint systems. Roof corners can only be addressed through fall arrest approach with anchor points at least 5 ft. high. Note: OSHA roofing standards state a 6 ft. or 10 ft. rule, depending on whether mechanical equipment is being used. The 12 ft. guidance is a practical measure adopted by some corporations.

Parapets or effective perimeter railings are vital, and must be designed in, for long-term safety of maintenance personnel who will be at the roof edge over the life of the building.

Aerial personnel lifts should be used by both employees and contractor employees to position under and reach up to lights and other high areas in foyers in lieu of stepladders or extension ladders. In addition to safe work practices, use of the proper equipment that can help engineer out height hazards is a critical cornerstone of building management safety commitment.

Guidelines for Consulting Engineers (Civil, Structural, Design, Project, Industrial)

Construction specifiers of buildings, bridges, dams, and other civil or industrial projects must show that construction at each stage can be done with reasonable access and reasonable fall protection. Anchorage strength design should minimally equal twice the maximum force of the fall system that will be attached to the anchorage. Designing for fall protection should tend to follow shock and vibration engineering of a 2:1 minimum factor for engineered systems, as opposed to the 5:1 or higher wear-and-tear factor frequently used in industry. Note: Be sure to evaluate for corrosion and misuse such as lifting points. Under most circumstances, a 5400-lb. anchor strength requirement is easily obtainable. However, where specific situations limit anchor selection or design, the strength can be engineered down to a minimum of 2:1.[3] For example, the existing structure around a valve may be capable of supporting 1200 lbs., not 5400 lbs. For a shock-absorbing lanyard that limits the arresting force to 600 lbs., this anchor point may now be suitable and the expense of new construction can be avoided. Other examples might include piperack horizontal lifelines, aircraft structures, aerial lifts, and antenna and radar tower parts.

Overall, establishment of an engineering policy to specify fall protection systems that limit arresting forces to an average of 650 lbs. is recommended. Yet, each system also must be detailed to suit a specific work method. Workers should have reasonably easy and protected work access, and availability of suitable fall arrest equipment.

In almost any aerial project where fall hazards exist, the first worker up assumes the greatest risk of falling. In addition, that worker is often responsible for attaching the fall arrest equipment that will be used by other workers and, perhaps, other trades. To accomplish this task without unnecessarily exposing the first worker up, a plan is required before the work begins. Workers should be involved in discussions on available systems and their work methods to determine the best-suited fall protection. Typical solutions in the construction industry could involve attaching lifelines at ground level to columns, beams or trusses and, with the assistance of hoisting equipment or cranes, raising them into place prior to climbing or walking in fall exposed areas.

Similarly, the last worker down can be exposed to a fall hazard after having detached the fall arrest equipment. Protection can sometimes be achieved by threading ropes though suitably rounded shackles.

This way, the end of the lifeline accessible at ground level can be used to pull the rope through when the work is complete. Alternatively, if the structure will be climbed in the future for maintenance, a permanent climbing system should be installed. Then the last worker down can use this system to remove temporary equipment before making the final descent.

The design of fall protection systems also must take into account the need for periodic inspection and maintenance. Appropriate materials should be specified for the environment and system components should be readily accessible for routine checks. Engineers also must make sure that additional hazards in using personal fall protection equipment are not introduced. For example, swing falls are of particular concern with retracting lifelines. See Chapter 7 for details.

Estimation of the strength of structural members as possible anchorage points, particularly by workers in the field, should be avoided. One person may be able to "tug" up to twice his body weight, or 300 to 350 lbs. Multiple persons pulling on a line may or may not get multiple values. The only way to field test an apparently stable anchor location is to pull it with a come-along and dynamometer. However, earlier predesignation and marking of anchorage points by structural engineers is best. Models sketched out for reference are the next best thing.

The duty to protect workers is transferred to the engineering firm or to the general contractor or contract manager if the owner is not knowledgeable of the hazards. The designer or civil engineer must know that people will be exposed to fall hazards in the building of his or her structure. The consulting engineer must know, too. To pretend these hazards do not exist is not reasonable. Designs must henceforth be reasonably safe for construction and subsequent maintenance.

A new planning skill for engineers is acrometry! Establishing the topography of the work place in order to plan fall protection security is essential.

Guidelines for Steel Fabrication Suppliers

You know with reasonable certainty the steel erection sequence. You know that workers need to position themselves for connecting and bolting the steel, and from your experience you know how they do it.

You need to do your part to assist in developing proper fall protection methods, such as by offering a hole location plan for post and lifeline support while walking the steel. You also should become aware of which edges on the steel you provide will cut wrapped lanyards in a fall, and then warn about the hazard and carefully apply this particular method of fall protection. (See Figure 2.6.)

As an encouraging press-time note, OSHA has committed steel erection fall protection to its Negotiated Rule-making process.

Guidelines for Corporate Counsel of Knowledgeable Principals

Attorneys should carefully review the company's bid documents. Wording should be added to require compliance with the company's safety rules, especially fall protection rules, so that standards can be maintained by contractors. Gone are the days in most jurisdictions when you could rely solely on the exculpatory contract wording, "Contractor must meet local, city, state, and OSHA safety rules," not because it is untrue but because it is incomplete. The knowledgeable owner must require contractors to fulfill these obligations to help avoid third-party tort claims.[4]

The knowledgeable owner also must know that many contractors will not follow "general safety rules" – they are presently exempt from responsibility under Workers' Compensation laws in most jurisdictions, and the insurance carrier will be made whole if the third party suit succeeds. He or she especially must aim to solve the most predictable cause of loss, which is from elevated falls. Even an indemnity clause signed by the contractor must at some stage be negotiated after the owner has spent months or even years preparing for trial at great expense, and possible public embarrassment. Your company's loss is guaranteed unless preventative measures are taken at the contract stage. Elevated work fall hazards no longer should be viewed as ordinary risk.

Educate supervisors and safety personnel in the "standards of care" required for a project. Teach doctrines of liability and the Restatement (second) of Torts as they apply in specific jurisdictions. Explain the legal tests for liability of parties. Do your part for preventive safety engineering.

Guidelines for General Contractors

☞ General contractors and contract managers should be seeking subcontractors for elevated work who can demonstrate an effective fall protection program that fits the general parameters for a safety program. Trades should indicate where anchor points and perimeter cables are needed and by when. Subcontractors should specify to the general contractor where they will need anchor points by examining the blueprints and explaining the anticipated work method. For groundlevel work where trenching is to be done, fencing or other barriers should be required. Shoring with elevated panels or posts to support a warning or perimeter cable are other methods to guard an existing trench.

The general contractor is the coordinator of work and safety.

Guidelines for Subcontractors

☞ For all your urgency to speed along with the job, finish and move on, you must take time to analyze your rising insurance costs and to consider the risk of falls by those who often are your friends. Bids for projects should be made showing adequate fall protection as a separate additional cost. This will help establish the need for roof-top anchorage points on buildings for building maintenance work, and it will help owners and general contractors to decide whether the low bid is omnipotent, without losing your opportunity to win. See whether they are serious about delegating safety and are willing to pay for this investment.

Your goal is to set the safety standard for your industry in your area.

Guidelines for Employers

☞ The terms competent person, qualified person and qualified engineer need to be defined, and standards of performance need to be developed around safety rules for fall protection. Chapters 5 and 6 specifically are designed for you after the principles of fall protection are understood. Your EMR – Experience Modification Rate – in future years needs active accident prevention now. Be the leader in your industry!

Guidelines for Owners

☞ The search for contractors with experience modification rates (EMR) trending below 1.0 over the three most recent years should be first choice for owners (refer to Business Roundtable, A-3, p. 20, 1982). If the owner is knowledgeable about industrial and construction practice and the danger of falls, he or she must

WHO NEEDS FALL PROTECTION?

SUCCESSFUL PRODUCT ENGINEERING INCLUDES
FALL PROTECTION

The following are examples of the many equipment, prefab, access and material handling manufacturers that
need to address on-site end-user fall protection while
designing and engineering their products.

Silos	Prefab Buildings and Structures
Bins and Boilers	Tanks and Elevated Platforms
Rigs	High Rack Storage
Outdoor Advertising	Hammerhead Cranes
Towers	Off–the–Road Vehicles

Printing Presses
Bucket Trucks – anchorage point for specified lanyard
Scissor Lifts – anchorage point for specified lanyard
Swinging Scaffolds – independent lifeline specified
Vessels/Scaffolds (Frame and Tube/Clamp)
Boatswain's Chairs – independent lifeline specified
Single Point Suspension Scaffolds – independent lifeline
specified

FIGURE 2.3

prepare bid documents indicating an active search for
an effective worksite fall protection program. Owners
not in the industrial or construction business must consciously delegate the responsibility for fall protection to
the general contractor. Asking a general contractor to
meet local, state and federal work safety requirements
will not protect the owner from inevitable lawsuits by
injured workers. Falls are the major cause of losses;
therefore, the issue of fall protection needs to be specifically addressed in the documents. This also makes it
fair to all contractors and allows fall protection to
become part of the various work methods. Finally, your
policy on fall protection should prohibit the purchase
of capital equipment that incurs fall hazards during
installation or maintenance.

Guidelines for Equipment and Prefab Manufacturers

☞ Those companies who make material handling or
access equipment are at risk if they have not considered
fall hazards and escape needs from buckets, platforms,
crane cabs and scaffolds, and during erection and
maintenance procedures.

The requirement of fall protection through warnings, which clearly depict falling hazards, is the first
line of awareness for workers or inspectors so exposed

to fall hazards. Going further to propose the method
of fall protection is an important goal for rig manufacturers.

A practical method should be proposed by rig and
scaffold manufacturers that mirrors the anticipated
work method. Anchorage points should be instructed
or provided to suit this anticipated need.

Examples of equipment and prefab manufacturers
who need to think out how their installers, equipment
users or maintainers should be protected from falls are
shown in Figure 2.3.

Scaffold manufacturers should detail erection fall
protection methods.

Scissor lift manufacturers, recognizing that workers
may use the mid-railings as a ladder rung to reach up
to and in between an obstruction, may decide that a
grating or mesh could be installed to limit this tendency to cause a fall hazard exposure. However, it also
makes sense to specify personal fall protection for over-
reaching or leaning over.

Lack of means of escape from these high work sta-
tions means that, in an emergency, the workers could
be trapped. For example, a slow-to-respond bucket
truck could be a problem if a swarm of bees attacks an
elevated operator and causes him or her to jump out.
The manufacturers should be able to address this type
of problem, once they become aware of even a single
occurrence or believe the scenario may occur. Oil
drilling and service rig manufacturers need to address
the problems of derrickmen in an emergency by detailing the types of controlled descent systems that are
practical and then making provisions for their installation.

Other types of rigs, such as yarders in the logging
industry, need to have climbing devices specified that
meet the needs of the work method. Yarders and
piledrivers experience vibration characteristics that
need matching with the capability of fall protection
devices in order for them to survive such long-term
vibration exposure.

Tank manufacturers need to address maintenance
work methods with practical access and fall protection.
Tank and vessel manufacturers must be sure to design
manways greater than 18 in. diameter to avoid trapping
both workers and rescuers; 24 in. minimum should be
considered. Maintainers of digester tanks in the pulp
industry in particular should have systems for access
specified, and should recommend practical fall protection and emergency retrieval systems.

☞ In summary, equipment manufacturers should
engineer fall protection to meet state-of-the-art technology and current or pending OSHA standards. Do
not ship fall hazards to your customers! This applies to
design, installation, inspection and maintenance.

What Is the Function of Insurance?

Owners, contractors and employers are currently insuring their way to safety at the finance end of corporations, in the absence of a policy for addressing or endorsing corporate rules for "no-fall-hazard" worksites. This policy can come about through a corporate president's "no-fall" endorsement letter to management. Otherwise, or in addition, it is the president or senior managers who must endorse the elimination or control of a rather obvious hazard. The degree of commitment by management is measured by how effectively the fall protection program is incorporated into each project's contract.

The insurance companies' underwriting departments seem to have no real stake in the outcome of this discussion, because workers' fall hazards are one reason insurers are in business. Naturally, their loss control engineers should warn employers about carelessness, poor habits, and other work practices they are aware of for the purpose of minimizing risk as they see it. But loss control has not yet taken the lead in promoting adequate fall protection on the job. Underwriting's role has been primarily to raise premiums when losses mount while seeking to be made whole from a third party. This subrogation amounts to a reimbursement of losses without any benefit to an already assessed client.

Insurers also attempt to limit the legal parameters for suits (such as time limits for filing), to minimize attorney fees, and to control awards through legislative action in order to obtain a reliable actuarial basis for setting premiums. This amounts to self-protection rather than accident prevention. Insurers provide a barometer to the cost of fall accidents, the number-one jobsite hazard, with their premiums.

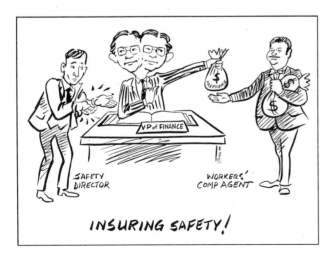

FIGURE 2.4

Increasing Premiums

Refer to Figure 2.5 to compare the Workers' Compensation and general liability premium rates for various industries with experience modifications of 100.

One can easily see that fall hazards from heights greatly add to costs for employers. Window cleaners, in recent years, because of their high visibility and urban exposure to publicity, have become very safety conscious. This degree of commitment is surprisingly successful in gaining the cooperation of building managers despite bids sometimes higher than those of their less safety-conscious competitors. The result is usually a vastly improved experience modification rate, which pays back those safety-conscious owners in the best way of all...cash savings!

On construction projects, insurance frequently now costs 10% of the price of the job.[6] That means that if payroll is 40% of the job, then insurance is 25% of payroll. Therefore, there is a lot of money to invest and save dealing with fall hazards, the number-one jobsite killer, with high expectations of a return on investment.

☞ In summary, loss control engineers can contribute much more to reducing the toll from workplace injuries.

What Level of Fall Protection is Adequate?

Because an accidental fall seems to occur so rarely, it often has been difficult for concerned managers to query a particular method of fall protection used by a worker until after it is too late and an accident has occurred. Managers have relied too much on workers to know where and how to protect themselves. Specific rules of equipment use by the employer that are diligently applied will help to diagnose potentially improper or doubtful use. To illustrate this point, examine the following list of questionable protection methods actually utilized and rationalized according to depositions and the author's first-hand experience:

1. New Bridge Construction –
   Protected access along an 18-in.-wide trestle bridge girder flange in the Pittsburgh area bolter-uppers consisted solely of a single 3-ft.-high hand-line at one side with an 80-ft. fall hazard to the river below.
2. Water Tower Painting –
   A rope lifeline was positioned "close by" to a single point scaffold in New Orleans, and was available for the water tower paint inspector, in his own words, "to leap and grab in an emergency should the scaffold fail".

		PENNSYLVANIA				NEW JERSEY				DELAWARE		
		'90	'91	'92	'93	'90	'91	'92	'93	'90	'91	'92	'93
Window	G.L.	9.72	9.72	21.229	15.731	91.70	91.70	10.351	10.351	9.72	9.72	8.947	8.830
Cleaning	W.C.	24.39	30.09	30.09	41.520	14.69	18.35	22.94	22.94	11.66	11.66	11.66	13.04
TOTAL		34.11	39.81	51.319	57.251	106.39	110.05	33.291	33.291	21.38	21.38	20.607	21.870
Roofing	G.L.	6.59	6.59	38.144	27.304	55.51	55.51	19.386	20.827	6.59	6.59	22.042	21.255
	W.C.	27.01	31.61	31.61	43.30	15.67	17.12	18.69	18.69	22.88	22.89	22.89	27.63
TOTAL		33.60	38.20	69.754	70.604	71.18	72.63	38.076	39.517	29.47	29.48	44.932	48.885
Steel	G.L.	6.55	6.55	29.61	18.139	50.57	50.57	13.457	14.187	6.55	6.55	15.417	13.103
Erection	W.C.	41.51	50.77	50.77	59.05	10.49	9.81	11.54	11.54	26.31	26.69	26.69	27.34
TOTAL		48.06	57.32	80.380	77.189	61.06	60.38	24.997	25.727	32.86	33.24	42.107	40.443
Masonry	G.L.	6.53	6.53	10.676	7.615	50.22	50.22	6.325	6.886	6.53	6.53	3.864	3.660
	W.C.	12.19	15.00	15.00	18.96	7.98	8.21	8.16	8.16	9.77	9.85	9.85	12.25
TOTAL		18.72	21.53	25.676	26.575	58.20	58.43	14.485	15.046	16.30	16.38	13.714	15.910

FIGURE 2.5

Sources: General liability information provided by Insurance Services Office, New York, NY. Workers' compensation rates provided by compensation and rating office for each state.

3. Two Point Swing Scaffold Window Cleaning –
Apparently no lifelines seemed necessary, since the scaffold was operating properly and there seemed to be no danger before it fell. In another case, when a lanyard was used it was attached to a horizontal line strung across the back of the scaffold regardless of potential severe swing collision injuries in a scaffold failure of one of the load cables. When both load cables failed in yet another case in Houston, Texas, both workers rode the scaffold 32 floors to the ground and were killed, along with a pedestrian.[7]

4. Boatswain's Chair Window Cleaning –
No lifcline was deemed necessary by a window cleaner in Boca Raton, Florida, since the rope used to position and suspend workers "constituted a lifeline," and if a separate lifeline was in fact to have been used, both lines were designed to go through the same variable speed control unit to which the chair was attached.

5. Attachment of Lanyards to Vertical Lifelines from Swinging Scaffolds Using a Hitch Knot –
This is a common occurrence regardless of the condition of the rope, its size compatibility or its material composition. This was interpreted as a work skill by an OSHA CSHO in Aurora, Illinois, and allowed after the worker demonstrated how it worked. (See Appendix A-4 for detailed discussion of knot-tying methods.)

6. Body Belt Worn Around Chest –
The wearer, an engineering inspector with a heart problem, felt he could survive a fall better from a swinging scaffold if the belt was worn under the arm pits rather than around the waist.

7. Lanyard Snaphooked to Rope Lifeline –
In an elevator shaft, several construction workers attached 10-ft. lanyards to the same vertical lifeline, which was knotted every few feet.

These methods obviously reflect a lack of adequate employer standards, or of sensible guidelines, or a meaningful attempt to meet federal or state regulations. They are ineffective solutions to fall hazards, and should be addressed point by point:

1. A hand-line is not adequate fall protection, even if the worker holds it. Many times a worker will carry tools or boxes of bolts without holding on to the line. Also, when an intermediate post is reached, no grip is feasible. Only when the hand-line is converted to a guard-rail cable with midcable and positioned on both sides of the girder, can it be considered as a candidate for adequate fall protection. For a limited number of workers, a hand-line might be upgraded to a horizontal lifeline. A worker's body support with a suitable lanyard, and a snaphook or device which automatically bypasses intermediate posts, could be a one-way access system for one of the girders. Yet, to make this particular method credible, effective fall protection for subsequent bolt-up of x-braces, for example, should be a fact. An erection method plan that considers early installation and use of the sub-deck inspection walkways (if applicable) could be the better means of access, providing fall protection with the final guard rails securely in place.

2. No rope or cable can be grabbed in a sudden fall; the notion is absurd. The fact that a person falls 16

feet in the first second of a fall, and it takes only 2 and 1/2 seconds to fall 100 feet, shows how devastating a fall can be. All single point scaffolds must be designed to allow independent lifeline systems that can arrest a fall automatically if a failure to the main load line suddenly occurs.

3. This overconfidence defies regulations and common sense for work at heights involving work surface suspension on cables. All above-ground scaffold work is dangerous and hazardous. A separate independent lifeline is absolutely necessary for each worker in case the scaffold fails at either end. For four point suspended scaffolds, the case for attachment to the scaffold itself becomes a reasonable consideration to help protect against falling off the scaffold. For four point scaffolds with railings around all four sides, and where falling accidentally over the railings is an unreasonable possibility, perhaps no personal-use fall protection can be considered because it might be argued as redundant. Emergency descent capability remains a question, however, to be answered.

4. Misunderstanding that a rope load line is in itself a lifeline shows lack of thinking through the application or is merely a desire to fox unwary employers and authorities with a specious argument. The best way to view boatswain's chair work is to have a totally separate, independent personal lifeline system for the worker and to avoid any common element with the suspension system.

5. The use of hitch knots is a questionable practice because of lack of ability to test that knot if a fall injury arises. OSHA General Industry and Construction rules require that the employer makes sure the employees' equipment or method is safe. Only the most advanced corporations can claim such a level of control over their work force, that they could guarantee the efficiency of every worker-tied sliding hitch knot now and in the future. There is no reason, however, to take such a gamble. The best approach is a rope grab system or self-retracting lanyard/lifeline device to suit the application.

6. Temporary suspension in a belt cinched around the upper chest for some can be more tolerable than when the belt is worn snugly and, as intended, around the waist. However, during a sudden fall, the larger chest diameter could allow the person to slip out of the belt. (See "The Safety Belt Question," Andrew Sulowski, *National Safety News*, February 1985.)

7. This work practice has several flaws from a safety viewpoint. The use of one lifeline per person is standard, unless a multiple-person fall system has been specially engineered. The use of overhand knots is a major weakening factor in rope strength. The rope would have to be 5/8 in. or 3/4 in. maximum in diameter to accommodate lanyard snaphooks, and thus would only be sufficient for one worker's fall (5000 lbs./worker). Attaching lanyard snap hooks to a rope above the knot, or to a cable above a wire rope clip, could result in catastrophic roll-out failure. If the worker fell, how would we know for sure that he had ever attached the lanyard in the first place? In addition, 10-ft. lanyards could exceed the 6-ft. OSHA fall limit and also be the cause of swing injuries. Based on these arguments, the consideration of rope grabs and retracting lifelines seems to be the responsible direction for improved fall protection in this application.

In summary, the acid test is that if you as manager are able to demonstrate that the fall protection methods chosen will reasonably suit all the foreseeable circumstances of a particular work need, then you may be able to show that you have looked at the work carefully, examined failure modes, and matched usable and acceptable fall protection systems to that particular work without relying solely on the individual worker's judgment or experience. Over time your diligence will show in the record that the methods of fall protection employed under your direction have been appropriate and that workers have been educated to use well-thought-out systems for personal protection. Only then can it be claimed that fall hazards are being controlled.

What's Wrong With Present Methods?

The typical philosophy has been to encourage workers exposed to hazards to tie off when stationary or when working. However, the choice is usually left up to the workers, especially, for example, in skeleton steel connecting.

Many employers regard fall hazards as a necessary occupational hazard, and overlook them, depending instead on workers' practical ability. The Ironworkers' training manual[8] encourages "ad hoc" fall protection in this manner, via belt and rope safety line. And yet there is no meaningful training in fall protection during apprenticeship, or published requirements for the employer to provide horizontal lifelines, or more complete safety details for workers to use. No wonder some ironworkers never use – and sometimes even cut off – this rope on their belts.

Different industries have progressed at different speeds, some taking their cue from others in the same or similar business to stiffen requirements as work methods become safer, thanks to one or more pioneering companies.

WHO NEEDS FALL PROTECTION?

But what's wrong with tying off? The answer is as follows:

1. By definition it means that the worker is exposed to a fall both before tie-off and after tie-off.
2. It means that untested, understrength anchorage points may be used, and the workers must judge the strength of any object.
3. The shape, sharpness, and contour of the points set up cutting action, which can be instantaneous and catastrophic in some falls.
4. It means invariably that the fall protection equipment must be wrapped around a structural member and then attached back to itself – a method rejected by fall equipment manufacturers and one that restricts mobility.
5. It encourages the use of knots in rope lifelines and lanyards for securing when in actuality bend knots can reduce strength considerably.

The warning provided by the Canadian Standards Association Fall Protection Committee in 1987, recreated in Figure 2.6, shows how urgently we need a radical re-think of this concept... now!

The Problems with a Tie-Off Concept

- Anchorage point is not approved for strength and reliability by an engineer; sharp angle-iron can be dangerous (see Figure 2.6).
- Not always overhead.
- Can give rise to 12-ft. falls with 6-ft. lanyard when attached at foot level, such as on the top of a piperack.
- Lanyard frequently knotted without regard for residual strength or for providing a provable system.
- Too much handling.
- Impedes the flow of required work task mobility.
- Responsibility sits entirely with the worker.
- Usually ends up being a policy in theory only and never applied (i.e., the belt is sometimes worn but the lanyard very rarely attached).

HAZARD ALERT
regarding
USE OF LANYARDS FOR FALL PROTECTION
Toronto, May 7, 1987

HAZARD

Some synthetic fibre lanyards may not arrest a fall when wrapped around rolled or welded steel structural sections with sharp edges.

BACKGROUND INFORMATION

It is common practice for a worker to wrap a lanyard around a structural steel section for protection against falling. It was discovered during laboratory testing that 5/8-inch-wide (16mm) 3-strand nylon lanyards lost up to 93% of their original strength when arresting a fall. The test was performed according to CSA Standard Z259.1-M1976. Similar tests on 7/8-inch-wide nylon web lanyards ended with no arrest at all. In both cases the lanyards' loss of strength was caused by the cutting action of the edges of the I-beam. The I-beam used was a W10x33 (rolled) manufactured approximately in 1984. Comparative tests with the nylon rope lanyards on an I-beam of the same nominal size manufactured in 1977 (approximately), all ended in arrested falls with little damage to the lanyards. The edges of the I-beam manufactured in 1984 were found to be up to three times sharper than the edges of the I-beam manufactured in 1977. Both I-beams were produced by a rolling process. The cause of the sharper edges on the new I-beam is being investigated. Please note that welded steel shapes have edges sharper than rolled shapes, therefore, the hazard of cutting the lanyard is even greater.

RECOMMENDATIONS

This problem is under investigation and the recommendations below are preliminary:

1. Avoid wrapping synthetic fibre lanyards around structural steel sections if better points of attachment are available.
2. If no other points of attachment are available, wrap a cut-resistant material around the steel section, and tie off the lanyard to that material rather than the steel section.
3. The use of a shock absorber between a safety belt (harness) and the lanyard has been demonstrated to prevent the loss of strength in the lanyard during the arrest of the fall.

Andrew C. Sulowski, PE
Chairman
CSA Technical Committee on Fall Protection

FIGURE 2.6

Exploding the Myths and Mysteries of Fall Protection

Do you enforce the use of fall protection? The answer to "fall protection by mandate" is to not let it reach that point in the first place unless it is a last resort. At the same time, the owner cannot argue with the contractor all along the way to job completion, without fall hazard exposure promptly addressed up front (Figure 2.7). Fall protection must be planned, reviewed at pre-bidder's meetings, and developed into workable methods. First, a reasonable access method must be established, and then a safe work practice. Equipment standards and regulations help provide the basis for planning.

☞ Employers are responsible for informing their employees about workplace hazards and providing appropriate protection. Live equipment training and video sessions can better help achieve the needed awareness and understanding of equipment capability and limitations, which words alone can never do.

What Do Workers Say?

- Falls are a problem in the workplace.
- More fall protection should be used–we see it in government jobs and the apprentice programs.

- They'll protect equipment falling with debris nets but not people with personnel nets.
- Management says it costs 25% of the job more if we use lifelines.
- I'd get fired if I insisted on fall protection.
- I never thought about it.

Workers either underestimate the severity of elevated falls or have been indoctrinated, or pressured, into "getting the job done" with the available tools. "Either do it, or we'll get someone else to do it," they interpret management's view. A few express concern to the employer while others are content to cynically bide their time and wait for an opportunity to sue someone. Many workers assume that their management has addressed elevated fall hazards by providing them with a belt and lanyard, and have accepted this partial form of safety. In legal proceedings following an accident, the worker most often states that nothing was provided, while the employer says available equipment was never used. The truth is probably that the employer did not enforce the safety rules, which he later asserts existed.

What Are the Manager's Trade-offs in Thinking About Tie-off?

- Let him find his own anchorage point.
- Everyone else in the industry does it this way.

FALL PROTECTION BY MANDATE?

THE EXCUSE

"If you want this building finished on time...!"

"The workers will get tired."

"We're going to have trouble with the workers."

"There's no place to hook up."

"We can only get them to hook up if we stop in one place for a short while."

"It's going to put the price up."

"There's one thing you forget. We gotta get this building built!"

THE REALITY

A threat to safety planning to be overcome early in the game.

They'll become more confident.

Not if they are trained and you are interested in their personal safety.

Often correct...without planning.

The whole system is not credible.

May appear to at first, but will cut premiums and lower costs very quickly. A budget of 1% of a construction job of approximately $1 million dollars seems reasonable for fall protection.

Without planning, this comment may well be heard and you may be pressured to compromise in the short run. But never give up the planning process! Don't give up.

FIGURE 2.7

WHO NEEDS FALL PROTECTION?

- It's better to let him fall 6 feet or so rather than 90 feet.
- Falling in a belt may hurt her, but it won't kill her.
- No one got killed using a belt and lanyard.
- We've always done it this way.
- You give a guy safety equipment and he doesn't use it!

- They'll never use it properly
- The time it takes to hook up is not worth the effort.
- She gets paid for working up high.
- It's too much trouble.
- The idea is great... but they'll never use it.
- It will tire them out.

MYTH VS. FACT

THE MISCONCEPTION

Hooking up below your feet is the best we can do!

Guard rails are O.K. to tie off to.

Hook off to anything solid.

Tie-off to a hand-line is O.K.

Ground-built scaffolds have no provision for tie-off during erection.

Tie-offs are more dangerous than doing the work, and we move so quickly.

There's nothing left to tie off to.

A worker is responsible in the end for his own safety.

Contractors want you to get the job done ASAP.

I'll take my chances and jump clear if the whole building goes down (same for wood poles, scissor lifts, bucket trucks, steel girders).

THE REALITY

Improper planning – it doesn't take much planning for waist-high or overhead anchorage.

Very few guard rails are designed for use as an anchorage point for lifelines.

The random anchorage responsibility put in the hands of a worker is irresponsible.

Provided that the cable has been designed and approved for fall protection.

A well-designed tube and clamp or frame scaffold erection will already have either the anchorage point at waist height minimally or, alternatively, railings from a push-up masonry-type outrigger.

Planning to get the work done with fall protection is better than last-moment decision making.

Planning sorts this one out fairly easily for a specific work method.

Must be true! What are we doing to make it easier to achieve usable anchorage points? What training is being done on fall protection?

This fall hazard issue must be tactfully raised. Practical solutions may include constructive proposals.

This is a bit like the argument for not wearing seat belts for certain types of automobile collisions. The question will remain until the individual concludes that being hooked in is an overwhelming safety advantage compared to the relatively remote question of surviving or not surviving a collapse with or without attachments. No person should be required to work on any structure that has not been engineered sufficiently to support him.

FIGURE 2.8

- You just can't predict where she's going to be.
- How do you get the equipment down after use?
- In our situation, you can't use fall protection.
- There's nothing to hook up to, unless you use a sky hook.
- They're always moving; that's why they can't hook up.
- A guy should be careful and not go up when weather is bad.
- Fall protection is no good unless they use it.
- The problem is they never use the equipment we provide them
- It's hard enough to get them into belts so getting them into harnesses is simply impossible
- Tie-off... it's the best we can do.
- We try to get them to tie off when they stop at one place long enough.
- We leave it up to the individual to decide if she wants to tie off.
- You can't be tied off all the time because sometimes you need to move quickly!
- We agree that connectors should be tied off when they are more than 30 ft. above a work surface (steel erector contractors).

In addition to these differing perspectives between workers and managers, there are differing opinions on the effectiveness of body support mechanisms. Figure 2.9 presents the most common myths – along with the real facts – about belt use.

Again, the most effective method of overcoming these, and any other, fall protection myths or objections is controlled live training. In the case of body support, it is not even necessary to free fall. Simple suspension plus videotape viewing of an articulated dummy in a series of fall arrests is all that might be necessary to help guide worker selection.

Should Existing Work Practices Set the Standards?

The illustration in Figure 2.10 is not for the purpose of poking fun at tree trimming work methods. Instead, it points out the need to plan fall protection to suit a particular work method before the job begins to avoid serious, if not fatal, accidents. However, far too often, and for this reason, an industry elects not to enforce the use of personal protective equipment, even though it may be kept at the jobsite. Erecting scaffolds and steel, or installing roof panels, for instance, involve some established work practices wherein many people think a belt and lanyard are "not worth the trouble" relative to the

time it takes to do a particular job, except perhaps when the worker might be stationary for a time. Then again, maybe a belt and lanyard alone are not the best available solution for fall protection.

More thought is required.

Can industry work practices be changed? It starts with one company in the industry with the desire to succeed and willingness to prevail. That company will set out to break the bonds of traditional, unsafe work practices and achieve effective worker protection. For example, a no-fall hazard means of steel connection has been developed and now is being practiced for exterior falls. This alternative is illustrated in Figure 2.11, which is described below.

A System for Connector Fall Protection

To begin, a vertical lifeline can be attached to the column at ground level before it is lifted into place. This enables the connector to attach at a lower level, then climb up with protection. The horizontal lifelines also have been attached at ground level while the beams are being rigged. The worker in the background of Figure 2.11 is still attached to his vertical lifeline, while the worker in the foreground has transferred to the horizontal line with a second lanyard and is positioned out of the way of the incoming beam. Once the beam is lowered into place, the workers move into position and make connections. The equipment also may be used for bolting-up operations and perhaps by other trades as well. It also can be lowered or transferred to another area. After decking is in place, other fall protection methods for consideration can be the decking of each floor before the floor above is decked, and attachment of perimeter cables through eyebolts on the columns as they are each lifted past the connector. Maypole installations of retracting lifelines have been used successfully for protecting deckers.[10] (See Figures 7.24 and 7.25.)

More New Concepts

A very helpful film showing erection of a multistory concrete office building complex with no fall hazard has been prepared and was shown at the National Safety Council Annual Congress in 1986.[11] This film demonstrates that fall protection can be worked out in virtually any situation.

Other fall protection videos have been produced, as well, including:

2. The Pin-hole Safety Connection[12] demonstrates techniques for eliminating fall hazards for steel erection and assembly of multi-tiered steel structures.

WHO NEEDS FALL PROTECTION?

2. A video by Ironworkers Local 711 in Canada[13] illustrates steel connection and bolt-up with various methods of fall protection.
3. Safety Post System[14] shows drop testing of a 300-lb. weight onto a horizontal cable attached between posts assembled onto I-beam flanges.

As an additional encouraging press-time note, OSHA has committed steel erection fall protection to its Negotiated Rule-making process.

Notes

1. "A Partial Revocation of the Legal License to Kill Construction Workers," Philo, H. and R.L. Steinberg. Trial Magazine, Vol. 15, No. 6, June 1979, pp. 24-28.

2. Products Liability–Design & Manufacturing Defects, Bass, Lewis. Shepard's/McGraw Hill, 1986.

3. OSHA 1910.66. Final Rule for Powered Platforms For Building Maintenance. Federal Register, Friday, July 28, 1989. US Department of Labor, Washington, DC.

4. Lawyers Desk Reference, Philo, Harry M., The Lawyers Cooperative Publishing Co., Rochester, NY, 1979, pp. 865-880. Also Lawyers Desk Reference, Philo & Philo, Clark Boardman & Callaghan, Thomson Legal Publishing, Inc., 1993. pp. 401-402.

5. B.G. Balmer Agency, Paoli, PA. November 1992, February 1993.

6. Ibid.

7. Pennzoil Place Scaffold Failure. Houston Chronicle, May 25, 1987.

MYTH VS. FACTS ABOUT BELT USE

THE MYTH	THE REALITY
Belts will "cut you in half" if you fall.	You may indeed be injured by a narrow belt in a long fall.
Belts are better than nothing (6 ft. versus 90 ft.).	This may be true... provided that the fall is approximately 2 ft. maximum and the operator can regain his position within 1 to 2 minutes.
Belts are lifesavers.	Belts have indeed saved lives but harnesses allow the credibility necessary for training.
You can't fall out of a properly fitted belt.	Should be true, but improper wearing, such as a loose fit to allow for attachment of tools, may also permit the wearer to fall out of the belt, head first or feet first depending on the type of fall or his center of gravity.[9]
The D-ring location does not matter.	Slow-motion films show the side D-ring and front D-ring attachment can be much worse than the back D-ring for a 6-ft. free fall, because of the pivoting action of the body. The upper back D-ring location produces the least limb movements.
Body pads do not matter.	Body pads do to some extent spread the shock load over the waist area and provide better support (provided the strap is 1.75 in. minimum width) but the effect is small.
Belts do not produce injury from fall arrest.	This was and clearly has been proven a fiction. Serious injuries have occurred as a direct result of falling in a body belt. There is a much greater chance of neck injury from a fall in a belt than in a harness, in addition to limb flailing injuries.

FIGURE 2.9

8. Orientation Manual for Ironworkers. International Association of Bridge, Structural, and Ornamental Ironworkers. 1980.
9. "The Safety Belt Question," Sulowski, Andrew C. National Safety News. February 1985. pp. 44-46.
10. "Protection System Preventing Falls from Metal Roof Decks." Shipley, Carl. National Safety Council Construction Section Newsletter. May-June 1981.
11. Pre-phase Planning: Job Hazard Analysis, video film produced by Michael Pennington, Hensel Phelps Construction Co., Greeley, CO.
12. The Pin-hole Safety Connection, video film produced by Dwight R. LeBow, Rald Industries, Freeport, TX.
13. Ironworkers Local 711, Montreal, Quebec, Canada.
14. Safety Post System, video film produced by Gerald Whitmer, Whitmer's Welding Service, Shenandoah Junction, WV.

Review Questions

1. Stepladders and extension ladders are typically used in your plant to access maintenance work in ceiling panels and piperacks. However, a recent series of falls among contractors produced several lawsuits against your company for negligence in requiring contract safety rules to be enforced. What should you do to reduce future risks from falls?
   a. Train people, both on ladders and step ladders
   b. Require use of elevating platforms.
   c. Devise fall protection or work methods without exposure to a fall hazard; review contractor proposed solutions.
   d. Do nothing because nothing can be done.
   e. Contract in future for indemnification by the contractor for all injury claims.

2. What liability does a principal potentially face if he or she contracts for elevated work and requires the contractor to meet local, state and OSHA regulations?
   a. Third party liability.
   b. Personal liability of the contract administrator.
   c. No liability.
   d. D & O liability.
   e. Workers' Compensation claims.

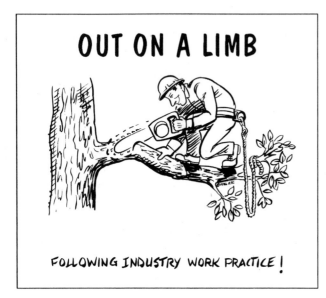

FIGURE 2.10
Too many incidents occur in this way, while topping trees, dismantling scaffolding, or removing guardrails. Planning proper work access is a key to the type of fall protection required. Random and incompatible anchorages contribute to needles fall fatalities.

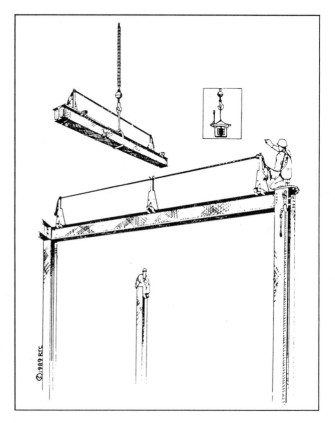

FIGURE 2.11
Connector Fall Protection – Lifeline Systems are attached after beams are shaken out and before hoisting. Direction to the crane operator is provided remotely, as shown. This avoids the consequences of possible damage to the connector's current fall protection system by swinging or misplaced loads. Note the vertical lifeline in place on the column on the right. The worker in the background, using his vertical lifeline, will seek protection behind the column as the beam approaches. Not shown: Ladder for access of the columns. Ladders are being used more frequently for this purpose.

3. What minimum anchorage strength to maximum arrest force should consulting engineers consider for design if 5400 lbs. is not possible?
   a. 5:1
   b. 20:1
   c. 10:1
   d. 2:1
   e. 6:1

4. "Belts do not produce injury from fall arrest...". The fact is that, compared with a full body harness, a fall arrest in a body belt has a much greater chance of injuring which region of the body?
   a. Chest
   b. Head
   c. Thighs
   d. Neck
   e. Spleen

5. How can existing industry work practices be effectively changed?
   a. Discussion prior to a job.
   b. Eliminate the use of personal fall arrest equipment.
   c. Design fall protection to suit the work task.
   d. Create new federal and local regulations.
   e. By-pass sole remedy of Workers' Compensa-tion laws.

WHAT ARE THE PRINCIPLES OF FALL PROTECTION?

Anyone who seeks to provide fall protection must first understand the principles.

- ❖ Slips: falls on the same level
- ❖ Trips: falls on the same level
- ❖ Stair falls: falls on one or more levels
- ❖ Slips/trips and fall signage
- ❖ Elevated falls: one level to another
- ❖ Elements of a fall hazard
- ❖ Prevention or fall arrest as a method of fall protection?
- ❖ Setting fall arrest equipment objectives
- ❖ The personal fall arrest equipment triangle
- ❖ Personal lifelines (backup) vs. positioning lines (primary)
- ❖ Confined space retrieval planning: avoiding multiple fatalities

Slips: Falls on the Same Level

As a person moves along a walkway, there is a relationship between the supporting surface and the opposing surface of the foot or foot gear. When the friction between these two surfaces is inadequate, a sliding motion – a slip – results. This slip, in turn, can lead to a loss of balance and result in a fall. In general, a number of design factors can contribute to a slip–fall, individually or in combination, including:

1. *Footwear:* the composition and condition of the sole, as well as its shape and style. Proper fit of the footwear. New leather soles and heels can be very slippery when dry, and especially so under wet conditions, until they have absorbed water sufficiently. The ASTM F13 (American Society for Testing and Materials) Committee on Safety and Traction for Footwear has addressed important frictional issues.
2. *Floor Surface:* the design, installation, composition and condition, gradient, modifications by protective coatings and cleaning/waxing agents, and illumination. Solutions include grooving or gritting, or adding matting and mats, to help deal with wet or slippery surfaces, floors and grating. Epoxy painting of concrete surfaces promotes slip resistance when the surface is wet or oily. For extreme friction, aluminum oxide coating can be used. Diamond plate designs vary greatly in their slip resistance properties. See Figure 3.1.
3. *Individual:* the physical make-up of a person, including disabilities, locomotion or gait characteristics, age, physical and mental health, emotional state, attentiveness, and agility.
4. *Work Task:* the lifting, reaching for or moving of objects. The important principle is that the individual must be reasonably able to maintain his/her balance at all times.

Trips: Falls on the Same Level

A trip is defined as a loss of balance due to the foot (or leg) contacting an object or obstruction. On occasion, too much friction between the foot or footwear and the walking surface also can cause a trip.

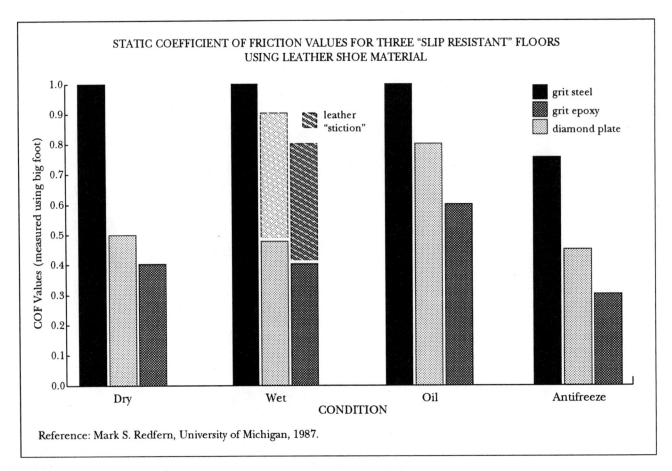

FIGURE 3.1
Grit surfaces have been shown to perform better than those of diamond plate.

Poor or inadequate housekeeping, such as blocked aisles, exposed cords and uneven rugs, are a few of the conditions that often produce trips. A poor physical layout can promote dangerous shortcuts. The emotional state of the individual also is a factor in trips; primary causes include inattentiveness and physical and mental health impairments.

A start towards quantifying the problem, which has been proposed by Robert O. Andres[1] and others, is the requirement for a static coefficient of friction of about 0.5 for the shoe/surface interaction for walking, but not carrying.

Stair Falls: Falls on One or More Levels

☞ In 1979, the National Bureau of Standards reported that in the USA 3,800 people died and more than 5,000,000 were severely injured within a single year from stairway falls.[2] A loss of balance can occur from a slip or trip while an individual is traveling up or down a stairway. The vast majority of falls on stairs occur when someone is moving downwards and not holding the handrail.[3] The additional danger of a stair–fall is that the victim can continue to move or "fall" down the remainder of the flight, potentially causing a multitude of injuries.

The significant factors that may contribute to a stair–fall could include:

1. *Stair Surface:* design, installation, composition and condition, stair width, riser height of 5 in. to 7 in. (J.A. Templer), tread width, illumination, visibility, and availability and use of a suitable handrail, ideally 1 1/2–in. diameter (J.L. Pauls), which may or may not be gripped.
2. *Stair Handrails:* The ideal shape of stair handrails for most hand sizes is round, 1 1/2 in. diameter (J.L. Pauls). Other shapes may also be firmly graspable. However, other shapes may only provide a pinch grip and are therefore unsuitable for maintaining balance. Figure 3.2 (NFPA sketch) illustrates several ideal as well as unsuitable handrails. Ideal stair handrail usage permits the hand to curl all around the rail and run smoothly down its entire length without needing to adjust the grip for any period. Stair users should be trained to use the "tennis racket" grip on stair handrails at all times whenever possible.
3. *Individual:* physical make–up or disabilities, locomotion or gait, speed or descent/ascent, age, physical and mental heath, emotional state, proper use, agility and physical location. For example, heavier individuals can suffer a severe disability if an ankle is turned while descending just one step.
4. *Work Task:* carrying of or reaching for objects, as well as type of clothing being worn and the individual's physical mobility. Carrying objects using both hands should be strongly discouraged so that handrails can be used. Use of elevators should be promoted whenever possible.
5. *Illumination on Stairs:* Lighting levels on stairs are important to the climber's concentration on personal stability, especially because so few people hold a graspable handrail.

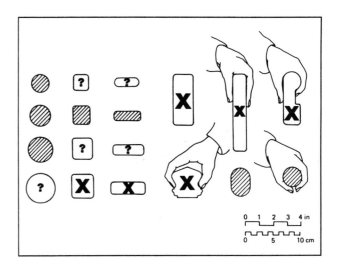

FIGURE 3.2
Acceptable (shaded), unacceptable (X) and marginal (?) handrail cross sections are illustrated in Figure 5-34 of NFPA 101 *Life Safety Code Handbook,* 1991, National Fire Protection Agency.

NFPA 101[4] gives lighting levels for stairs used under emergency conditions. A minimum of one foot candle is generally required. J.L. Pauls[5] has addressed illumination, color and pattern contrast on leading edges.

William English[6] addresses stair design, and especially for short flights advocates highly visible handrails by way of color or contrast. He emphasizes that step nosings with illuminated strips embedded in their top surface for dim environments; a spot light above the top landing; and spots illuminating the steps from just below the handrails can be important visual cues. The author believes these are also valuable criteria for longer flights and in industrial environments.

J.A. Templer[7] reported 12.3 inches as the ideal tread depth for the fewest mis-steps, and a 4.6–in. to 7.3–in. rise and additional 33 degrees pitch for ideal energy savings in human effort for stair climbing. (See Figures 3.3.a and 3.3.b for recommended stair dimensions.)

The handbook published by the Society of

Illuminating Engineers[8] is a useful resource beyond code requirements[9]. Another reference resource is *Slip and Fall Practice*.[9] And *The Slip and Fall Handbook, Volume 2*[10] gives a summary of current code wording on illumination and cautions that attorneys look first at illumination deficiency in many slip–fall cases.

A step or sudden change in floor level of one or two inches up to a foot or more, that is not guarded or clearly identified, can lead to many foreseeable falls and should especially be avoided in high-traffic areas or around equipment where operator traffic is high. Color contrast at a leading edge can help promote high visual awareness, provided added illumination is maintained.

More on Slips and Trips

Motor oil, water, snow, ice and spills need to be frequently and rapidly removed from floors, doorways, entrances, walkways, and other areas where employees or the public will travel. Floor mats can ripple and slide if they are not heavy duty or recessed. Grooving and gritting can help with wet or slippery steps, and grating helps in other cases.

Spills or slow drip leaks can be controlled with absorbent materials (such as pillows and socks), dikes, and loose materials. This type of spill control is only effective when immediate clean-up is intended for floor areas and the source of the spill is controlled.

Robert Pater[11] brings the experience of martial arts to industrial slip and trip training with his safe falling practices teaching seminar, and with his advice on how to walk more safely on slick surfaces. "Walk like Groucho!" says Pater when dealing with icy surfaces.

Escalators should be considered for replacing high-traffic stairs and elevators should be considered for multiple floor access to reduce fall exposure on stairs.

Slips/Trips and Fall Signage

Administrative controls often are needed when sudden slip, trip and fall hazards occur and before they can be eliminated or controlled. Signs warning of these hazards can be very helpful if used sparingly and on a very temporary basis.

On the other hand, signs placed next to fixed ladders, scaffold access points, and on suspended scaffolds can provide a continuous warning to workers to use fall protection provided, at least until it becomes second nature.

Pictorials have been standardized by ANSI Z535.3–1991 for slip, trip and fall warnings, and are shown in Figure 3.4.

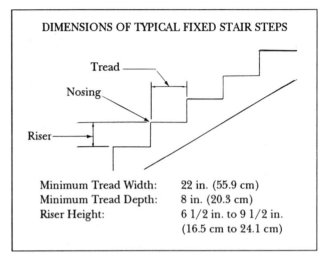

FIGURE 3.3A

From the *Federal Register*, Vol. 55, No. 69, Tuesday, April 10, 1990, Proposed Rules.

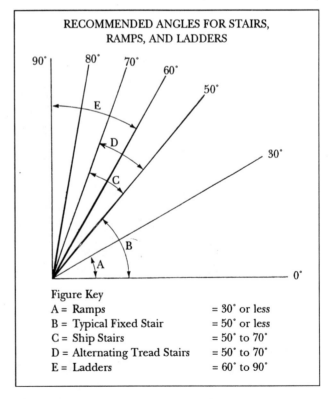

FIGURE 3.3B

From the *Federal Register*, Vol. 55, No. 69, Tuesday, April 10, 1990, Proposed Rules.

WHAT ARE THE PRINCIPLES OF FALL PROTECTION?

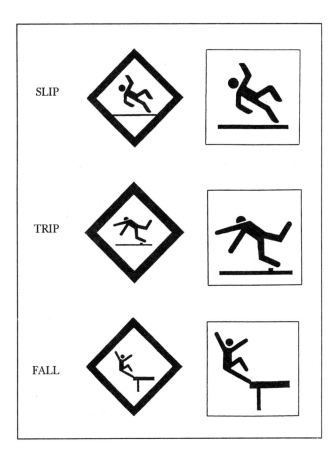

FIGURE 3.4
Warning pictorials for slips, trips and falls have been standardized by ANSI in its Standard Z535.3-1991.

Elevated Falls: Falls from One Level to Another

A momentary loss of balance resulting from a slip or trip can often lead to an elevated fall. Grabbing on to something to catch oneself after balance is accidentally lost is rare. For this reason, a hand-rail, or worse, a hand-line, cannot be an acceptable substitute for guardrails[12] on either side of a leading edge, including mid-rail.

Unlike many workplace hazards, few, if any, "near-miss" incidents help people learn to appreciate the seriousness of elevated falls.

"Close calls" or "near misses" that do not result in an incident – such as an automobile cutting in front of you on the drive home, a slight slip on a wet floor, or a trip on a stair – can serve to increase awareness which, in turn, generally leads to greater caution. However, once a person loses his or her balance and falls from elevation, whether it is 10 ft. or 200 ft., serious or fatal injury usually results. In fact, the worst elevated fall hazards are from potential sudden collapse and from potential walking into holes left after temporarily-placed covers have been lifted.

In 1989, NIOSH issued a Hazard Alert to industry concerning the severe hazard resulting from roof and floor openings, such as skylights or air conditioning duct holes. All holes and floor or roof openings must be either guarded or covered securely. Covers must support the intended loads and be securely attached. They must be clearly labeled, warning OPENING: DO NOT REMOVE. Concrete slabs should have holes covered before shipment.

A Note on Ladders

Use of ladders was the number-one cause of injurious falls in 1992, according to an OSHA Training Institute study of OSHA investigations.

Ladders are designed as a means of access only, provided three-point contact is used and maintained by the climber at all times. The shorter the distance of ladder climb, the safer the access should be for limited use by workers. Unless secured, these climbing devices can upset or slip if they are not used according to manufacturers' instructions. The fall risk is greatly increased if work is done from the ladder. Raised hand-rails and steps for secured ladders increase safety for access and permit consideration of fall arrest equipment use. Guidance for portable ladder manufacturers and users is found in the ANSI A14 Ladder Standards. Further discussion of ladders is found in Chapter 9.

Elevating personnel platforms or buckets and positioning portable stair towers on reasonably flat and stable ground further reduce risk and allow work to be conducted if over-reaching is not a reasonable foreseeability. However, if the possibility exists for climbing on the mid-rails of, for example, aerial lifts, and stretching outside the protection of the railing or barrier, then fall protection must be considered in addition to training workers in how to use access equipment properly or in the use of other equipment such as scaffolds. (Refer to Chapter 6 for discussion of permanent access means.)

Elements of a Fall Hazard

If we consider that a hazard is the potential to incur harm, what is it about falling that makes it so dangerous? Many wags are quick to point out that "it's not the fall that hurts you, it's the sudden stop!" That sudden stop at the end, or lack of adequate shock absorption at impact, is one of the three main elements of a fall hazard. Other clues are "The tallest tree has the greatest fall" and "The heavier they are, the harder they fall!"

Here is what makes falling so hazardous:

Elements of a Fall Hazard
1. Free–fall Distance
2. Shock Absorption at Impact
3. Body Weight

1. Free–fall Distance. As was pointed out earlier, if falls on the same level can produce injury, certainly each foot above the working level increases that likelihood geometrically. Therefore, the free–fall distance becomes a critical element of the hazard. Free–fall distance refers to the uncontrolled length of travel before the person either reaches grade level or his fall arrest equipment is activated. Free fall is most easily measured from foot level before the fall to foot level after the fall; this is OSHA's measurement and the easiest to use for planning. A 6–ft. lanyard, for instance, attached at foot level or below could result in free falling 12 ft. before the equipment is activated. Since free falling is a transfer from potential to kinetic energy, the longer the free–fall distance, the higher the forces generated on impact.

OSHA measures free falls as unrestricted free falls. Thus a fall from a church steeple may not count as a fall, except from the eave of the roof. Free–fall distance can be argued to be measured from foot level, waist level, shoulder level, or head level, but for strict planning purposes, it always should represent the worst case... and the worst case is usually when the head receives an injury.

It should be noted that head injuries occur in approximately 10% of free falls. When illumination is decreased, such as at dusk or when a worker is coming out of bright sunlight and into a darker area, head injuries dramatically increase for same–level or lesser–level falls.

The Chaffing Report to OSHA of March 1978 recommends physical barriers and protection beyond 4 ft. of free fall, because this distance in a backward fall is worst case and when the head is subject to maximum impact with a lower object below foot level.

Deceleration distance using equipment and fall distance differ from free–fall distance, as clarified in Figure 3.5.

How far should a worker fall? The free–fall and total fall distance should be limited to the point that injury can be avoided from:

- high arresting forces
- collision with an obstruction or grade level
- pendulum–like swing falls and subsequent collision
- no capacity of swift post–fall self–recovery

Limiting the free–fall distance to less than 2 ft. is the most effective way to avoid the above–mentioned consequences.

2. Shock Absorption at Impact. Shock absorption can vary considerably. A World War II pilot that was able to walk away from a parachute failure, having landed in a snowbank, is quite a different situation from a fall onto cement or gravel at a plant site. Shock absorption between different types of personal fall arrest equipment also can vary considerably. (See Figure 3.6.) For example, falling to the end of a 6–ft. rope lanyard while wearing a body belt is likely to produce injuries, whereas a shock–absorbing lanyard and full–body harness combination not only can substantially reduce the probability of a compounding injury but also can permit users to experience an actual fall arrest in a live training session.

3. Body Weight. The third element that makes falling so hazardous is the weight of the worker. This is of particular concern at heights for those workers who weigh in at more than 300 pounds. The concern stems primarily from the need to support the body properly during a fall arrest. Overweight users tend to have larger stomachs and waist lines that "disappear," which makes adjusting a body belt properly between the pelvic girdle and rib cage extremely difficult if not impossible. Most of these users tend to push the body belt down around the hips, which causes them to be

Fall Arrest Term	Definition
Free-fall Distance	The distance of the fall from the point of the attachment to the activation of the equipment, e.g., a 6-ft. lanyard at waist level, can result in a 6-ft. fall.
Deceleration Distance	The equipment from the activation of the equipment to a complete stop – slowing down or breaking to a stop – e.g., one type of shock absorbing lanyard may tear open 12 in. to absorb the energy of a fall depending on the free-fall distance and bodyweight.
Total Fall Distance	The combination of the two above, plus any other condition, such as a sliding D-ring on a harness or the reversible elongated stretch of a rope.

FIGURE 3.5

The difference between deceleration and free-fall distances.

WHAT ARE THE PRINCIPLES OF FALL PROTECTION? 39

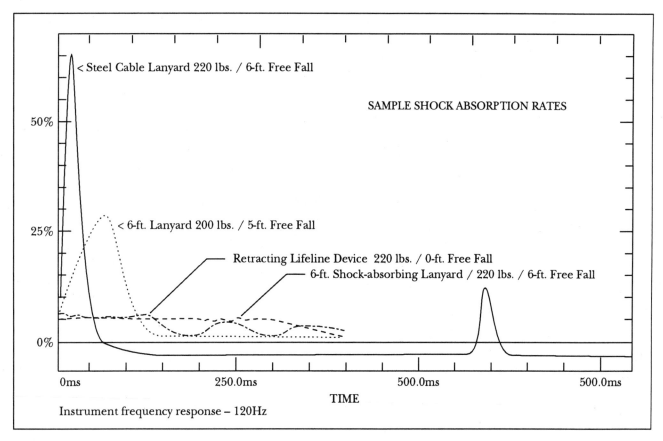

FIGURE 3.6
Courtesy of RTC, Wilmington, DE.

"top-heavy." Catastrophic fall-out thus can be the result if belts are used. Same-level and stair falls also are usually much more severe and disabling for heavier persons. Post-fall suspension in belts, including harnesses with belts, is much more distressing for heavier persons.

Prevention or Fall Arrest as a Means of Fall Protection?

When exposure to a fall hazard cannot be practically prevented during access to a work task, or at a work task, through such measures as floors, walls, aerial lifts, bucket trucks, guardrails, perimeter cables, crane-suspended work platform (manbasket), scaffolds, or planking, then personal fall arrest equipment can be selected to control a fall or provide a reliable means of escape.

In general, personal protective equipment is designed as a backup safety system for an individual during a work task. In the event of an emergency, the equipment should function automatically to help protect the worker from harm. A personal fall protection system should, therefore, provide continuous and complete protection without interfering with required work task mobility. Many ask whether this can be done on an economical or practical basis. Properly used equipment can often provide the most protection for the least cost.

Safety nets are an option if fall arrest equipment has not been shown to be practical. OSHA calls for nets where the potential fall distance exceeds two stories, or 25 ft., in multi-tiered building construction.

Setting Fall Arrest Equipment Objectives

☞ Fall hazard control begins by setting specific objectives based on the elements of a fall hazard (see Figure 3.7). To control the energy generated through a fall, the free-fall distance should not exceed 2 ft. Additionally, reducing the total fall distance (free-fall plus deceleration distance) can help decrease the possibility of striking an obstruction within the fall path.

Where free falling cannot practically be held below 2 ft., adequate shock absorption and proper body support become more critical, along with rapid rescue techniques.

For shock absorption at impact, the objective should be to limit the potential forces on the body during an arrest. OSHA limits forces on the belt to 900 lbs. This force level is significantly lower than the potential forces with belt and lanyard or with lifeline combinations presently used in many industries. For example, a fall arrest with a steel cable lanyard following a 6–ft. free fall can result in forces exceeding 10 times body weight. This might mean a worker weighing 200 lbs. could experience more than 2000 lbs. of dynamic force. Automobile lap belt studies have concluded severe or fatal injury occurs close to or at this threshold level. Studies on anesthetized dogs in 1952 in a project produced by the American Society of Safety Engineers (ASSE) documented the nature of internal injuries reported from fall arrests in straps, and showed heart damage could be severe if force exceeded 2000 lbs.[13]

Maintaining average arresting forces around 650 lbs. not only keeps the potential for compounding injuries to a minimum: It also allows people to train with fall arrest equipment. This critical first–hand experience can help promote confidence and enable users to develop an understanding of the capabilities and limitations of various systems. Knowing the capabilities and limitations of available equipment is essential to thinking out which equipment fits in with the work method.

☞ As opposed to a narrow body belt around the soft, vulnerable mid–section, a full body harness is designed to distribute arresting forces primarily over the buttocks and to some extent over the thighs, chest and shoulders. It can provide proper body support during an arrest as well as during suspension after a fall. A harness also helps eliminate the excessive whipping of the neck associated with long free–fall arrests in a body belt.

For heavier or overweight workers, the body belt is difficult, if not impossible, to fit properly between the pelvic crest and rib cage. An improper or loose fit may result in the worker falling out of the belt as his or her center of gravity (heavier upper body) tips forward during an arrest or suspension. Also, breathing will be very difficult as the belt constricts the diaphragm, which could result in suspension of breathing (winding) during the fall arrest or asphyxiation while awaiting rescue. Finally, for retrieval from a confined space, the upright suspension of a harness – particularly one with a shock–absorbing, sliding back D–ring – can allow the victim to be raised up directly through the opening.

Elements of a Fall Hazard	Equipment Control Objectives
1. Free-fall Distance	1. Minimize to less than 2 ft.
2. Shock Absorbtion	2. Aim for 650 lbs. or lower average force
3. Body Weight	3. Support properly with a full-body harness

FIGURE 3.7

The Personal Fall Arrest Equipment Triangle

Once the equipment control objectives have been established, how are the pieces put together to provide continuous and complete personal protection?

The three basic components – The ABC's of Fall Protection – of a fall arrest system are easily illustrated through a conceptual triangle. As illustrated in Figure 3.8, this Personal Fall Arrest Equipment Triangle consists of an Anchorage, Body Support, and the Connecting Means. Here's a closer look at each of these basic components.

Anchorage

This first component of the triangle makes fall protection equipment unique among most other forms of personal protective equipment. Unlike hard hats, glasses or safety shoes that are issued to the workers and

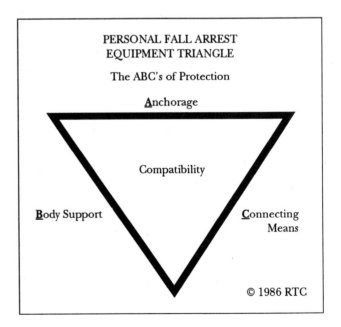

FIGURE 3.8

WHAT ARE THE PRINCIPLES OF FALL PROTECTION?

allow them to walk away "protected," fall arrest equipment must be attached to something. And that something is a part of your plant, building or structure. Therefore, the anchorage point must be carefully planned into the job in order to provide continuous and complete protection during the work task, including travel to and from the elevated workstation. Skyhooks should not be mythical; they should be real.

Considerations in the selection of an anchor point should minimally include:

1. **An independence of the work surface whenever possible.** For example, instead of tying off to the back rail of a two–point swing–scaffold, attach a separate lifeline to a suitable independent anchor point on the structure overhead. Then, should a support cable fail, thereby causing the swing scaffold to drop down, the worker would not be pulled down in a potentially lethal swing fall with subsequent injurious collisions.

    In those situations in which it is necessary to attach to part of the work surface, first consider using the structural location that is not likely to fail catastrophically. If this part is still arguably a hazard because it appears flimsy, an independent means of anchorage must be designed. Situations such as 1) tripods over manholes, 2) four–point suspended scaffolds, and 3) work platforms and certain building structures may provide suitable anchorage points for both load lines and fall protection. If you have no access to an engineer, always consider a worst–case scenario to help you make a reasonable judgement for adequacy in the field.

2. **Anchor points that can be identified for workers by a qualified person and are clearly marked.** Paint all approved locations and configurations a bright orange or yellow so workers know exactly where to hook up their equipment. The members of a roof truss, for example, should be calculated and tested for ultimate strength and modeled. The same applies to railing, tower struts, and overhead pipes. If the general rule is that "nearly all" markers may be used as an anchorage, then labels or signs or markings should indicate what is not to be used, and why.

3. **A waist–height minimum attachment for belt–lanyard combination, shoulder–level for a harness–lanyard combination, and overhead for devices.** For a belt and 6–ft. lanyard, a waist–height minimum attachment helps to ensure that the worker does not free fall farther than 6 ft., thus staying in compliance with most OSHA regulations, unless a lower free–fall distance is mandated. Remember that shock–absorbing lanyards will be needed to meet the OSHA force limit of 900 lbs., and that only harnesses are recognized by the ANSI Z359.1 industry fall arrest systems standard. For devices, however, it is essential to ensure installation overhead to eliminate dangerous lifeline slack that might contribute to excessive free fall and higher force levels.

    In all three cases cited here, the objective is to keep the free–fall distance to a minimum.

    Equipment manufacturers need to engineer anchorage points to meet these criteria. Anchorage points at waist level or below may be easier to engineer, but they are probably not going to be adequate except for restraint. This means designing a system to prevent reaching the fall hazard. One example is a calf–height horizontal lifeline, installed parallel to and 6 ft. back from the leading edge of a new deck, along which railings are being erected, and where all leading edge work is done in the kneeling position. In this case, a belt and 6–ft. lanyard may provide adequate restraint, yet allow sufficient mobility. For an aerial lift or scissor lift, a floor–mounted anchorage point may not provide the required mobility without excessive potential free fall. For proper documentation, an engineering drawing showing and stating requirements is necessary. Therefore, in this case, the anchorage point must be higher.

4. **Sufficient strength based on federal or local requirements and manufacturer's guidelines.** The needed anchor strength for a fall arrest system depends on the potential forces on that point along with an acceptable safety factor. In some

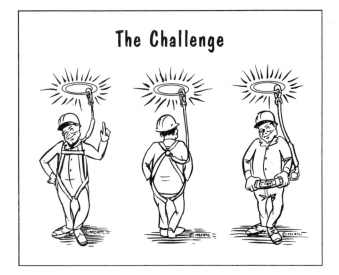

FIGURE 3.9
How to meet the fall protection challenge.

cases, required strengths can be reduced to increase consideration of other potential anchor points; careful collaboration with the manufacturer on each specific system is imperative. The recent OSHA 1910.66 Appendix C regulation (see Appendix A-6) allows anchorage point strength based on twice the anticipated dynamic load (maximum arrest force) for engineered systems.

5. **Horizontal lines for lateral protected mobility.** To move laterally away from a fixed anchorage point and to fall can produce a dangerous pendulum-like swing fall. The danger of such a fall results from the force levels being generated through the swing being the same as those generated by a fall through the same distance vertically, but with the additional hazard of striking an obstruction. Horizontal lifelines are designed to enable the device or attachment point to remain overhead so that a fall arrest occurs within a vertical plane. For further detail on swing-fall hazards, refer to Chapter 7. And for an engineering treatment of horizontal lifelines, see Appendix A-3.

6. **Minimum clearance requirements established above grade or any obstruction.** Each fall arrest system involves different total fall distances. For instance, a 600-ft. section of rope lifeline will have a considerable elongation stretch factor; this must be accounted for within the minimum clearance requirements in addition to the free fall and deceleration distances.

   Figures 3.10, 3.11 and 3.12 illustrate several different fall arrest situations and how to calculate their personal fall arrest system requirements.

7. **Self-recovery that is possible within a few seconds.** A worker experiencing a fall arrest should be able to recover his or her position quickly enough to relieve any stress on the body that might be caused by post-fall suspension. This is of greatest concern with a body belt.

Body Support

This is the second component of the Personal Fall Arrest Equipment Protection Triangle (page 40).

For almost all applications, the full body harness is preferable over the body belt because of its ability to spread arresting forces primarily under the buttocks, as opposed to concentrating them to the soft, vulnerable mid-section. Prolonged suspension in an upright manner without restriction of breathing is also possible with a full body harness. And, of particular importance, the full body harness with a sliding back D-ring helps to avoid excessive whipping of the neck during an arrest.

Harness Selection. Not all harnesses are alike, therefore, several critical design factors should be considered:
a. **An absence of an integral waist belt.** An unneeded belt around the mid-section (diaphragm) could

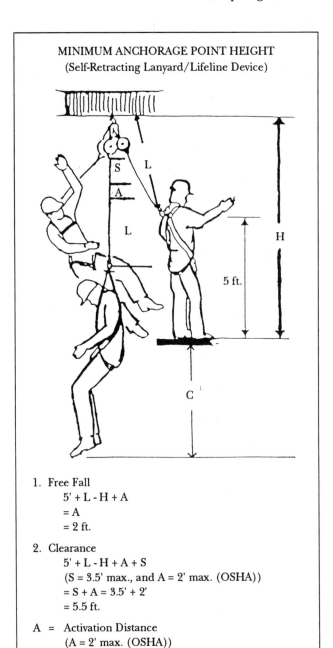

MINIMUM ANCHORAGE POINT HEIGHT
(Self-Retracting Lanyard/Lifeline Device)

1. Free Fall
   5' + L - H + A
   = A
   = 2 ft.

2. Clearance
   5' + L - H + A + S
   (S = 3.5' max., and A = 2' max. (OSHA))
   = S + A = 3.5' + 2'
   = 5.5 ft.

A = Activation Distance
    (A = 2' max. (OSHA))
C = Clearance
S = Deceleration Distance

Note:
H = 5' + L   for harness users
H = 3.5' + L   for belt users

FIGURE 3.10
© 1992 Dynamic Scientific Controls

WHAT ARE THE PRINCIPLES OF FALL PROTECTION?

interfere with proper breathing during suspension. When required for performing the work task, tool belts or climbing/restraint belts can be worn over top of a light-weight harness.

b. **A seat strap that can distribute arresting forces more suitably over the buttocks.** This extra strap can be adjusted to fit under the seat and serves to comfortably cradle the individual both during and after a fall arrest without cutting circulation.

c. **A sliding back D-ring.** This serves to provide additional shock absorption and to position the body in a proper, upright manner for suspension and retrieval through narrow openings. Additionally, it enables the harness to be adjusted for a comfort-

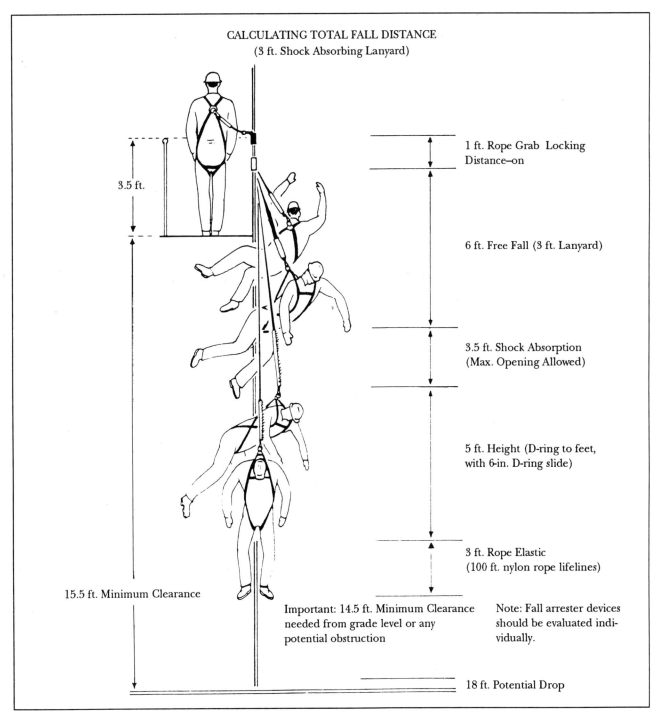

FIGURE 3.11
©1992 Dynamic Scientific Controls

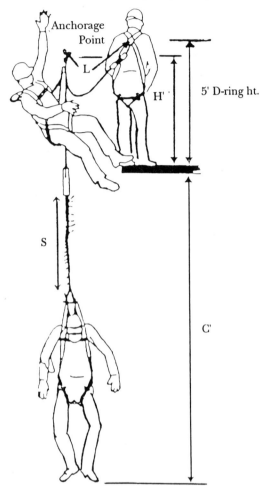

FIGURE 3.12

MINIMUM ANCHORAGE POINT HEIGHT
(Shock-absorbing Lanyard)

1. Free Fall
   $5' + L - H$
   $= 6'$ max. (OSHA)
   So, if $L = 6'$
   Then $H = 5'$ (min. anchor height)
2. Clearance
   $5' + L - H + S$
   ($S = 3.5'$ max., and $A = 2'$ max. (OSHA))
   So, if $H = 5'$
   $S = 3.5'$ max. (OSHA)
   $L = 6'$
   $= 9.5'$ Minimum Clearance

C = Clearance
H = Anchor Point Height
L = Distance Between Anchorage Point and D-ring
S = Deceleration Distance
5' = Harness D-Ring Height

Note for Belt Users:
Free Fall = $3.5' + L - H$
Clearance = $3.5' + L - H + S$

---

able, proper fit with the D-ring centered between the shoulder blades. However, the D-ring should not be able to migrate lower on the back, which can permit shoulder straps to fall off the shoulder when stooping.

d. **Color coding of the top and bottom straps.** Coding helps to make the harness quicker and easier to put on.
e. **Lightweight and soft webbing material.** This makes for comfortable, all-day wear if necessary.

Belt Selection. One fall arrest application for a body belt would be for climbing fixed ladders with climbing protection systems. Here a front D-ring is required to permit the device to quickly sense a free fall and begin fall arrest. Body belts should have the widest body pad possible, perhaps up to 6 in., to provide the greatest comfort and support possible. For example, brief suspension in a 4-in. belt is slightly less painful than in a 2-in. belt. This difference is magnified for persons over 200 lbs. Many safety directors will be choosing harnesses for all fall arrest applications and relegating belts to work positioning.

Selection of the Appropriate Body Support. Proper selection of body support is determined by its anticipated use in conjunction with the work task, namely a fall arrest system. The American National Standards Institute, in its A10.14-1975 Standard (since replaced by ANSI Z10.14-1991), classified body support mechanisms into four major categories according to use:[14]

Class I: Body Belts (work belts), used to retain a worker in a hazardous work position and to reduce the probability of falls.
Class II: Chest Harnesses, used where there are only limited fall hazards (no vertical free fall hazard) and for retrieval purposes, such as removal of a worker from a tank or bin.
Class III: Body Harnesses, used to arrest the most severe free falls.
Class IV: Suspension Belts, independent work supports used to suspend or support the worker.

However, just because body support mechanisms are broken down into four separate categories does not mean that the use of a single belt or harness constitutes a complete personal fall arrest system. When any piece of safety equipment is used to complete part of a work task, it becomes a tool and is, therefore, no longer backup personal protection – for example, leaning out, against a lanyard attached to the structure, to read a valve. Moreover, upon closer inspection of the ANSI categories, it is apparent that Class III Body Harnesses are the only type indicated for vertical free-fall arrest.

When does a body support become a tool? First, let's take a closer look at how specific body support mechanisms are designed for use. Figure 3.13 defines the five

WHAT ARE THE PRINCIPLES OF FALL PROTECTION?

main functions of body support and which mechanisms best achieve them.

Body support mechanisms are equipped with D–rings or O–rings for the attachment of a connecting means, that is, a lanyard or other device. The location of these attachment points is designed to meet the anticipated use of the body support. Specifically, body belts and full body harnesses with a front D–ring (10 o'clock in Figure 3.13) are designed for climbing with fixed climbing protection systems. The close orientation between the front D–ring and the rail or cable climbing system is essential in enabling the device to quickly sense and arrest a free fall. A saddle belt with two front O–rings also is used for climbing fixed ladders on oil derricks and rigs. The subpelvic strap of the saddle belt supports the body as the counterweight system lifts the body weight like a personal elevator.

Full body harnesses with a back D–ring (6 o'clock) are intended for free fall arrest. Six o'clock is the most suitable location for supporting the body during the arrest to minimize compounding injuries. Additionally, it keeps the attachment of the connecting means behind the worker so as not to interfere with the work task. If prolonged post–fall suspension is probable, a full body harness will keep the victim upright and more comfortable, and will aid in retrieval.

Supporting the body in an upright manner for retrieval from a confined space is achieved through attachment to a back D–ring on a full body or chest harness. If the use of breathing apparatus conflicts with

THE BODY SUPPORT PENTAGON

FALL ARREST
- Full Body Harness with Back D–ring (6 o'clock).
- Fall Arrester Required

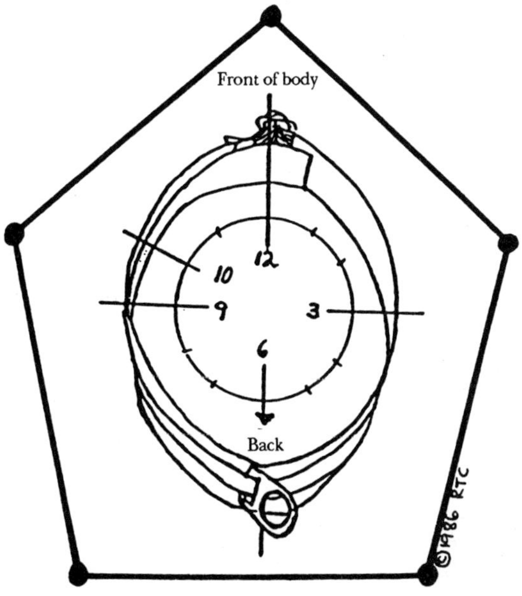

CLIMBING PROTECTION
- Body Belt or Full Body Harness with Front D–ring (10 o'clock or 12 o'clock, depending upon center or side mount).
- Saddle Belt with Front O–rings.
- Carrier rail or cable required.

RETRIEVAL
- Full Body Harness with Back D–ring (6 o'clock) or Two Shoulder Rings.
- Wristlets (truly a last resort!).
- Winch required.

(WORK) POSITIONING
- Saddle Belt with Front O–rings (12 o'clock).
- Lineman belt (3 o'clock and 9 o'clock D–rings).
- Boatswain's Chair.
- Tree Trimmer Belt.
- Full Body Harness with Work Positioning Belt.
- Strap with adjustable lanyard, or rebar chain and hook, required.

RESTRAINT
- Body Belt or Full Body Harness with Side D–rings (3 o'clock and 9 o'clock).
- Limited–length lifelines required.

© 1986 RTC

FIGURE 3.13
Five protection tasks are addressed by the Body Support Pentagon concept.

attachment to the back D–ring, a spreader bar yoke and two shoulder D–rings can be substituted for easy vertical retrieval.

Wristlets are a last resort. Not only do they usually mean hazardous exposure to the rescuer who must go down in the space to hook up the victim, but also they can cause physical damage to the shoulders and arms of the unconscious victim. If it is necessary to lift the victim's arms over his or her head in order to fit the victim through the opening, a full body harness should be used to lift the body weight, leaving the wristlets to simply hold up the arms. As a rule, if a worker is exposed to a free fall hazard when entering a confined space, fall protection should be worn. This can eliminate the need for the rescuer(s) to enter the space for hook–up and thereby subject themselves to the same harmful conditions, increasing the risk of multiple fatalities.

Finally, positioning refers to work positioning access and, in some cases, to emergency escape support. The two front O–rings of a saddle belt in conjunction with the subpelvic strap are designed to cradle and maintain the body in a comfortable sitting position. A tree trimmer belt is a good example of such body support for work positioning. Similarly, the body is comfortably supported during an emergency descent from an elevated workstation.

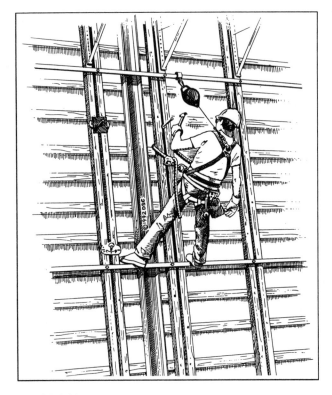

FIGURE 3.14
This form worker is wearing both work positioning equipment and personal fall arrest body support.

Should Backup Fall Protection Be Used?

Use of Body Support	Free Fall Hazard Exposure?	Fall Arrest Equipment Required
Restraint	Should Not Be	If practical
Suspension (escape)	Yes	No (except for training)
Retrieval Only	Yes	No (except for training)
Positioning	Yes	Yes

FIGURE 3.15

☞ Restraint involves using the body support to lean against while performing an elevated work task. Fall arrest is designed to "catch" a person once he or she falls, whereas restraint systems are designed to keep the free fall from occurring in the first place. A lineman's pole strap and belt with side D–rings (3 o'clock and 9 o'clock in Figure 3.13) are a form of work positioning. In such cases, a body support becomes work positioning when it is used for leaning and the worker is off–balance. In such cases, additional fall protection is required. For example, see Figure 3.14. This worker, wearing a saddle belt while being lowered down the side of a tank via a cable winch so that he can paint, is using a work–positioning system. If the winch mechanism connections or cable fail, does the worker have a backup fall arrest safety system?

A separate fall arrest system consisting of a full body harness with a back D–ring and an independent lifeline could provide the needed protection. The chart in Figure 3.15 provides some guidelines for considering when backup fall protection or equipment is imperative.

Connecting Means

This is the third component of the Personal Fall Arrest Equipment Triangle forming the ABC's of Fall Protection, shown on page 40.

Whether to use a device or a lanyard as the connecting means is often dictated by the nature of the work. The choice is the key to controlling the fall hazard.

Connecting means are roughly broken down into climbing protection and emergency escape systems, of which there are only a few, as well as vertical lifelines, horizontal lifelines, and emergency retrieval systems, of which there are numerous alternatives. (Chapter 7 provides greater detail on these types of systems.)

To provide complete and continuous protection, the connecting means should:

1. **Keep the free–fall distance to a minimum, preferably to 2 ft. or less.** The idea is to choose the

WHAT ARE THE PRINCIPLES OF FALL PROTECTION?

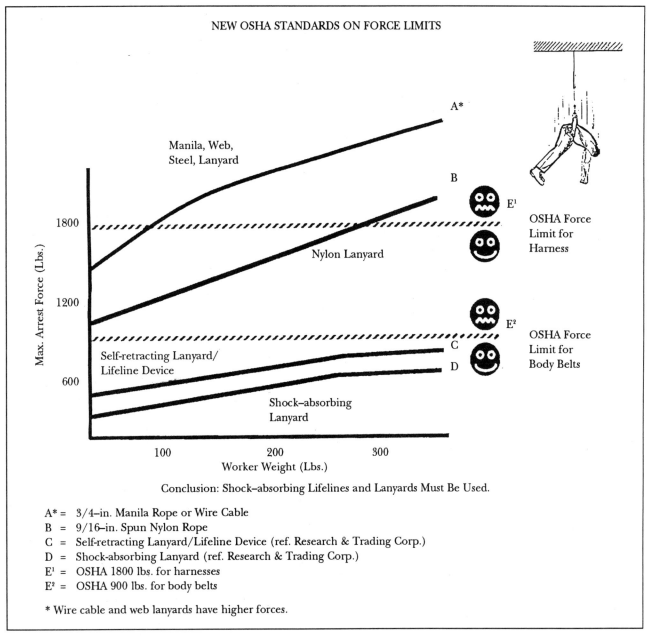

FIGURE 3.16
Arrest force limits must be maintained to new OSHA standards.

method that can provide the least possibility of injury should a fall occur.

2. **Maintain arresting forces at an average of below 650 lbs.** to minimize compounding injuries and to enable first-hand live training.

See Figure 3.16 on force limits set by new OSHA Standards.

3. **Not create prolonged suspension after a fall arrest when an automatic, controlled descent system is feasible for use.** Rather than using equipment that arrests a fall but also could create the need for a difficult and costly high-level rescue, workers should use a lifeline system that automatically lowers them at a constant rate following a fall. This is especially advantageous for external applications without obstructions below and for large confined spaces with a lower (bottom) means of egress such as a generating or recovery boiler. Post-fall analysis is essential to solving such problems completely and often indicates the need for substitution with controlled descent systems.

4. **Eliminate creation of dangerous pendulum-like swing falls that can result from a worker's falling after moving away from directly under a fixed**

anchor point. Horizontal lifelines used in conjunction with the connecting means – a device or lanyard depending on required vertical travel – can provide continuous protected mobility.

5. **Allow ease of retrieval after a fall.** For instance, in confined space entry, attaching a lifeline to the worker before he or she enters eliminates the need for a rescuer to go down to hook the victim up.

6. **Make possible continuous and complete protection.** The device or lanyard, used individually or in combination with other appropriate systems, should permit needed mobility to complete the work task effectively, but with protection.

☞ Reference back to the Personal Fall Arrest Equipment Triangle, shown in Figure 3.8 on page 40, shows that compatibility is the one thing that binds together the three components. The anchorage, body support and connecting means must be compatible with one another in order to create a fall safety system with maximum effectiveness and continuous protection.

Personal Lifelines (Backup) vs. Positioning Lines (Primary)

Similar to body–support mechanisms, when a fall arrest lifeline is used for positioning at a work station(s), that lanyard or device becomes a work tool. For instance, if a worker locks a self-retracting lanyard/lifeline device and leans out against the line, that worker has forfeited his or her backup protection. If a situation such as form work calls for a work tool, then a second, separate fall arrest system is required.

If a worker uses a primary positioning line and a backup lifeline, a second anchorage and body support are required. In principle, safety systems and work tools should be completely independent of one another. In some situations, however, this may not yet be practical. An exception might be when a portable tripod with adequate strength is used to anchor both lines because of the need to keep the lines directly overhead and centered in the opening. If harnesses are used to lower a worker through a narrow opening, the same D–ring may be used. Yet when a saddle belt or boatswain's chair is used, a separate full body harness is required because most saddle belts are worn loosely for comfort and the wearer may fall out if a fall occurs.

Manual vs. Automatic Equipment

☞ It is important to keep in mind that fall arrest equipment is safety equipment. And safety equipment is ideally designed for fail–safe backup, to reduce the possibility of injury in the event of an emergency. Requiring a worker to manually operate or manipulate a safety device during a panic situation introduces a significant potential for human error. Such error should be designed out. A fall arrest system is not mountaineering or fire rescue equipment, nor a restraint tool, nor for positioning. The latter require tremendous levels of skill that are only obtained through extensive amounts of initial and periodic training. Safety equipment that functions automatically can be more reliable for fall arrest and emergency escape. It's important to remember Alphonse Chapanis' admonition, "To err is human, to forgive, design!"[16] Keep fall arrest and work positioning separate.

Confined Space Retrieval Planning: Avoiding Multiple Fatalities

As was alluded to earlier, rescuing someone in a confined space introduces the additional danger of the rescuers being overcome and trapped as well, particularly if they are entering through a small upper opening. It is not uncommon for a number of would–be rescuers to go down before one realizes that there is a serious problem.

A person entering a confined area that involves exposure to a vertical free–fall hazard or that may contain toxic air or an insufficient oxygen supply should be hooked up to a lifeline. Should that person be overcome, a co–worker should be able to retrieve the victim without further need for hook–up. The retrieval mechanism should have a minimum mechanical advantage of 4:1, such as a manually operated winch, because of the great difficulty of lifting dead weight vertically through a small opening. A rope attached to the worker for the purpose of "hauling him out" in an emergency, regardless of the number of rescuers, is simply not efficient or reliable. At best, it indicates lack of planning.

Architects and engineers should be strongly encouraged to design or redesign manway openings with no less than a 24–in. diameter clearance to facilitate prompt emergency retrieval. Many workers would ask for a minimum of 36 in. An opening of 18 in. or less promises a much more delayed rescue time, which could prove to be the fatal factor.

Summary

☞ Although many of the principles discussed in this chapter may seem basic, the high number of injuries due to workplace slips, trips and falls indicates they are not sufficiently applied as common knowledge. Only when these principles are applied will industry hope to achieve 100 percent fall protection.

Notes

1. "An Ergonomic Analysis of Dynamic Coefficient of Friction Measurement Techniques," Andres, Robert O., Ph.D., with Keith Kreutzbert, M.S.E., and Eric M. Trier, B.S.E. (Center for Ergonomics, College of Engineering, The University of Michigan, Ann Arbor, January 1984).

2. "Guideline for Stair Safety," NBS Building Science Series 120, Archea, J., Collins, B., and Stahl, F. (National Bureau of Standards, Washington DC, 1979).

3. "Injuries Resulting From Falls on Stairs," Bulletin 2214 (US Department of Labor, Bureau of Labor Statistics, US Government Printing Office, Washington DC 20402, August 1984).

4. *NFPA 101 Life Safety Code Handbook* (National Fire Protection Agency, 1991).

5. Pauls, Jake L. National Research Council on Canada. Article in *Building Standards*, May–June, 1984, presented at National Safety Council, October 1985, New Orleans.

6. *Slips, Trips and Falls*, William English, CSP, P.E. (Hanrow Press, Del Mar, CA. 1989).

7. Templer, J.A. "Stair Shape and Human Movement". Doctoral dissertation, Columbia University, New York, 1974. Highlights included in an article co–authored with J.M. Fitch and P.Corcoran, "The Dimensions of Stairs". *Scientific American*, Oct. 1974, pp 82–90.

8. Handbook from the Society of Illuminating Engineers, 345 E. 47th St., New York NY.

9. *Slip and Fall Practice*, Turnbow, Charles E. (James Publishing Group, Santa Ana CA).

10. *The Slip and Fall Handbook*, Rosen, Stephen I. (Hanrow Press, Vol. 1, 1983; Volume 2, 1992; Supplement 1993).

11. "Don't Fall For It," Pater, Robert (*Nation's Business*, December 1985. Reference: FallSAFE, Inc., Portland OR).

12. "A Model Performance Standard For Guardrails," NBSIR 76–1131, Fattal, S.G., et. al. (US Depart-ment of Labor, OSHA, Washington DC, July 1976).

13. "Final Report on the ASSE Research Project: Safety Belts, Harnesses, and Accessories." Funded by the National Safety Council and produced by the American Society of Safety Engineers, Chicago IL, 1952.

14. ANSI A10.14–1975, "Requirements for Safety Belts, Harnesses, Lanyards, Lifelines and Droplines for Construction and Industrial Use" (American National Standards Institute, 1430 Broadway, New York NY 10018. Withdrawn December 31, 1987 and replaced by ANSI A10.14–1991).

15. "A Study of Personal Fall–Safety Equipment," NBSIR 76–1146, Steinberg, H.Z. (Product System Analysis Division, Institute for Applied Technology, National Bureau of Standards, Washington DC, June 1977).

16. "To Err Is Human, To Forgive, Design". Chapanis, Alphonse, Ph.D. (Speech given at the American Society of Safety Engineers Professional Development Conference, New Orleans, LA, June 1986).

Review Questions

1. What is a fall arrest system?
   a. A body belt and lanyard.
   b. An anchorage, fall arrest device and a body support.
   c. A lifeline, body belt and a lanyard.
   d. An anchorage and a fall arrest device.
   e. A harness and shock–absorbing lanyard.

2. What is deceleration distance as defined in OSHA Standard 1910.66 App. C?
   a. Distance from fall arrest equipment activation to a complete stop.
   b. Distance from foot level to a complete stop.
   c. Distance from D–ring position before the fall to where the fall arrest equipment is activated.
   d. Distance from D–ring position before the fall to a complete stop.
   e. Distance from equipment activation to momentary stop before rebound.

3. What anchorage point criteria are vital for successful use?
   a. Height, location.
   b. Location, size.
   c. Strength, height.
   d. Strength, location.
   e. Size, strength.

4. What is the proper use of a full body harness (single back D–ring)?
   a. Restraint.
   b. Climbing, fall arrest, retrieval.
   c. Leaning, retrieval.
   d. Positioning, fall arrest.
   e. Retrieval.

5. On what parts of the body should fall arresting forces be distributed?
   a. Waist, shoulders, thighs and buttocks.
   b. Chest, thighs.
   c. Waist, chest.
   d. Shoulders, thighs and buttocks.
   e. Chest, pelvis.

WHERE IS FALL PROTECTION NEEDED?

To say that a thing has never yet been done among men is to erect a barrier stronger than reason, stronger than discussion.

-THOMAS B. REED

❖ Are there fall hazards in every industry?

❖ Fall protection needs

❖ Can one fall protection system meet the needs of a work task?

❖ What does fall protection protect against?

❖ Fall protection by worker activity

❖ Risk: Should every fall hazard be controlled?

❖ A role for the unions

Are There Fall Hazards in Every Industry?

Nearly every industry at one time or another engages in work at elevation. It could be as simple as using a 10-ft. step ladder to change a light bulb, or operating a powered platform 185 feet up inside a generating boiler, or climbing 600 feet up a flare stack ladder. The short six-month BLS (1984) study of approximately 77 elevated fall injuries showed a variety of industries involved.[1]

Although injuries in the construction industry were predominant in this survey (41%), nearly one-fourth of the victims were employed by manufacturers. Forty-four percent of the injured workers were craftworkers, including carpenters (10 percent), and mechanics/repairers (6 percent). A large portion, 24 percent, were working as laborers, while 12 percent were employed as operators. Other victim occupations included clerical and sales workers, managers and transport equipment operators.

Certain industries, of course, require much more elevated work. For instance, frequent elevated work tasks associated with transmission and distribution operations in the utility industry are significantly different than operations within a microchip processing plant. For those industries with a lot of activity at elevation, the probability of a fall is consequently higher.

During Work. Elevated work tasks can be an integral part of a job or trade. Scalers, for example, whose job it is to remove built-up residue from tanks, digesters or vessels, are often exposed to fall hazards on an ongoing basis. Other examples, often associated with construction or maintenance, include roofing, painting, sandblasting, pipe welding, masonry or bricklaying, and utility service work. Steel connectors also commonly work at great elevation.

During Access. In other cases, exposure to a fall hazard occurs simply while the worker is accessing an elevated work station. A repair of a valve located in the upper tier of a chemical processing piperack may require that the worker use a fixed ladder 25 to 100 yards away, then walk the pipe to the valve. Some trades, such as scaffold builders, serve to provide a local means of access. However, fall protection for these workers during erection and dismantling should not be ignored. Temporary systems can be brought to the site and removed by the contract scaffold company. Alternatively, access/fall protection can be provided by the principal/owner and later used by other employees throughout the job.

Quite often, contractors are brought in to perform elevated work tasks. It could be a maintenance contract that requires the contractor to climb unprotected towers and stacks to change aviation warning lights, or a complete repair project involving a number of people.

It is not unusual to hear a company executive respond, "Oh, we don't send our people up there – we contract that out!" This means handling elevated work tasks at a particular worksite can be reasonable, provided the contractor's employees are well-trained, well-equipped, and guided by solid requirements in the bid document and contractor rulebook to provide protection from falls. This is especially important to the owner because of the third-party legal relationships.

Fall Protection Needs

Although personal fall arrest equipment is designed to control a fall, and thereby minimize the potential for injury, there are different worker needs. Fall protection may be needed as follows:

Backup Protection. In most cases, personal fall arrest equipment is designed and should serve as back-up protection – that is, it is "passive" until a fall occurs, at which time it either arrests the fall or acts to lower the falling individual in a controlled manner. This protection must fit in with the mobility requirements of the work task to 1) remain passive, and 2) provide continuous protection. It also must take into account other variables, such as obstructions below the workstation.

Restraint/Positioning Suspension. What is commonly referred to as fall protection may only be a means of restraint prevention from reaching an edge or support necessary to complete the work task. Equipment, such as a lineman's belt and pole strap, and rebar belt with rebar hook assembly, are designed to enable workers to position themselves to prevent a fall from occurring. Since this usually involves moving or repositioning the equipment, an independent backup lifeline should be considered where possible. Any time a worker's balance is substituted by belt and lines, a backup fall arrest system is needed. Restraint systems are particularly difficult to design because of workplace geometry and human factors. If the restraint system is too short, the worker will detach near the edge; if too long, long free falls can be expected; and if leaning occurs near an edge, a backup system is required.

Means of Retrieval. In certain instances, such as vertical entry into a confined space, fall protection equipment also can be used for emergency retrieval. When a lifeline is worn by an entrant for protection against a vertical fall hazard while entering a space, then rescuers should not have to go inside the space to hook up the victim for retrieval. This reduces the emergency response time considerably, and doesn't subject rescuers to the same harmful conditions that overcame the first worker. NIOSH reports show that 60 percent of confined space fatalities occur among "would-be" rescuers.[2]

Means of Escape. Workers at elevation may become trapped due to a medical problem or a sudden emergency, such as fire or an explosion. Exits such as stairs may be blocked and ladders may be unreliable because of the potential of falling during a panic descent. Controlling either a fall or a descent automatically through an emergency escape device can be simple for users and provides a reliable means of escape vertically or at an angle to ground or grade level. Some equipment can serve for both fall protection and emergency escape; for instance, a retracting cable lifeline with controlled descent feature.

Can One Fall Protection System Meet the Needs of a Work Task?

In some situations, yes. In others, more than one system may be required to provide a worker with continuous fall protection.

☞ **Transition Points.** An operator climbs to the top of a ladder and moves across to a platform. An inspector steps over an extended walkway onto the top of a tank truck to attach her lanyard to a horizontal cable. A maintenance worker uses the overhead pipe for an attachment while traveling down a piperack until he reaches a perpendicular structural support beam. These are all examples of points of transition. Too often these transitions are made without protection. Fixed ladder climbing systems should have an extension that enables the climber to move onto the guarded platform before disconnecting his climbing protection sleeve. In some applications, a second lanyard or lifeline system may be necessary. The objective is to not permit unprotected exposure while traveling to or returning from the workstation as well as while tasking.

☞ **Multiple Users.** Elevated work tasks that require more than one person to complete must be planned carefully. Most horizontal lifeline systems accommodate two or more workers. (See Appendix A-3 for multiple user discussion.) Independent lifelines may be suitable depending on available anchorage points and an ability to keep the lines from entangling. For large numbers of workers, measures such as personnel nets, perimeter cable protection, or catch platforms might be more efficient means of guarding.

Multiple Fall Hazard Control Measures. Personal fall protection equipment alone may not be adequate to provide continuous protection. A combination of fall arrest and prevention may be necessary. Aerial lifts can be used for access and personal fall protection while stationary at the elevated workstation. Workers on sloped roofs can use a combination of horizontal and vertical lifelines for two-dimensional protection.

However, should the worker fall off the gable edge of the roof, a dangerous pendulum-like swing fall can result that could lead to striking an obstruction. Therefore, after fall hazard analysis, perimeter guarding or catch platforms are needed to prevent exposure to these additional fall hazards.

Framed boxes brightly painted can help guard small vertical openings and skylight openings on roofs. Skylights themselves should be protected with rigid wire canopies.

☞ In December 1989, NIOSH published an Alert on deaths and injuries from falls through skylights accounting for 8% of all occupational deaths from trauma – DHHS (NIOSH) 90-100[3].

What Does Fall Protection Protect Against?

As stated in previous chapters, preventing exposure to an elevated fall hazard is the primary objective. Access must be reasonable before personal fall protection can be applied. Additionally, the walking and working surface should be at least 18 in. wide, stable, reasonably skid-resistant and free of tripping hazards such as bolts or tools. No personal fall arrest equipment system can guarantee that a victim will not sustain injury. However, when used properly and inspected regularly, this equipment can significantly reduce the chance of severe injuries resulting from fall impacts. Low system force levels, simple and automatic equipment, as well as selection of the appropriate system(s) for the work task, all are essential to ensuring minimal risk of injury. Anchorage points must have integrity for worker confidence.

☞ No anchorage structure must ever collapse due to inadequate design, meaning each point must be structurally sound and approved for its intended use. Anchorages can be modeled, tested and documented on engineering drawings. Scaffold structures and aerial lifts must be secured or outrigged to reduce any chance of tipping. Foundations, ladders, railings, etc., must be analyzed for corrosion and deterioration before these structures are used as anchorage points.

Fall Protection by Worker Activity

The importance of designing fall protection systems to suit the work method cannot be overemphasized. The misapplication of preventive or protective fall hazard control measures will rapidly defeat a program. The multitude of elevated work activities can be overwhelming when you consider the diversity of operations within an industry. However, worker activities at elevation can be broken down into fundamental groups to simplify the design of fall protection systems. Several examples follow.

- Climbing/Traversing: includes climbing fixed or temporary ladders as well as temporary and permanent structures (e.g., fixed ladders on towers, chimneys, buildings, ships, tanks or vessels; temporary structures typically under construction including buildings, vessels, bridges, precast concrete and roofs; and permanent structures such as piperacks, tanks, boilers and antennas).
- Mobile Work Positioning Systems: involves the use of some type of suspension equipment to position a worker such as a winch and boatswain's chair or single and multiple point powered platforms (manual or mechanical). A backup lifeline is needed in the event of a suspension line failure or equipment collapse.
- Aerial Lifts: manlifts, scissorlifts, bucket trucks, suspended platforms or work baskets that are used to access an elevated workstation or to position for work. For access, a fall protection system may or may not be necessary, depending on the frequency of access, materials of construction, and attachment method to the boom – if questionable, a lifeline/lanyard should be used. For work positioning use of such platforms, fall protection is always needed, because workers tend to overreach, which can lead to a fall. Alternatively, workers can be thrown from the bucket due to unforeseen impacts. Aerial lifts and other platforms are sometimes stabilized by applying forces to the platform railings under a truss or next to an exit point. This can lead to weakening of the platform attachments. It is better to tie the structures together to minimize platform movement.
- Horizontal Travel: work that requires horizontal mobility, such as walking along crane runways, piperacks or elevated catwalks, and unguarded platforms or mezzanines.
- Two-Dimensional Travel: access and work can often require travel in both vertical and horizontal directions, necessitating two-dimensional protection. Tank car loading and unloading, tank truck cleaning, water cooler tower construction, water treatment facilities, and work on dome and sloped roofing are examples.
- Escape: for workers who may become trapped at elevation, an emergency means of escape vertically or at an angle away from additional hazards may be needed (e.g. on overhead cranes, grain storage silos and oil derricks).
- Confined Entry and Retrieval: exposure to a vertical fall hazard often arises when climbing down

or being lowered into tanks, vessels or below fixed structures. In an emergency, these workers may have to be retrieved. Lifting dead weight up against gravity requires adequate mechanical advantage that can be achieved via a block and tackle arrangement or with mechanical retrieval devices (manual or powered). The lifting stroke and ratio must suit diverse weight and size characteristics of both worker and attendant, including potential emergency responders.

Chapters 5 and 6 provide techniques on analyzing these and other elevated fall hazard exposures.

☞ Risk: Should Every Fall Hazard Be Controlled?

This may seem a blue sky impossibility from many companies' perspectives. Yet, once a plant manager digs into the fall hazards and upgrades many of the work methods, particularly access to the elevated workstation, the problems seem to melt away. Certain types of maintenance work performed once a year or less frequently still pose the question: "Does the cost justify the end?" The answer is that despite the time-weighted low exposure, the exposure itself is very real, and every attempt should be made to focus on that very time period of exposure, when the work is being done, to provide protection as soon as possible. Deferred maintenance and deferred safety don't pay. No worker wants to become a statistic in the consequences of a known hazard. No manager would admit he or she had applied such statistics following a fall accident.

☞ Can anyone know if a serious or fatal fall will occur in the first few seconds of a worker's career or 30 years later in the last five seconds? Professionally, our safety approach must assume the first few seconds, and immediately act to control a fall hazard, which is likely to result in serious or fatal injury if the fall occurs.

What about Qualified Climbers?

These are workers, for example, who climb different towers every day consistently and thus arguably "do not need" protection, because it is not cost-justified, based on low accident incident rate over a period of years. Worker training and skill level is an argument to excuse the hazard and allow it to exist.

The argument is based on the assumption that a worker will not lose his or her balance while climbing, and that when stopped for work, he or she can keep hands free through work positioning. Three-point control is an excellent principle for climbing (three of the four human limbs attached securely to the climbing structure while moving). The fact remains that little or no backup safety exists either for climbing or working fall hazards.

The problem with falls is a bit like the problem of hitting the jackpot at Las Vegas. You never know when you will do it, if ever in your lifetime. But if you do, then it is not unheard of to strike once more or even twice more in rapid succession. In the case of falls, how many deaths or paraplegics will a company allow before it is statistically required to control the fall hazard? Statistically averaged, there should not be a fall incident over one's supervisory career. But that does not change the fact that the severe fall hazard still exists and should be controlled.

All persons who work at heights or in confined spaces should be physically qualified by a doctor and should train for anticipated hazards, in addition to receiving fall protection.

☞ Although the qualified climber concept has been met with great applause by electric utility and outdoor advertising managers, the author believes the program, if instituted, to be an administrative nightmare which will, in time, void all affordable fall protection for affected workers.

The quality concept that 99.9% reliability is not good enough should be adopted. Managers know that when faced with a death or serious injury involving an actual worker coming from the 0.1%, no argument for an exemption is reasonable. The only argument left is to blame the worker for his or her loss of balance, and therefore his or her contribution to the injury.

A Role for the Unions

Labor supplied by union halls poses a special problem for companies seeking to avoid or control elevated fall hazards. The encouragement for development of union apprenticeship training programs and certifications for high work, to include a curriculum for physical safety at heights, needs to come from major contractors through agreement with the large national unions. The teamwork required and so vital on the job should not excuse the fall hazard from being addressed. Construction associations are beginning to fill this training void.

When workers understand that the issues go beyond simply keeping a job or a high pay scale, then roofers, overhand bricklayers, steel connectors, and others will look for better access and for safety from the fall hazards that threaten their livelihood.

The United Auto Workers Union (UAW) has contributed greatly to controlling fall hazards at automobile plants in recent years by a willingness to research the solutions, write procedures, and train the work force. The unions will have a very special role in abatement of fall hazards at the worksite in the years ahead.

Notes

1. Injuries Resulting From Falls From Elevations (Bulletin 2195), June 1984. U.S. Department of Labor, Bureau of Labor Statistics. U.S. Government Printing Office, Washington, DC 20402.

2. National Institute of Occupational Safety and Health. DHHS (NIOSH) Publication No. 86-110. January 1986.

3. "Preventing Worker Death and Injuries from Falls Through Skylights & Roof Openings." National Institute of Occupational Safety and Health. DHHS (NIOSH) Publication No. 90-100. December 1989.

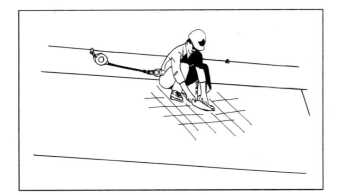

FIGURE 4.1
Roofing Fall Protection. Example of a two-dimensional fall protection system used during sloped roof maintenance. Note the wire rope clamp on the horizontal line that prevents the worker from reaching the side edge of the roof and falling with severe swing injury potential. (Anchorage stanchions not shown.) Note: OSHA requires that all horizontal lifeline systems be engineered for their intended purpose.

Review Questions

1. In addition to being needed while working, where is fall protection often overlooked?
   a. The workstation.
   b. Only needed while stationary.
   c. Egress.
   d. Travel to and from workstation.
   e. Planning.

2. Under which circumstances does a personal fall arrest system not serve as backup protection?
   a. Leaning out against a lanyard to reach a valve.
   b. Emergency retrieval from a confined space.
   c. Using controlled descent for emergency escape.
   d. Climbing with a permanent climbing protection system.
   e. Lineman's belt and strap for climbing a pole.

3. Where should fall protection requirements be detailed for effectiveness?
   a. Employee handbook.
   b. Bid documents.
   c. Contractor bid documents and company rules.
   d. Contractor bid documents, company policy and rules.
   e. Union apprenticeship program.

4. What types of personal fall arrest equipment can be used for reliable emergency escape?
   a. Most fall arrest equipment can be easily disconnected for escape.
   b. Fall protection equipment with a builtin shock absorber.
   c. Lifelines with an automatic controlled descent feature for vertical or angled escape.
   d. Fall protection is not suitable for emergency escape.
   e. Rappelling devices.

5. What fall protection measures can be used in conjunction with personal fall arrest equipment?
   a. Catch platforms.
   b. Aerial lifts.
   c. Perimeter guardrails.
   d. All of the above.
   e. Flat walking surfaces.

HOW TO ORGANIZE A 100% FALL PROTECTION PROGRAM

Any organization that neglects to provide employee protection from known hazards deserves the consequences.

❖ Should fall protection always be provided?
❖ What is 100% fall protection?
❖ Can 100% fall protection be achieved?
❖ Developing an effective fall protection program
  • Establishing policy and developing rules
  • Conducting a fall hazard analysis
  • Determining appropriate hazard control measures
  • Orientation, personnel selection and training
  • Inspection and maintenance
  • Program audit and feedback
❖ Additional considerations for confined entry operations
❖ Return on investment

Should Fall Protection Always Be Provided?

If we start with the objective of 100% protection and then work toward that goal, it will be achieved. The effectiveness of protection is usually dependent on the degree of planning that occurs before the job begins. Fall incident experience should decrease in proportion to the planning commitment. Such planning and the resulting work practice experience should decrease in proportion to the planning commitment, and can lead over time to the control or elimination of elevated fall hazards within a particular company or trade work-practice. For trained workers, fall protection ultimately becomes as simple as "hooking up".

An excellent principle to follow is that fall protection must be provided when a fall hazard could result in serious injury or death.

What Is 100% Fall Protection?

100% fall protection means that no exposure to an elevated fall hazard is permitted without backup protection. It means continuous protection. Exposure can be prevented by 1) establishing walls, floors and guard-rails; 2) using work platforms and aerial lifts, 3) implementing an operational change or 4) restricting workers' travel. Hazardous areas can be determined by warning lines 6 or more feet from an exposed edge.

When the prevention of fall hazard exposure is not practical to the work method, personnel nets or personal fall protection equipment can be designed to mitigate the effects of elevated falls.

A written policy commitment by top management to work toward and achieve this goal is necessary for success in any organization, and for building credibility among workers. The underlying message is that management really intends to protect them. Contractor safety rules written by the owner are a good place to start to reduce the probability of a substantial loss, and to learn how to field "you show me how" type objections before revising the employee safety rule book.

☞ Figure 5.2 shows several examples of general fall protection policies. Although specific rules are continually being developed, a strong general policy represents an initial proactive approach to effectively support controlling elevated fall hazards.

☞ Figures 5.3, 5.4 and 5.5 present three real-life fall protection programs.

Can 100% Fall Protection be Achieved?

Achieving 100% fall protection begins by planning the specific work methods through a collaborative effort between managers, foremen and workers. This should minimally include an analysis of the work task, including travel to and from the worksite and the proper selection of equipment, supplemented by initial and ongoing training, knowledgeable supervision and regular maintenance. In other words, 100% fall protection can be achieved through a complete systems approach to each potential exposure before work begins.

Exemptions for some trades by OSHA may be temporarily expedient because the fall problems have not been tackled seriously. Some exceptions seem economically justified, such as making inspections for the purpose of estimating roof work to be done. However, no

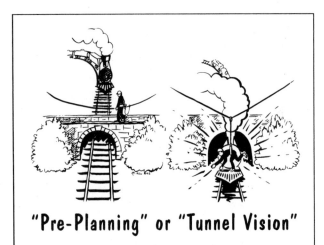

FIGURE 5.1

SAMPLE FALL PROTECTION POLICIES

It is the policy of this corporation to provide a workplace free from recognized elevated fall hazards.

or

We will not create, tolerate or fail to recognize a work method in which a fall hazard occurs, no matter for how short a time, that we will not eliminate, prevent or control.

or

If we cannot work without a fall hazard, then we shall not do the work.

FIGURE 5.2

blanket exemptions will solve the fall problem. If steel erection connectors were exempted to 30 feet, does that mean that they would be protected on exteriors or over open stairwells? This is analogous to an argument requiring use of auto seat belts only when exceeding the 55 mile-per-hour speed limit.

It is essential to develop the habit of designing fall protection based on a complete analysis before beginning each job. Installing a fall protection system that fits the requirements of one situation may not be appropriate in another, even though the situations are apparently similar. Each work method and elevated work task should be examined thoroughly. Outside of specific personal fall arrest equipment and its anchorage, planning what to do after a fall occurs is often overlooked or left up to a "rescue" operation. Much can be done to eliminate the injuries incurred after a worker falls, as well as devising methods that afford the worker self-recovery.

Developing an Effective Fall Protection Program

To facilitate a collaborative effort, a joint committee comprised of employee representatives, superintendents, supervisors, foremen, upper management, purchasing, and safety professionals should be established. This "fall protection committee" should then become familiar with available technology for controlling elevated fall hazards. Once a reasonable level of understanding is reached, an employee awareness program should be initiated immediately. This may be through various means, including signs, posters, reference materials or hard hat stickers. Hazard awareness alone can begin to reduce the probability of an incident as much as 20% to 50%. However, this awareness must be maintained.

The actual development of the program begins with establishing a policy for management commitment and developing rules to guide countermeasure efforts. The fall hazard analysis reveals details on elevated work tasks essential for determining appropriate hazard control measures. Control can be achieved either by preventing exposure or by providing personal protection. Initial orientation and ongoing training are imperative for effectively implementing countermeasure programs. The need for inspection and maintenance of personal protective equipment should be all too obvious. However, these vital tasks are often minimized or neglected altogether. Finally, auditing the program provides a means of continual improvement.

Establishing Policy and Developing Rules

The success of controlling elevated fall hazards is strongly dependent on sound policy guidelines. It is critical that this commitment and all subsequent rules apply not only to employees, but also to contractors, so that fall protection becomes part of the job. The purpose of a fall hazard control policy could be stated succinctly as follows:

Purpose: To establish a means to analyze elevated work tasks and determine appropriate personal protection against elevated fall hazards.

The scope of the program should address all elevated work involving exposure to an actual or potential fall hazard, both above and below ground. It also should cover elevated fall hazards as they pertain to entering confined spaces and emergency escapes. For example:

Scope: When exposure to an elevated fall hazard cannot be prevented through such measures as floors, walls and guardrails, then personal fall arrest equipment shall be used to control a fall.

Two specific rules can be used as a foundation to building procedural guidelines. The first rule is:

☞ Rule 1: Personal fall arrest equipment shall be used when a free fall hazard exceeds "X" feet.

"X" could be almost any height to suit an industry standard. Existing U.S. regulations call for protection in the steel erection industry at 25 ft. or more for multi-level structures and general industry at 4 ft. Almost everyone in industry and construction knows that you're not supposed to free fall more than 6 ft. on a lanyard, so why not 6 ft. or less if there are obstructions? Also, for fall protection in construction, OSHA Std. 3-3.1 recognized a 10-ft. height requirement for fall protection until October 1992, when it was withdrawn. OSHA would like to standardize on a 6-ft. rule.

The idea is to establish a height as a guideline to tackling exposures with complete and continuous protection. A good place to start would be 6 ft., and then tackling all the exposure problems on a prioritized basis above this height. Then, as rules are tightened by the company, this height should be lowered to about 4 ft. to include those sometimes more difficult exposures, such as applications presently served by step and extension ladders.

The second rule applies specifically to proper body support, both during and after a fall arrest.

☞ Rule 2: Wear a full body harness if you can free fall more than 2 ft. with your equipment and where immediate post-fall self-recovery is not possible.

For example, a worker using a 6-ft. lanyard attached at waist level 80 ft. off the ground can still "free fall" more than 2 ft. The long-term, costly injuries associated with long free-fall arrests and prolonged suspension

Continued on page 63

3.1 FALL PREVENTION PROGRAM

3.1.1 Purpose

To provide guidelines for maximum protection for all personnel against falls.

3.1.2 Goal

Achieve 100% fall protection for all personnel when working above ground level.

3.1.3 Responsibility

Project management and front line supervision are responsible for supporting and enforcing this program to ensure 100% compliance by all personnel. The Project Safety Department shall have full authority to ensure 100% enforcement of the program. The Safety Department's primary responsibility, however, will be to support crafts and to monitor the program for compliance and advising project management.

3.1.4 Total Safety Task Instruction (TSTI)

Total Safety Task Instruction is to be given to each person assigned work in elevated areas. Supervisors must analyze all elevated tasks as to fall protection needs and to ensure adequate fall protection systems are provided. After analyzing the tasks, supervisors shall instruct personnel involved in the specifics of the fall protection measures to be used.

3.1.5 Procedures

All personnel on this project will be required to wear an approved full body harness and shock absorbing lanyard or an approved safety belt with a shock absorbing lanyard.

Crafts/departments shall make maximum use of primary fall protection systems such as scaffolds, aerial lifts, personnel hoists, etc. These systems shall be equipped with complete working/walking surfaces free of floor openings, standard guard rail systems and a safe means of access.

Personnel traveling or working in elevated areas where a fall exposure exists shall make use of secondary fall protection in securing their safety lanyard at all times to a structure, lifeline or approved fall arresting device capable of supporting 5400 pounds.

Personnel working from or traveling in powered work platforms or personnel lifting/hoisting devices shall also properly secure their safety lanyards as noted in procedures below.

NOTE: PERSONNEL TRAVELING IN CONSTRUCTION ELEVATORS ARE NOT REQUIRED TO SECURE SAFETY LANYARDS.

Fall protection devices such as lifelines, safety harnesses/lanyards, etc. shall be inspected on a regular basis for damage and/or deterioration. Defective equipment shall be removed from service and destroyed or in some cases repaired.

Fall protection devices subjected to shock loadings imposed during fall arresting shall be removed from service and the Project Safety Department notified.

Fall protection devices and systems shall not be used for any other purpose other than employee safe guarding.

Subcontractors shall comply with the requirements set forth in this program as a minimum for fall protection.

3.1.6 Fall Protection Devices

3.1.6.1 Primary Fall Protection Systems. These systems provide walking and working surfaces in elevated areas which are free from floor openings and are equipped with standard guard rail systems on all open sides and with closure apparatus for ladder openings or other points of access when required. These systems include but are not limited to: scaffolds, pencil boards, aerial lifts (JLG, scissor lifts, etc.), and other approved personnel hoisting devices.

Standard guard rail systems consist of a top rail of 2 x 4 lumber or equivalent material approximately forty-two inches (42") above the walking/working surface, a mid rail at approximately twenty-one inches (21") above said surface and a four inch (4") tall toe board mounted at the walking/working surface. Upright support post spacing must not exceed eight feet 8') and the entire system must be capable of supporting 200 pounds force in any direction with minimum deflection. These systems are used to guard open sides of floors, platforms and walkways in elevated areas.

Floor opening/hole covers are used to close openings and holes in floors, platforms and walkways. These covers must be capable of supporting the maximum potential load they may be subjected to. The cover must completely cover the opening/hole and be secured against accidental displacement. These covers must be marked "HOLE COVER–DO NOT REMOVE".

3.1.6.2 Secondary Fall protection Systems–Safety Harness/Lanyard Systems. These systems must be worn and used as a backup to Primary Fall Protection Systems noted above and in the absence of Primary Systems.

Only safety harnesses/lanyard systems furnished by Brown & Root may be used on this project. Personal safety harnesses/lanyard systems may not be used.

Subcontractors shall provide appropriate fall protection equipment to their employees.

Lanyards must be of the shock absorbing type when used for fall protection.

The fall protection lanyard shall be attached to the D-ring located in the middle back of the safety harness.

D-rings located at the waist may only be used for positioning and with rail type ladder climbing devices.

Work positioning lanyards are to be attached to D-rings at the waist belt location and be supported by an appropriate work belt. Positioning lanyards need not be of shock

continued on next page

FIGURE 5.3

From the Brown & Root Safety & Health Reference Manual (January 1991). Reprinted with permission.

HOW TO ORGANIZE A 100% FALL PROTECTION PROGRAM

absorbing type and must not be used for fall protection. The positioning lanyard must always be backed up by a properly secured shock absorbing fall protection lanyard.

3.1.7 Lifelines

Lifeline systems are points of attachment for fall protection lanyards and must be capable of supporting at least 5400 pounds. Lifelines may be mounted either vertically or horizontally and are generally intended to provide mobility to personnel working elevated areas.

Horizontal lifelines must be made of at least thee-eighths inch (3/8") wire rope cable properly supported to withstand at least 5400 pounds impact. Alternate materials for specific cases (e.g. use of synthetic fiber rope) must be okayed by the Project Safety Department.

Horizontal Lifelines should be positioned so as to provide points of attachment at waist level or higher to personnel utilizing them.

Lifelines shall not be used for any purpose other than fall protection.

Horizontal lifelines shall be installed and maintained by the project rigging/structural department. (NOTE: Other crafts must obtain Safety Department approval to install alternate material lifeline lines noted above.)

Vertical lifelines are used for personnel fall protection when vertical mobility is required and may be comprised of static lifelines made of synthetic fiber rope or cable which are equipped with approved sliding rope grabs or they may consist of self retracting reel type lanyard/lifelines which are attached directly to a safety harness.

Static rope lifelines with rope grabs are required for personnel working from spiders/sky-climbers and two point suspension scaffolds. These types of lifelines can also be used to provide fall protection for other operations such as scaffold erection and structural steel erection where tie off points are limited and vertical mobility is required.

Sliding rope grabs approved for the size rope used are the only method for securing a safety lanyard to a vertical lifeline. Lanyards shall not be attached to lifelines by means of knots or loops.

Rope grabs shall be positioned on the lifeline at least above the shoulders of the user.

Other devices which can be used are:

- Safety Nets. Safety nets may be used in some situations as secondary fall protection. Use and installation of nets when required will be under direction of the Project Safety Department. The Structural/Rigging Department is responsible for net installation when required.

- Connectors Toggles. These devices lock into structural steel bolt holes to provide an attachment point for a safety lanyard. These devices are to be used by structural iron connectors and bolt up personnel during steel erection.

- Concrete Form Tie-Offs. These devices attach to patented concrete forms to provide an attachment point for safety lanyards. These devices are to be used when placing concrete forms at elevations where a fall exposure exists.

3.1.8 Lifeline Placement/Installation

3.1.8.1 Horizontal Lifelines. All horizontal lifelines placed in skeletal steel structures (e.g. pipe racks, etc.) shall be three-eighths inch (3/8") cable as a minimum and shall be secured on each end by at least two (2) cable clamps. Intermediate supports shall be adequate to minimize sag and vertical deflection under loading.

Horizontal lifelines shall be installed and maintained by the Rigging/Structural Department.

Priority shall be given to lifeline placement as structures are erected.

Lifelines shall be arranged to provide adequate mobility in all areas of the structure while maintaining 100% fall protection for personnel.

Lifelines should be arranged to provide tie off points at least waist high for personnel using them.

Lifelines shall not be used for any purpose other than fall protection.

Personnel installing lifelines shall be protected from falls at all times by use of retractable lanyards or tie off to structural steel, etc.

The Rigging/Structural Department shall schedule regular documented inspections of all lifelines at least weekly.

3.1.8.2 Vertical Lifelines/Retractable Lifelines. Vertical lifelines and retractable lifelines will be used as follows:

> **3.1.8.2.1** Static Rope: Static rope lifelines shall be of synthetic fiber rope approved and maintained by the Project Safety Department.
>
> Static rope lifelines must be used with approved rope grabs for lanyard attachment.
>
> Static rope lifelines must be anchored at the top by means capable of supporting 5400 pounds.

NOTE: SOFTENERS SHOULD BE USED WHERE LIFELINES CONTACT SHARP EDGES SUCH AS BEAM FLANGES.

> Static rope lifeline/rope grabs will be placed for each person working from or riding in spiders/sky-climbers or two point suspension scaffolds. Each person must have an individual lifeline.
>
> 3.1.8.2.2 Retractable Reel Lifelines: Retractable lifeline devices shall be attached to support capable of withstanding 5400 pounds impact loading.
>
> Retractable lifeline devices shall be secured by means of shackles and wire rope chokers or synthetic slings. ROPE (synthetic or natural fiber) SHALL NOT BE USED TO SECURE THESE DEVICES. *Continued on next page*

FIGURE 5.3 (continued from page 60)

Each retractable lifeline device shall be equipped with a rope tag line for extending the device to elevations below the point of attachment.

Retractable lifelines shall be placed at the top of every temporary construction ladder which is to be used for repeated access/egress to elevations.

Retractable lifelines shall be placed at the top of every temporary construction ladder which is to be used for repeated access/egress to elevations.

Retractable lifelines shall also be used to provide fall protection to structural iron workers during erection prior to installation of other fall protection systems.

3.1.9 Ladders

Permanent caged structural ladders may be ascended or descended without additional fall protection.

Temporary construction ladders shall extend at least thirty-six inches (36") above their uppermost landing and be secured against displacement.

When ascending or descending ladders, personnel shall use both hands. Materials or tools shall not be carried in hands while using ladders.

All temporary construction ladders placed for repeated access/egress to elevations shall be equipped with retractable lifelines. Personnel using these ladders shall secure the retractable lifeline to their safety harness while ascending or descending the ladder.

Retractable lifelines reels shall be secured above the highest point of access to applicable ladders and be equipped with a tag line of one-fourth inch (1/4") synthetic fiber rope extending from the lifeline reel to the ground when the reel is fully retracted.

Portable ladders (e.g. extension ladders, step ladders, etc.) do not require the retracting lifeline when they are used for access to an elevation to perform a single task. When using these types of ladders in this way, the following must be complied with:

- Personnel using the ladder must receive specific TSTI concerning the use of portable ladders and associated fall protection techniques.

- Personnel climbing ladders which are not tied off at the top must have another person hold the ladder at the bottom until it can be secured. This includes the last trip down after untying a ladder at the top.

- Upon climbing to the elevation where the task is to be performed, the person on the ladder shall properly secure their safety lanyard before doing anything else. Next, the ladder must be tied off before work can begin. When the task is complete, the process is reversed with the safety lanyard being the last protective device released prior to descend.

- Absolutely no objects, tools, or materials are to be carried in hands while climbing or descending ladders.

3.1.10 Temporary Work Platforms/Walkways (Scaffolds and Pencil Boards)

Every effort shall be made to ensure all temporary platforms/walkways are equipped with solid decks free of openings and standard guard rail systems.

Personnel working from temporary platforms or travelling on temporary catwalks shall have their safety lanyard secured at all times to a lifeline or structure capable of supporting 5400 pounds impact loading.

Every temporary work platform or walkway must be provided with a safe means of access/egress which allows personnel to remain tied off at all times. Retractable lifelines shall be used to achieve fall protection while ascending or descending access ladders to temporary work platforms or walkways.

3.1.11 Personnel Lifts/Hoisting Devices

3.1.11.1 Aerial Lifts (JLG, Scissor, Snorkel, Etc.). Personnel riding in or working from these lifts must secure their safety lanyard to the lift basket at all times.

Lifts shall be placed on solid level surfaces so as to eliminate possibility of overturning.

3.1.11.2 Spiders and Sky-climbers. Personnel riding in or working from these hoisting devices shall each be provided an independent lifeline and rope grab to which their lanyard shall be secured at all times when aloft.

3.1.11.3 Crane Hoisted Personnel Baskets. Use of these devices shall comply with the safety procedures set forth in the Project Procedures Manual.

Personnel riding in or working from personnel baskets must have their lanyard secured to the basket at all times when aloft.

3.1.11.4 Elevators. Personnel riding inside enclosed elevator cars are not required to secure their safety lanyard.

3.1.12 Skeletal Steel/Open Structures

This section deals with fall protection when personnel are required to gain access to travel and work in skeletal steel/open structures such as pipe racks. This includes traveling on or working on any elevated surface which is not designed as a personnel work surface or walkway (e.g. pipe, cable tray, etc.).

Personnel working or traveling in elevated skeletal steel/open structures shall secure their lanyards to a lifeline or structure capable of supporting 5400 pounds at all times (100% fall protection). NOTE: THIS INCLUDES BOTH HORIZONTAL AND VERTICAL TRAVEL.

Personnel working or traveling in skeletal steel/open structures shall have two (2) safety lanyards at all times in order to achieve 100% fall protection. One of the lanyards must be secured at all times.

Continued on next page

FIGURE 5.3 (continued from page 61)

From the Brown & Root Safety & Health Reference Manual (January 1991). Reprinted with permission.

HOW TO ORGANIZE A 100% FALL PROTECTION PROGRAM

Adequate lifeline system will be provided in skeletal steel/open structures to allow 100% fall protection for personnel working or traveling in these structures. The Rigging/Structural Department shall be responsible for installation and maintenance of these lifelines.

Vertical travel in these structures shall consist of properly placed and secured access ladders equipped with retractable lifelines. Personnel climbing or descending these ladders shall secure these retractable lifelines to their safety harnesses while using the ladder.

In lieu of lifelines, personnel may secure safety lanyards to substantial structural steel members, pipe and pipe supports. Personnel shall avoid securing lanyards to cable tray, conduit and small bore screw pipe.

3.1.13   Permanent Structures/Stairs/Caged Ladders

All Brown & Root and subcontractor personnel are required to wear an approved full body safety harness and shock absorbing lanyard or an approved safety belt with a shock absorbing lanyard. THIS REQUIREMENT INCLUDES COMPLETED PERMANENT STRUCTURES.

Personnel working or traveling in incomplete permanent structures where fall protection exist, such as floor openings and open sided floors, must be properly tied off when within six feet (6') of any fall exposure.

Priority shall be given to installation and securing of permanent floors and walking surfaces and all guard rails and other permanent fall protection devices.

When required, temporary guard rails and floor coverings shall be installed to eliminate fall exposures.

Only personnel of the Rigging/Structural Department responsible for steel erection are allowed on elevated floors and with fall exposures, such as floor openings or open sided floors.

Permanent stairs when completed shall be used to access or egress elevated work areas.

Caged ladders do not require secondary fall protection as the cage is a fall protection device. Personnel climbing ladders must keep both hands free for climbing at all times.

3.1.14   Structural Steel Erection

Personnel erecting structural steel shall achieve 100% fall protection through use of safety harnesses/lanyards, retractable lifelines, connectors, toggles and aerial lifts (JLG, snorkel, etc.).

Access to structural steel shall be obtained by use of ladders, aerial lifts or other approved personnel hoisting devices. Climbing of structural steel members such as columns and diagonal braces shall not be allowed.

Prior to and during horizontal lifeline placement, structural personnel shall crawl (coon) steel members with lanyards secured around said members. Retractable lifelines secured at elevations above the point of operation may be used in some applications to provide fall protection prior to availability of horizontal lifelines.

When lanyard lengths longer than standard are required due to large steel members, the Project Safety Department shall be contacted to approve methods for obtaining the additional length.

3.1.15   Reinforcement Steel/Concrete Form Work

Personnel working on rebar walls, piers and on concrete form walls must have fall protection 100% of the time they are off the ground.

This fall protection can be achieved through the use of retractable lifelines, static lifeline and rope grabs or use of double lanyards.

Personnel working rebar or formed walls and elevated piers generally require a work positioning lanyard (cannot be used for fall protection) and a fall protection lanyard.

On vertical rebar walls, the safety lanyard shall be secured at a point above the workers head, either to a lifeline or a horizontal section of rebar.

On form walls, personnel shall use patented construction form tie-off attachments or lifelines to secure their safety lanyards. These persons shall receive specific TSTI on the equipment to be used and the fall protection practices to be used.

3.1.16   Rigging/Crane Assembly and Dismantling

Crane assembly-dismantling operations pose a challenge to the 100% fall prevention program. However, through thought an planning, maximum protection can be achieved.

Fall protection shall be obtained during these operations through the use of retractable lifelines, safety harnesses and lanyards and minimizing movement in elevated areas by using ladders and in some cases personnel lifts.   □

FIGURE 5.3 (continued from page 62)

continued from page 59

in a body belt should provide adequate impetus to use full body harnesses instead of belts in almost every application. Note that in the 1990s it may be easier to require harnesses for all fall arrest methods at a worksite.

Finally, it is up to each employee performing a work task at elevation to assume responsibility for evaluating the need for a personal fall arrest system as an integral part of the job. The evaluation process should occur before the work is started and must include travel to and from the workstation.

Each user should check his fall arrest system before using the equipment. This means checking parts for cuts, distortions, and wear, particularly with snaphooks. Any questions concerning the proper application of a

continued on page 67

Safety Standard No. M-71
FALL RESTRAINT SYSTEMS

I. SCOPE

This standard covers the requirements for the use of Fall Restraint Systems.

II. DEFINITIONS

A. Class I body belt is a device worn around the waist to which a lanyard or lifeline grabbing device is attached.

B. Class III body harness is a harness system designed to spread shock load over the shoulders, thighs and seat area.

** C. Lanyard is a flexible line that secures the wearer of a harness to a vertical or horizontal lifeline or a fixed anchorage.

** D. A lifeline is a component consisting of a flexible line for connection to anchorages either vertically (vertical lifeline), or horizontally (horizontal lifeline).

** E. Fixed anchorage is a secured point of attachment and not part of the work surface.

F. A Motion-Stopping-Safety (MSS) System is a system providing fall protection by using the following equipment singly or in combination: guardrails, scaffolds or platforms with guardrails; safety nets; and body belt/harness systems.

G. A Warning Line System is a temporary rope, wire, or chain and supporting stanchion erected not less than six feet from the edge of a roof and flagged at no more than six foot intervals with high visibility material. The lowest point of the line, including sag, must not be less than 34 inches or more than 39 inches from the roof surface. If mechanical equipment is being used, the warning line must be not less than six feet from the edge if the equipment is being operated parallel to the warning line, and ten feet from the edge if it is operated perpendicular to the warning line. The warning line stanchion supports must be able to withstand at least 16 pounds force 30 inches above the roof surface without tipping. Minimum tensile strength of the rope, wire or chain must be 500 pounds. The rope, wire or chain must be secured to the stanchion in such a manner that slack is not created when pulling on a section between stanchions.

H. Safety Monitoring System is a system in which a competent person monitors the safety of all employees in a roofing crew and warns them when it appears to the monitor that they are unaware of the hazard or are acting in an unsafe manner. The competent person must be on the same roof and within visual sight and voice communication of the other employees.

I. Low-pitched roof is a roof having a slope less than or equal to four in twelve.

J. Mechanical equipment - all motor or human propelled wheeled equipment except for wheelbarrows and mop carts.

** K. Working within confines of a ladder is defined as an employee maintaining their mid-body area within the ladder side rails.

L. Work areas include all surfaces except ladders, vehicles and flatbed trailers.

** M. An anchorage point must be capable of resisting twice the force created by the fall of a 250 lb. person a distance of six feet and stopped by a lanyard with a built-in shock absorbing device. See attachment.

III. PROCEDURES

A. USE

** 1. A fall restraint system with continuous attachment shall be used by personnel in work areas not protected by guardrails where there is a danger of employees falling from a distance of six feet or greater. (Distance based on elevation where person is standing or sitting.)

2. The primary fall restraint device shall be a Class III body harness. The lanyard anchorage point must be such that the maximum fall distance is four feet or six feet if the lanyard is used in conjunction with an ANSI approved shock absorber.

3. The use of a Class I body belt must have approval of the department head and the free fall distance must be restricted to two feet or less.

** 4. Personnel shall be trained in the correct use of fall restraint devices. NOTE: "Fall Protection," #88-1357 is a videotape that may be used for training. Department head will determine the frequency for retraining.

** 5. Approved safety lanyards shall be a minimum of 1/2 inch thick nylon or equivalent. Lanyards will have double locking snap hooks.

6. If a lanyard made of synthetic fibers is subject to come in contact with hot surfaces, such as uninsulated steam lines, valves, or hot furnace stacks, an insulated cover, either on the lanyard or on the hot surface, must be used for protection. Lanyards must be protected against sharp surfaces.

7. Fall restraint devices exposed to impact loading shall be removed from service and destroyed.

8. When personnel are working off portable ladders and the work requires them to be outside the "confines of the ladder," a fall restraint device must be used.

continued on next page

FIGURE 5.4

From the Dow Safety Standard M-71. Reprinted with permission.

HOW TO ORGANIZE A 100% FALL PROTECTION PROGRAM

9. Personnel working from or riding in any aerial lift device shall wear a fall restraint system with the lanyard attached to the boom or basket.

** 10. In erecting or dismantling scaffolds, the person on the top level of a scaffold is allowed to work without an attached lanyard when there is nothing adjacent to the scaffold that a lanyard can be properly anchored to at a higher level or at the same level, to provide fall protection. This does not apply to suspended scaffolds.

** 11. When vertical lifelines are used, each person shall be provided with a separate lifeline.

** 12. A Lineman's belt and a Pole Shark (which is manufactured by Scepter) utilized for climbing and working on poles are acceptable fall restraint devices.

13. Personnel engaged in roofing work on low-pitched roofs shall be protected from falling by using one of the following systems:

    a. A Motion-Stopping-Safety system (MSS system).

    b. A Warning Line System erected not less than six feet from roof edges not having other means of fall protection where there is danger of personnel falling. If personnel are working outside the warning line system, an MSS system or a safety monitoring system must be used.

    c. A Safety Monitoring System on roofs 50 feet or less in width where mechanical equipment is not being used or stored.

14. Personnel engaged in roof work must be trained in the fall hazards of working near a roof perimeter, the erection and use of the MSS System, the Warning Line and Safety Monitoring Systems, and job procedures required for roof work.

    ** Exception:

    When personnel are on roofs only to inspect, investigate or estimate roof level conditions, they are exempt from requirement 13 above.

15. Personnel engaged in work on low-pitched roofs other than roofing and more than ten feet from the edge do not need to have a fall restraint system.

B. INSPECTION AND TESTING

1. Fall restraint devices shall be visually inspected for defects by user prior to use.

2. Fall restraint devices shall be inspected by owner when new and every six months thereafter. Inspect for cuts, burns, excessive wear, loose splices, defective hardware and distorted thimbles. The date of each inspection shall be recorded on an inspection tag and permanently attached to the harness.

ATTACHMENT

** **Minimum anchorage points for attaching lanyard for fall restraint systems.**

** **Anchorage Points**

MINIMUM SIZES AND CONDITIONS

**1 Pipe

2" schedule 10 carbon steel or nickel. These metals must be identified with a magnet. Pipe not attracting a magnet shall not be used except 2" schedule 10 stainless. This pipe must be identified by its owner. Span (between pipe supports) must not be greater than 20 feet for any size pipe.

** 3" or greater of any metal pipe may be used if in good condition.

The pipe length must be continuous for at least two supports on either side of the attachment.

Do not tie off to insulated pipe of any size unless permission is received from the owner.

** Do not tie off to any plastic pipe.

Do not tie off to electrical conduct of any size.

**2 Structural Steel

2-1/2" x 2-1/2" x 3/8" angle. Span must be 20 feet or less.

** Guardrails are not to be used as anchor points.

**3 Lifelines

3/8" diameter; silicon-tin-bronze cable, alloy 13, 7 strand, ASTM B-105 (Refer to Engineering Specification 38-012 for support and attachment.)

** 3/8" diameter galvanized steel space-lay as manufactured by Mac Whyte).

** Lifeline cables that are part of a climbing protection device are acceptable. (Ex-RTC-2700 Series Retractalok™).

** NOTE:

When securing to an anchorage point, the user must take into consideration the deflection of the pipe or cable, (which could be up to 24" for 2" pipe), and for the amount of lanyard that would be lengthened from the shock absorber unstitching, plus an individual's leg length. Also check the anchorage point for corrosion.

** If the situation occurs that the above conditions cannot be meet as an anchorage point, the person will contact his supervisor who will determine that the selected anchorage point meets the requirements of this standard. Contact the Civil Engineering Group Leader for assistance. This group has issued fall restraint anchorage guidelines.

** Denotes 1991 changes   □

FIGURE 5.4 (continued from page 64)

FALL PROTECTION POLICY
H. B. ZACHRY COMPANY
HOUSTON DISTRICT OFFICE

I.   **INTRODUCTION - WHY "100 PERCENT?"**

II. **COMPANY POLICY STATEMENT**

   A. OSHA Regulation

III. **MECHANICS**

   A. Basic Equipment Requirements

   B. Rescue & Retrieval Considerations

   C. Swing Fall Potential

IV. **ENFORCEMENT POLICY**

   APPENDIX:

   1) Fall Distance Interpretation

   2) Travel Path Lifelines

   3) Lifeline Anchorage

   4) Temporary Anchorage

   5) Personal Fall Protection

100% FALL PROTECTION

I.   **INTRODUCTION - WHY "100 PERCENT"?**

   A. Falls are the second leading cause of accidental death in the nation, second only to motor vehicle accidents.

   B. Federal Occupation Safety and Health Administration (OSHA) 1.29CFR 1926.105 Safety Nets.

   1. Safety nets shall be provided when work places are more than 25 feet above the ground or water surface or other surfaces where the use of ladders, scaffolds, catch platform, temporary floors, safety lines or safety belts are impractical.

   2. Basic/literal interpretation is: if the work place is more than 25 feet above any surface, you must be protected by some means.

   C. H. B. Zachry recognizes the danger of being exposed to an unprotected fall of six (6) feet or more saying, "100% FALL PROTECTION WILL BE USED ANYTIME THE FALL EXPOSURE IS 6 FEET OR MORE".

II. **COMPANY POLICY STATEMENT**

   A. The policy requires the strict enforcement of the following:

   1. An approved safety belt/harness and lanyard shall be worn at all times while working more than six feet above ground and/or floor elevations to include but not limited to:

   a. a building/structure that has incomplete construction activities presenting potential fall hazards;

   b. all ladders, elevated platforms and vessels under construction, and scaffolds regardless of completion status.

   2. The lanyard must be tied off when working more than six feet above the immediate work surface where a fall hazard exists. This includes but is not limited to ladders, lifts, elevated platforms and scaffolds regardless of completion status.

   3. Anyone moving about outside of a handrail area (i.e., pipe racks, structural iron) must have two lanyards securing oneself from a fall at all times.

   4. There will be no walking on open iron or pipe, unless you secured to the iron or pipe, or a lifeline.

   5. Lifelines are to be used for continuous protection. Lifelines may be horizontal, or vertical. If you anticipate working in an area with no apparent structure to tie off to, or you will be moving about, contact your supervisor to have a lifeline put up.

   6. Project management will establish disciplinary action for this project for those employees who fail to comply with this policy.

   B. A 100% Fall Protection Policy means that no exposure to a fall hazard shall be permitted without protection.

   1. A work place fall is an accidental loss of balance that permits an uncontrolled drop from one level to another.

   C. 100% Fall Protection can consist of the following:

   1. Removing the hazard exposure by establishing walls, floors or railings.

   2. Restricting/barricading the travel possibility to the fall hazard.

   3. Using personnel fall protection equipment to arrest an accidental fall.

   4. Using safety nets to safely catch an accidental fall.

III. **MECHANICS - MAKING IT WORK**

   A. Basic Equipment Requirements

   1. Lanyard

   a) Lanyards used for fall protection will, as a minimum, have:

   1. Double locking snaphooks

   2. Built-in shock absorbing devices

Continued on next page

FIGURE 5.5

From the H.B. Zachry Company Fall Protection Policy. Reprinted with permission. [Editor's Note: Appendix materials for this policy have not been included in this sample.]

HOW TO ORGANIZE A 100% FALL PROTECTION PROGRAM

2. Harness/Body Belt

a) Through a Class "C" - Full Body Harness is preferred, those projects still allowed to use a single body belt must document training on proper fit and use.

1. Snug fit, in manufactured grommets, just below the belt line.

2. Once secured to anchorage point, the "D" ring being utilized must be repositioned to the back of the waist area.

B. Rescue and Retrieval Considerations

1. Never put a person in a situation where, in the event of a fall, prompt rescue would be impractical/impossible.

2. Consider equipment such as:

a) Basket stretcher (Stokes) with lifting bridal

b) Aerial lift (JLG) availability

c) Systems which include self rescue/controlled decent

C. Never work more than 6 feet off the ground or see APPENDIX 1 for: Fall Distance Interruption.

D. Never unhook your safety belt lanyard once you get 6 feet off the ground or see APPENDIX 2 for: Travel Path Lifelines.

E. Don't do the smaller jobs where decking and lifelines would not be practical or see APPENDIX 3 for: Specialty Devices.

C. Swing-Fall Potential:

1. When not tied off directly overhead (i.e., worker moves away from lifeline anchorage point), a swing-fall hazard can exist in the case of an accidental fall.

2. The arc of a swing fall will produce as much energy as a vertical fall through the same distance.

3. The impact on the side of the body can be a serious result of the fall being arrested.

IV. **FALL PROTECTION ENFORCEMENT POLICY**

Due to the severity potential of all falls, even from 6 feet, the following policy will be strictly enforced on all HDO projects:

A. Verbal Warning

1. During new hire orientation, all prospective and newly hired employees will be given the basic philosophy of the Company 100% Fall Protection Policy.

2. They will sign a statement acknowledging understanding of the policy and receipt of the "verbal warning".

B. First Violation

1. When observed by a supervisor (any craft foreman or above) to not be in compliance, the employee will receive three (3) days off without pay.

2. A record shall be made of this action.

C. Second Violation will result in termination of employee!

1. If within one year (12 months) of the recorded first offense.

2. The termination shall be for "safety reasons" with not eligible for re-hire for "30 days" from termination date.

D. Documentation

1. Documents produced from A, B, or C above shall be maintained for job duration or 5 years.

V. **I M P O R T A N T - USE NOTICE**

* * * The products described in the following appendices (1, 2 and 3) are for informational and idea purposes only * * *

Before using any of these systems consult your H. B. Zachry safety representative AND closely follow the manufacturers instructions for installation/use limitations and care. ☐

FIGURE 5.5 (continued from page 66)

continued from page 63

system should be brought to the immediate supervisor, fall protection committee, or safety department, depending on the existing communication lines.

Conducting a Fall Hazard Analysis

An analysis of elevated work begins by individually identifying the fall hazards that can occur during the work task as well as while traveling to and returning from the worksite. A video camera is an invaluable asset for this purpose. A careful look at the required work task mobility is important. What may be an industry work practice or a job that lacks a set pattern or sequence of movement, may necessitate a change to meet the capabilities and limitations of the available equipment. Scaffold erection, for example, varies considerably depending on the facilities or structure around which the scaffold is built. However, certain patterns of movement could be used to assemble the pole or frames without entangling lifelines suspended from above.

An appraisal of each exposure may serve to provide a rationale for reducing the risk level. Overall, the primary objective would be to minimize the probability of a loss by controlling the most frequent elevated work task with the highest potential severity.

Classifying related work tasks, particularly in terms of their required mobility, can facilitate the preplanning of anchor points, foreseeing maintenance, and determining environmental or facility influences. For example, the methods for entering vertical confined spaces may be similar in storage tanks, process vessels, vaults or sewers.

Once classified, specific work tasks can be prioritized. The fall hazard height set in Rule 1 (discussed above) can help indicate which exposures to address first. However, the frequency, duration, environmental conditions and potential severity of an incident should also be considered. Some situations, particularly those that have been ingrained as an "industry work practice" may require additional planning. These can often be tackled concurrently with exposures that are relatively straightforward.

The key to effectively controlling fall hazards with personal protective equipment is to ensure that the system is designed to fit in with the work method. Fall arrest equipment should simply act as a backup and provide mobility with protection when selected and installed properly.

Determining Appropriate Fall Hazard Control Measures: Prevention or Fall Arrest?

☞ Once an elevated fall hazard has been analyzed, an appropriate control measure must be selected. Exposure to a fall hazard can be either eliminated or prevented, or when prevention is not practical, then personal fall arrest equipment can be used to control a fall.

Elimination. Where fall hazard exposure is predicted, careful planning can eliminate the bulk of the exposure. For example, a multitiered plant structure can be assembled tier by tier, moved a short distance onsite, and then lifted into place using the pinhole method. In this way, approximately 95% of the aerial exposure can be eliminated.

Prevention. Preventive measures typically involve the installation of floors, walls, nets or fixed platforms and walking surfaces with the appropriate guardrails, midrails, and toe boards. These measures usually consist of permanent, passive systems, but all require substantial engineering and installation efforts. Scaffold-ing with temporary floors and appropriate guarding may be suitable; however, the fall exposure during erection and dismantling must be addressed. Also, personnel may be denied access to a location where they may be exposed to a fall hazard. Restricted access can be achieved through the use of chains, barricades, tape or signs. For example, tapes or cables can be used to warn workers to keep away from the edge of a roof or skylight.

As mentioned above with regard to scaffold erection and dismantling, permanent preventive measures almost always involve fall hazard exposure during the installation process. Therefore, personal protective equipment may be needed to control a fall during the installation or dismantling/demolition process. This often can be achieved with overhead or portable anchorage points. A secondary method is the use of the scaffold members as part of an engineered fall arrest system. The objective is complete and continuous protection. Outrigger brackets equipped with cable railings snapped together one at a time could provide side protection. Tying in the scaffold approximately 5 ft. to 6 ft. above grade will overcome the critics' objection about scaffold tipover.

Finally, the availability of guarded bucket trucks, scissor lifts, crane-suspended work platforms and other personnel lifts is increasing. These devices can offer a means of access to a workstation or can be effectively

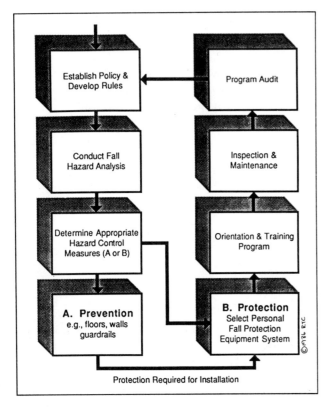

FIGURE 5.6
The steps of fall prevention and protection.

used for the installation of a preventive or personal fall protection system. When aerial lifts are used for access only, that is, getting to a workstation, personal fall protection may or may not be needed depending on the construction and reliability of the basket/lift. However, transition to and from the workstation requires protection. When aerial lifts are used for work positioning, a personal fall arrest system is definitely needed because of overreach out of the basket and continual operational use. A full body harness and a shock absorbing lanyard that can be anchored to the boom or another suitable location, preferably overhead, serve as fall protection. NOTE: Aerial lift fall protection must be engineered, tested, and documented on an engineering drawing.

Fall Arrest Systems. When prevention is not economically feasible due to location or work sequence, or practical in the sense that a specific work task is only to be performed once a year or less, personal fall arrest equipment can be used to control a fall. The overall objective would be to minimize the potential for the user to sustain injury due to the fall arrest. Careful consideration should be given to the performance of the system and its ability to not interfere with the work task and required mobility.

Personal fall protection is not designed to be used as a tool for positioning or restraint. Rather, it should serve as a backup to a worker's balance, and to comfortably arrest a free fall or automatically lower the victim at a constant rate to a suitable location. Systems should be selected using a careful set of criteria that have been determined through the fall hazard analysis process and that are within the scope of the program.

☞ A personal fall arrest system must include not only the device and all the accessories, but also the service, repair and comprehensive instructions required for proper use. For instance, how would you know a fall arrest device is fully operational and reliable after several months or even years of service?

Orientation, Personnel Selection and Training

☞ **Orientation.** The need for training cannot be overemphasized! Training is the first step to increase awareness and to develop an understanding of the capabilities and limitations of available equipment. Initial training of the safety committee by a qualified person is needed to properly perform the fall hazard analysis. Then, supervisors or foremen can be trained on fall protection principles, techniques, and equipment performance. The "training of the trainers" forms the basis of an in-house, live training team. Ongoing training is as critical as the initial overview. Periodic training for trainers and end-users can serve

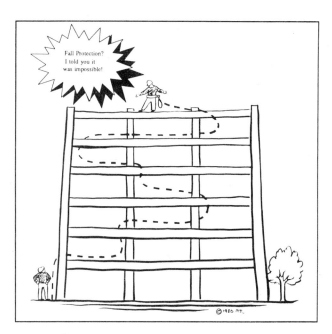

FIGURE 5.7
Planned access leads to planned fall protection.

to reinforce proper equipment use and care as well as provide an opportunity to review new technology. Training is the key to making workers aware of the danger and how to hook up the proper equipment, once anchor points have been selected. A fault tree analysis will disclose the equipment hazards to be closely watched for.

Personnel Selection. Climbing or working at heights is not a normal, routine job. The selection of workers who will perform elevated work tasks should be minimally based on the following:

1. No history of back or internal medical problems.
2. Not on medication.
3. A check of references on previous elevated work.
4. A willingness to be involved in planning the use of protective equipment during the job and to set a safety example for others.

☞ Employers should encourage local union shops to train and certify trainers and users. Workers should be trained first hand or, minimally, watch a live training session, then be tested.

Who should be trained and how? In all cases, fall arrest equipment is designed for people, and therefore people should have the opportunity to train with their personal protective equipment to learn its capabilities and limitations. The objective of training is to determine what additional skill, knowledge or understanding an individual or group needs to perform their responsibilities with maximum efficiency and effectiveness...without incidents. An understanding of the equipment and its limitations enables workers to work out simple sequences of moving with protection. Product warnings and instructions should be carefully read. Actual live, first-hand classroom or on-site experience is invaluable in a well-organized program.

Historically, and for obvious reasons, fall protection training with a 6-ft.lanyard and body belt has been limited to inspection and a few points on tying off when stationary. No trainer would ask workers to wrap a 1 3/4-in. strap around their waist and then drop 6 ft. to the end of an unforgiving rope or cable lanyard to find out exactly what their equipment will do when they need it. Training without experience is much like trying to teach a person to swim without entering the water. This is particularly important with life-protecting personal equipment. Consider the amount of performance training done with respiratory protective equipment. Why should fall arrest equipment be an exception?

Many arrest protection systems are now available with 1) low arresting force levels, and 2) an automatic function that does not require user manipulations. These systems can provide an opportunity to personally try out arrest protection equipment in a supervised training session with minimal risk of injury.

As with all personal protection equipment, training helps all workers understand the value of their equipment. This includes auto seat belts. The National Safety Council's "Convincer" program has been extremely effective in increasing each participant's appreciation not only of the hazard, but also of the protection provided by the "seat-harness." The forces that drive people horizontally through windshields are not that different from the incredible forces that develop during a vertical free-fall.

At the worksite, the more experienced workers need to be encouraged to use fall protection as an example to the more "unsafe" new and younger workers, so that fall protection norms can be instilled.

Among other general requirements for safety educators/trainers/instructors, a supervisor should also have the following capabilities and qualifications:

1. Plan fall protection for a project.
2. Perform (and enjoy) live, physical demonstrations.
3. Carefully supervise and exercise control.
4. Know the workers' expected behaviors.
5. Anticipate the objections and surmount them.
6. Fully understand the capabilities and limitations of the equipment based on product instructions.

FALL PROTECTION CONNECTOR INSPECTOR GUIDELINES

Checklist for snaphooks:
It is critical to inspect snaphooks regularly especially if they are kept exposed to the elements in order to keep them functional. Heavy wear and tear can also disable the lock over time through handling, abuse, misapplication, incompatibility or abrasion.
Snaphooks must close and must lock each and every time for life safety effectiveness.

Recommendations:
1. Check function regularly. Each hook must open and when pressure is released, close FULLY and lock RELIABLY each and every time by close observation of the user and by audit of a Competent Person designated by the employer or owner (OSHA 1910.66 Appendix C).
2. Avoid leaving equipment in areas exposed to dust, powders, dirt, salt, vegetable matter, salt atmospheres. Keep under cover if possible. After contamination, wash with water to loosen particles.
3. Check hook parts for wear/cutting or lock/abrasion/tampering with screwdrivers or other tools, use as a hammer, other forms of damage or disabling. Withdraw from use and destroy this equipment. Educate and train users.

4. Check spring
   a. in place
   b. fully functional in closing and locking
5. Check for damage
   a. bent
   b. jammed
6. Wash and clean hooks regularly. Oil or grease if hook will not attract dusts/powders, etc. Make sure that oil/grease has correct temperature range for location; generally use 100 degrees to +250 degrees F silicon sprays. Aim lubrication at rivet pivot points.
7. Check application: snaphooks are best connected to harness D-rings or other fall arrest attachments which cannot bring pressure to bear on the snaphook gate. Use anchorage connectors.

SUMMARY: Snaphooks must be fully functional at all times during usage, achieved through preventive maintenance programs.

WARNING! Malfunctioning snaphooks can accidentally and suddenly disconnect from attachments, resulting in catastrophic falls to a lower level, resulting in serious or fatal injury from almost any height.

FIGURE 5.8

HOW TO ORGANIZE A 100% FALL PROTECTION PROGRAM

7. Have experience in the field or be in the field.
8. Be satisfactorily tested on the principles of fall protection.

Fortunately, the younger workers are often more aware of hazards and are willing to participate in methods of protection. Video training tapes tailored to specific needs can be an effective medium for training. They represent an efficient way to convey information to short-term and long-term contractors to help them meet on-site fall protection requirements.

☞ Each plant or construction department should consider designing one or more videos to suit their specific work methods. You will find your work methods becoming much more efficient.

Finally, an area that is far too often missed is to ensure that the manufacturer's equipment instructions get to each and every user and remain accessible for periodic review. A checklist and "certified user" system could be used to identify who has had an opportunity to read and understand the instructions, as well as to train with the equipment.

Inspection and Maintenance

Like all equipment at a worksite, fall arrest systems need to be inspected and maintained regularly. Moreover, because they are safety systems designed to prevent serious or fatal injury, visual inspections before each use and periodic inspections and maintenance are vital. This should be done in accordance with the manufacturer's guidelines and written plant procedures.

Visual inspections before each use generally require a check for cracks, cuts, dents, distortion and excessive wear as well as for proper operation. If defective or questionable conditions are found, the item should be immediately removed from service, tagged and replaced. See Figure 5.8 for snaphook inspection guidelines.

Periodic inspection and maintenance by a qualified person would typically involve a closer and more thorough visual examination and appropriate cleaning. Permanent anchorage points should be periodically inspected by a qualified engineer and immediately following an accidental fall arrest.

Manufacturers should offer a reconditioning and recertification program for equipment. Many devices are intentionally sealed and must be worked on only by trained personnel. Taking regular advantage of an available manufacturer's program can help ensure management and user confidence in the device, by providing recertification of an "as new" condition. Other in-house programs, such as using color-coded tags to help monitor ownership or length of time in the field,

also can be developed.

Adequate provisions should also be made for the storage of fall protection and emergency escape equipment. An uncluttered, cool and dry location that is accessible to users is most suitable. For certain systems that remain outdoors continuously, depending on the materials of construction, a weather resistant cabinet can enhance reliability and help ensure that the equipment will be available to the user when needed. (See Chapter 7 for more information.)

Program Audit and Feedback

To continually improve any program, a means to gather feedback is important. This can be achieved in a number of ways, including formal conversations, questionnaires, interviews or suggestion boxes, to name a few. This evaluation is necessary to check that the elevated fall hazard control employed is working properly, and is the most suitable for the job. It also can serve as a means of addressing other exposures at the site.

Overall, an audit (of which there are numerous types published) can be used to assess the effectiveness of the fall protection program. It is an opportunity to see if previously set objectives have been met, and what changes need to be made.

☞ Since a fall protection program often flounders early on due to a mass of details left unanswered, an audit committee is essential to point out weaknesses and focus on removing blockages to progress.

Additional Considerations for Confined Entry Operations

In addition to addressing vertical fall hazards associated with confined space entry, a means of retrieval in an emergency must be preplanned. Confined space operations using personal fall protection control measures are outlined in table in Figure 5.9.

The selection of a confined entry and retrieval system should minimally include the following criteria:

1. Determine vertical distance of travel and method of access (fixed, temporary or mechanical).
2. Specify method of retrieval and allotted rescue time (mechanical or power).
3. Designate rescuers.
4. Determine suitable anchor point/design system (e.g., portable or permanent).
5. Evaluate other confined space aspects (e.g., opening, respiratory apparatus, multiple users, horizontal movement).
6. Sketch out fall protection and emergency retrieval

equipment usage.
7. Select compatible equipment.
8. Training, inspection and maintenance.

Return on Investment

Experience shows that a serious or fatal injury occurs on an average of every two to three years in companies where workers are regularly exposed to elevated fall hazards. Although this number may seem low relative to other injuries, fall accident severity is usually very high, perhaps the highest of all types of injuries, which are multiple in scope.

The cost of instituting a comprehensive fall protection program is negligible in comparison to the economic benefits an employer receives. Because the severity of a single fall incident is so high, whatever the existing general insurance and compensation insurance program coverage, relief from the crippling costs

of fall disabilities and death benefits should be immediate. With fewer or no elevated falls, there will be fewer payouts and fewer lost workdays, both of which translate into increased productivity.

Improved protection can enhance employee morale through a more secure feeling while working at heights, as well as enabling workers to share common goals and objectives in developing a valuable safety program.

By reference, the DuPont Safety Management Services Newsletter, Winter 1987, projected an average drop in lost workday cases of 86% after the fifth year for highly committed companies. DuPont has worked on safety programs for more than 16 years. The cost of a lost workday averages $18,650, according to the National Safety Council.

Construction projects using a fall protection policy requiring 100% fall protection have shown an average of 35% labor savings and lower material handling costs due to planning efficiencies.

CONTROL MEASURES FOR CONFINED ENTRY OPERATIONS

Confined Space Entry and Retrieval Operations	Control with personal fall protection.
Method of Vertical Access (either fixed or temporary)	Backup fall protection is needed.
Vertical Retrieval Method	1) Manual mechanical means suitable for up to 50 feet.
	2) Power mechanical means (with manual backup) may be more suitable over 50 ft.
	3) Minimum of 4:1 mechanical advantage; 6:1 or 8:1 preferable to allow one standby person to retrieve a victim.
Retrieval Time	Should be under 4 minutes to help avoid permanent brain damage (cardiac and respiratory arrest victims) unless alternate life support means are established.
User With Respiratory Equipment	A spreader bar and yoke configuration attached to shoulder D-rings avoids interference and enables vertical lifts through smaller openings.
Fully Body Harness	Can provide proper support during suspension and can position the body vertically for retrieval through the opening. Can be combined into work suits to help keep harness clean.
Narrow Openings	If a small opening diameter requires the arms to be overhead, wristlets can be used to hold up the arms, but a harness should always be used to lift the body weight, to avoid the possibility of arm dislocation. Some openings are so small they should not be entered even by a small worker, in case he or she needs to be rescued. OSHA is recommending a 24-in. opening as a minimum size for entry.

FIGURE 5.9

Review Questions

1. Workers have worn belts for years at a chemical plant but they rarely attach them to the structure. You have seen a film that shows how suspension in a belt after a fall can be a serious hazard to worker health. You decide to:
   a. Show the film to your workers.
   b. Discuss the merits of belts and harnesses.
   c. Show the film and statically suspend workers in a belt and harness.
   d. Since you haven't had a fall in years, nothing is needed.
   e. Route the film to your boss and purchasing.

2. You recommend a fall system which costs $2000/worker, as opposed to the $50 system they are presently using. Your ideas are rejected by management on a cost basis. Your next step is:
   a. Continue to use the same protection.
   b. Gather and present fall incident statistics from your industry.
   c. Develop and submit new policy guidelines, hold a live training session, build support.
   d. Attempt to get the price of the fall system down and resubmit.
   e. Start by purchasing one system for trial.

3. What maximum time limit should be planned for the rescue of a victim from a confined space to either the outside or to a refuge area?
   a. 1 minute
   b. 3 minutes
   c. 4 minutes
   d. 6 minutes
   e. 20 minutes

4. Everyone agrees with you that your company needs to control fall hazards and put a fall protection program in place. You organize it by separating work fall hazards and submitting solutions to engineering for approval of anchorage points. Engineering rejects your proposal for scaffolding because they cannot find a 5400-lb. anchorage point. What do you do?
   a. Exempt scaffolding from your fall protection requirements.
   b. Seek fall arrest systems with low arresting force levels that require less anchorage point strength.
   c. Build independent anchor structures.
   d. Require workers to tie off when stationary.
   e. Go over the engineering department's head.

5. You are a new Safety Director of a medium-size construction company. You have found it widespread practice for company managers, foremen and workers to pay lip service to a policy controlling exposure of workers to fall hazards in elevated areas for a good part of the time. You want an effective 100% fall protection policy; however, you understand there have been no falls during the past two years. What do you do?
   a. Evaluate fall hazard exposure and probability of a loss in order to focus your program.
   b. Recognize that falls are not a serious problem and continue with present program.
   c. Give an orientation program on fall protection methods with actual live experience.
   d. a and c.
   e. Observe and try to get workers to tie off.

INTRODUCTION TO FALL PROTECTION, SECOND EDITION

FALL HAZARD ANALYSIS

"Nowhere to fall but off,
nowhere to stand but on."

THE PESSIMIST, BENJAMIN KING (1857-94)

"It's bad luck to even discuss
fall hazards!"

STEEL ERECTOR FOREMAN, WILMINGTON,
DELAWARE, NOVEMBER 1986.

❖ How are fall hazards analyzed?

❖ Identifying hazardous exposures

❖ Appraising risk

❖ Classifying related tasks

❖ Prioritizing control measures

❖ Providing needed personal protection

❖ The engineering of anchorage points

❖ Interpretation of dynamic peak loads in fall
   arrest systems tests

6

How Are Fall Hazards Analyzed?

A hazard is defined as the potential to incur harm. The analysis of elevated fall hazards is a systematic process; it entails gathering pertinent information on work tasks that involve exposure to a potential fall from one level to another. Locating and evaluating those hazardous exposures that are most likely to result in a fall or that could have the highest severity are essential in developing effective control measures. Since an elevated fall usually results in a serious or fatal injury, a proactive approach is imperative.

OSHA's Instruction Standard STD 1-1.13 for General Industry is a minimum standard that distinguishes between what is predictable and regular fall hazard and what is not. For example, regular maintenance on a specific platform once every week, or four work-hours per month, would be classified as a predictable and regular fall hazard exposure. This is used for the application of the 1910.23(c) OSHA regulation. Less frequent exposure is covered under the 1910.132(a) personal protection equipment regulation.

Work method analysis should consider not only the location at which the task is performed, but also the required travel to and from that workstation. The objective is to gather enough information to determine the most practical means of continuous protection without reducing productivity. Data may be gathered through onsite observation, questionnaires, interviews and a review of literature.

Individual perceptions of what is involved in the completion of a work task, as well as what might be the appropriate means of personal protection, vary considerably. The architect's or engineer's idea of what is needed could be vastly different from how the worker might actually perform the work task and select protective equipment. Figure 6.2 illustrates this quandary.

Only collaborative effort between upper management, supervisors, foremen, employee representatives, and the safety department will achieve the most meaningful results.

Identifying Hazardous Exposures

☞ Fall hazard analysis begins by listing the work tasks that involve or could involve exposure to an elevated fall hazard. It is important to reemphasize that this should include travel. For example, a valve located in an elevated piperack that must be monitored regularly requires vertical and horizontal mobility for access and egress, but the actual work task may be stationary. Other elevated work, such as painting or sand blasting, may require more mobility.

Workers at an elevated workstation who, in an emergency, may become trapped, should not be overlooked. In this case an emergency escape system may be necessary as a primary or secondary means to automatically control descent for emergency egress.

When a task is considered an "industry work practice" with an accepted high level of risk, the usual reason is that no one has taken the time to analyze the job. More and more unsafe, so-called "industry work practices" are challenged every day. For instance, a no-fall-hazard steel erection process has been developed for both utility towers and building construction, both of which were once considered high risk occupations. A careful analysis can normally indicate the need and the means for modifying processes, facilities, operations, or work tasks.

A plant or facility can be broken down into sections or areas to help organize the identification process. Assigning a superintendent, supervisor or foreman who is familiar with all operations in a specific section will expedite a comprehensive review, using a local fall protection task group. Work tasks should be identified at a minimum by name and location.

Appraising Risk

Qualitative Risk Appraisal

☞ After identifying the individual elevated work tasks, appraising each exposure against a specific set of criteria

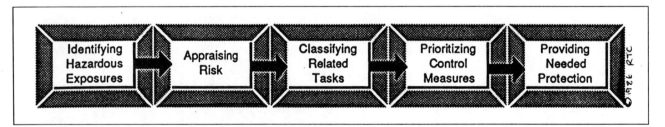

FIGURE 6.1
Analyzing a fall hazard takes these five steps.

FALL HAZARD ANALYSIS

enables the assessment of the relative risk. The appraisal should at a minimum include:

- A breakdown of vertical and horizontal movement.
- The number of workers involved.
- How often the task is performed.
- The length of time typically spent on the task.
- A general description of the workstation, with particular attention to potential obstructions in the fall path(s).
- A post-fall analysis to review expected self-recovery or the possible need for retrieval and rescue.
- Identification of influential environmental conditions, such as icy or wet surfaces.

Overall, the objective is to pinpoint the work tasks with the highest potential severity that are the most frequent. Assigning a value to each criterion and then ranking them all may represent an effective means to prioritize exposures for control measures.

Quantitative Risk Appraisal

To some extent, the risk of falling may be quantified for the purpose of prioritization. However, the seeming

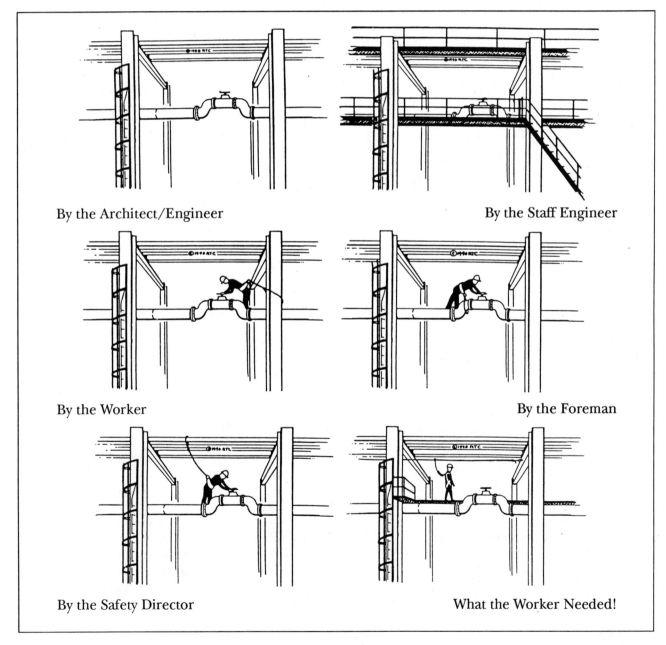

FIGURE 6.2
The classic story, as applied to identifying a fall hazard and achieving fall protection.

remoteness of risk does not eliminate the risk of falls, or justify ignoring the hazard. The big question to answer is, what is the worst-case consequence of ignoring a particular fall hazard? In the case of an elevated fall hazard combined with human error, the answer is obvious. Almost any accidental elevated fall over two stories is predictably fatal if the head, neck or spine are impacted, or the body is impaled. Yet almost any sudden impact on the body from any height can produce severe or fatal injuries. Conversely, a lucky landing into a snow bank, piled empty cartons, empty paint cans or soft ground, combined with landing on a suitable fleshy body part, can result in negligible injuries.

However, such an escape from injury cannot be relied upon. Compare this with the worst-case error of a punch press operator. In this example, the most severe foreseeable injury is limb and nerve damage, but not predictably a loss of life.

Falls, then, must be associated with the threat of loss of life or injury of catastrophic severity. The error impact for falls must always be very high. For general purposes, Alphonse Chapanis has analyzed workers' error probabilities, as shown in figures 6.4, 6.5 and 6.6.[1]

Figure 6.7 notes the criteria of risk appraisal.

When an error probability level of 3 or 4 is multiplied with an error severity level of 3 or 4, the result can be a risk level exceeding 13 points, meaning unacceptable. If the risk level is over 9 points, it certainly indicates a serious problem. Elevated fall hazards must be addressed by either measure of risk level – probability or severity – prior to any fall incident or lack of previous accident experience.

Note that although a similar appraisal of risk is made by OSHA Compliance officers, the trend in the U.S.A. is to emphasize the severity rating (error impact) as much more important than the modifying frequency rate (error probability). Therefore, any foreseeable exposure to a fall hazard needs to be addressed urgently in planning.

The chance of making an error resulting in an elevated fall is usually very low for those frequently exposed to high hazards, yet quite high for those where climbing and working in high places is often incidental to their occupations (e.g. sheet metal workers, painters, and mechanics).[2] Interestingly, the average age of the 210 ironworkers who lost their lives between 1981 and 1985 was 40[3]. This indicates greater complacency or errors as experience grows with members of this group, who are normally accustomed to working at heights. The big problem is that whether a worker is experienced with heights or not, that worker only has to make one major mistake in his or her career for his or her life to be permanently changed.

☞ Errors by skilled workers in trades are often related to unusual conditions, which combine to sneak up on a normally careful worker's lack of situational awareness. One example is a carpenter who was assisting in attaching slings to remove a 10-ft. column form at the edge of a concrete hotel/condominium complex 30 stories up. While signaling the tower crane operator to lift, he stepped back off the 6-in. slab and fell between the unguarded post-tensioning cables, left exposed because the tensioner had failed. He could not hold on to the greased cables long enough to be helped and fell to the ground. In another example, ironworkers may need to complete a lift at the end of the day, and they take short cuts. The sure-footed connector who usually "'coons" the beam may walk or run on top of the girder to catch the steel instead, and trips on a bolt placed on a beam. A gust of wind may catch him unaware. Also, epoxy-painted steel, dew patches in the shade, ice or dust all appear at various times of the day throughout the year to catch the unwary ironworker off-guard.

The time of day of ironworkers' accidents, according to a 1981-85 study, is usually just before noon,[4] just after lunch, or just before quitting time, when workers' personal guard is lower. The Air Force has similar statistics in a 1970-77 study.[5] These human fallibilities point to

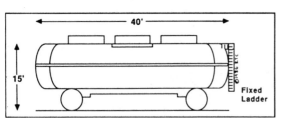

Outlined here is an sample analysis of a tank car/railcar work task that involves exposure to elevated fall hazards.

Situation: A tank car loading and unloading operation requires a worker to ascend the fixed ladder at the back of the car, traverse the top of the car, open each hatch, insert a hose, then return along the same route.

Required mobility: Vertical and horizontal.

Frequency: Job is performed regularly on a daily basis.

Fall hazard:
1) Falling from ladder, access platform or car (may be up to 25 ft.).
2) Falling inside the car tank or hopper.
3) Long falls and bouncing down the side of the car with traditional long lanyards.
4) Swing falls after moving horizontally away from a fixed anchorage.

FIGURE 6.3
Sample analysis of an elevated work task.

FALL HAZARD ANALYSIS

ERROR PROBABILITIES (CHAPANIS, 1986)

Probability	Frequency of Occurrence	Example
6 Frequent	A typical person is likely to commit this error frequently. Up to 1 in 100	Fail to attach a seat belt before starting to drive.
5 Reasonably Probable	A typical person is likely to commit this error several times a year. Up to 1 in 1,000	Slip in a bathtub.
4 Occasional	A typical person will likely commit this error several times during his lifetime. Up to 1 in 10,000	Drive the wrong way on a one-way street.
3 Remote	Although a typical person is unlikely ever to commit this error, it is possible for him to do so. Up to 1 in 100,000	Swallow poison by mistake.
2 Extremely Unlikely	One may reasonably assume that a typical person will never commit this error. Up to 1 in 1,000,000	Fall out of the second-story window of a house.
1 Impossible	It is physically impossible for a typical person to commit this error. Up to 1 in 100,000,000	Activate a microwave oven with the door open.

FIGURE 6.4

Common safety errors and their probability of occurence. Courtesy Alphonse Chapanis, 1986.

the need for a more disciplined work procedure, designed to be more error-tolerant.

Figures 6.8, 6.9 and 6.10 illustrate the results of several studies in ironworker fatalities.[6]

Classifying Related Tasks

Classifying related work tasks can assist the development of elevated fall hazard control measures. Like in the appraisal process, a list of criteria is compiled. "Climbing on fixed structures," for instance, could be used to group all fixed ladder climbing, regardless of whether the ladder was on a building, piperack, tank or chimney. Similarly, vertical confined space entries with fall hazard exposure are classified together because of

the additional need for emergency retrieval capabilities. Other considerations, such as horizontal movement, frequency, plant location, type of trade, multiple workers or the need for emergency escape, often represent additional essential criteria.

Prioritizing Control Measures

Once they are classified, exposures are prioritized for control measures. To begin reducing the probability of a loss, those elevated work tasks that have high risk and are reasonably straightforward are tackled immediately. For example, in the erection process of skeleton steel, the first fall hazard to be attacked is the exterior fall, perhaps using perimeter cables or nets during the lay-

ERROR IMPACTS (CHAPANIS, 1986)

Severity Level	Consequences	Example
4 Catastrophic	Almost certain to cause death or severe loss.	Touching a bare high-voltage wire.
3 Critical	May cause severe injury or major loss.	Diving into too-shallow water.
2 Marginal	May cause minor injury or occupational illness or damage.	Stumbling on a level sidewalk.
1 Negligible	Will not result in injury, occupational illness, or material damage.	Misdialing a telephone number.

FIGURE 6.5

Common safety errors and their severity of impact. Courtesy Alphonse Chapanis, 1986.

Actions Appropriate to Level of Risk (Chapanis, 1986)

Probability Level (Figure 6.4) x Severity Level (Figure 6.5) = Risk Level

Risk Level	Action
13+	This level is unacceptable and requires immediate changes in design or abandonment of the project, product, or procedure.
9 - 12	This level identifies potentially serious problems requiring innovative redesign and careful testing.
5 - 8	Although this level is not expected to cause serious problems, design changes should be made if they are technically and economically feasible.
1 - 4	Although redesign is not required at this level to reduce risk, design changes may still be recommended to improve usability or operability and to reduce user annoyance.

FIGURE 6.6
Courtesy Alphonse Chapanis, 1986.

Appraising Risk

Qualitative:

- A breakdown of vertical and horizontal movement; sketch out work task.
- Number of workers involved?
- How often is the task performed?
- Required work tools? (Including access)
- Length of time typically spent performing task?
- Determine obtainable anchor point strength.
- Set criteria for fall arrest equipment system.
- A general description of the workstation with particular attention to potential obstructions in the fall path(s); calculate fall distance.
- A post-fall analysis to review expected self-recovery or possible need for retrieval/rescue.
- Identification of influential environmental conditions such as icy or wet surfaces.

Quantitative:

- Error probabilities.
- Error impacts.
- Actions appropriate to level of risk.

FIGURE 6.7

out of the erection sequence. A new steel girder bridge over a river could have a sequence of erection where nets and horizontal lifelines are installed on to beams at barge level.

The fall hazard height limitation established within the fall protection policy as Rule One (see Chapter 5) also could be used to prioritize control measures along with frequency, duration and potential severity. For instance, a work task that is performed at height over 10 ft., performed weekly, takes more than 4 hours to complete and has a number of obstructions below the workstation, should be at the top of the list.

Work tasks that do not have any apparent sequence of movement, or those that have been ingrained as an "industry work practice" (such as certain roofing practices) may require additional analysis and planning. However, these should not be left until last, but be addressed concurrently with the more straightforward applications.

Providing Needed Personal Protection

The analysis of elevated work tasks is intended to determine the most suitable match between required worker mobility and the capabilities of the fall protection system. Whatever is selected should minimize the potential for personal injury without sacrificing productivity.

Consider our previous tank car loading and unloading operation (Figure 6.3), which requires a worker to ascend the fixed ladder at the back of the car, traverse the top of the car to the main center hatch, insert a hose, then return along the same route. A two-dimensional fall protection system that can be quickly accessed at ground level could provide continuous protected mobility, both vertically and horizontally.

The Engineering of Anchorage Points

Fixed stairs, fixed ladders, railed platforms, railed walkways and other standard means of access should always be considered in plant design for elevated workstations. For example, remote valve controls, manways and access panels that may be accessed once every 5 years should be designed with standard access means. Retrofitting suitable access should be considered for any elevated workstation visited once a year or more frequently (refer to Chapter 3) for temporary solutions to elevated access.

☞ We must end the blind eye to the use of railings, ladder rungs, and C-clamps (the "ironworker's widowmaker"). An engineering link to safety must be organized in recognition that workers will use anything they can find for anchorages unless they are instructed otherwise. Facilities engineers, project engineers, and plant engineering staff play a vital role in providing fall protection safety. Memos exchanged between the Safety Departments and Engineering Departments should clearly indicate the mutual intention and responsibilities. The desired work method

FALL HAZARD ANALYSIS

Ironworker Fatalities

	Steel Construction Fatalities	Precast Concrete Construction Fatalities	Total Ironworker Fatalities
1985	86	5	91
1986	61	5	66
1987	67	6	73
1988	65	4	69
1989	70	8	78
TOTAL	349	28	377

FIGURE 6.8

Relation Between Construction Activity and Fatalities

Activity	Number of Fatalities	Percent of Total Fatalities
Buildings and Plants		
• setting/connecting	45	12
• welding, bolt-up	52	14
• moving iron		
(includes rigging and crane service)	66	17
• decking	93	25
Rebar	7	2
Towers	24	6
Bridges	17	4
Precast	28	7
Miscellaneous	45	13
TOTAL	377	100

FIGURE 6.9

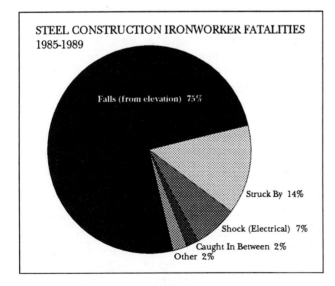

FIGURE 6.10
Steel construction ironworker fatalities.

Figures 6.8, 6.9 and 6.10
© Hardesty, Charles, Charles Culver and Fred Anderson. "Ironworkers' Fatalities in Construction." Occupational Hazards Magazine (June 1993).

must be established and documented in a fall protection plan, where the anchorage points are approved and incorporated into engineering drawings.

Engineers look for the long-term reliability of proposed anchorage points and for their use in presently unforeseen ways. They are likely to want to over-engineer for this reason. Therefore, where anchorage points are necessarily below 5,000 lbs. per person for vertical lifeline anticipated use, such as on antennas, order pickers, wood roof ridges, and many other places, engineers must know the criteria for the fall equipment to be used. Company or plant rules, which limit fall equipment force levels to 600-650 lbs., are very useful in guiding operating management and purchasing in what they should be buying. To prevent specific anchorage points from being used for attaching hoists and powered come-alongs, they should be painted yellow or orange and clearly tagged with their

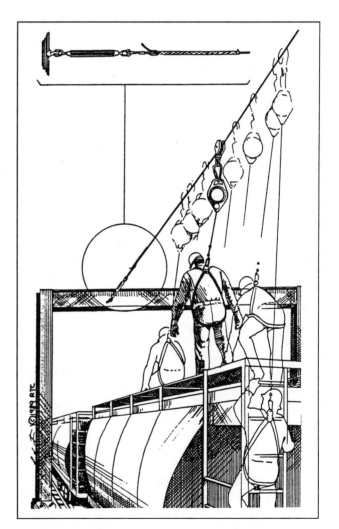

FIGURE 6.11
Note how the anchorage point (circled) for this fall protection task is designed with the worker's methods in mind.

ANCHORAGE POINTS STRENGTH REQUIREMENTS, OSHA 1926

	Current	Proposed
Vertical Lifeline for use with rope grab	5,400 lb.	5,000 lb.
Retracting Lifeline	N/A	3,000 lb.
Emergency Escape Controlled Descent Device	N/A	N/A (1,800 lb.)
Boatswain's Chair Loadline	5,000 lb.	5,000 lb. (or 6 X max. intended load)
Rescue Ropes	2,650 lb.	3,000 lb.
Special Engineered System for Fall Arrest	N/A	Static strength must be twice max. arrest force of fall device
Restraint or Positioning Systems	N/A	3,000 lb. (except boatswain's chair, 5,000 lb.)

NOTE: Check your local OSHA Office for regional requirements.

FIGURE 6.12
OSHA has established requirements for anchorage points strength.

usage rating – for example, "3,000 lb. load capacity for personal fall arrest attachment use only."

Specifically, let's deal with the engineer's key questions.

- What forces are your present fall protection systems seeing? (Refer to Appendix A-2)
- What forces must you design for in horizontal lifeline systems? (Refer to Appendix A-3)
- What must be done to prepare a worksite for installing fall arrest equipment? (Refer to Appendix A-4)
- What fall protection is outdated? (Refer to Appendix A-5)

If you design 1,200-lb. anchorage points for receiving a maximum of 500-600 lb. forces, you must require using the correct fall equipment in the correct way. Thus, a very close working relationship is needed between the safety director, the engineer and the purchasing department, especially for temporary systems. When you design anchorage points for a construction project or repair job, you should consider the topography of the work site and how workers move around, and preferably review videos of previous work methods (See Figure 6.11).

If the anchorage points are not strong enough, do not neglect your responsibility to help the safety director find a practical solution to the problem, which only you can do. Then, carefully document your solution.

Interpretation of Dynamic Peak Loads in Fall Arrest Systems Tests

The shock absorption properties of a fall arrest system must be measured and reported accurately if they are to be of value. Proper reproducible testing is vital. Traditionally, a sandbag has been used to simulate the movement of the human body in testing a lineman's belt and pole strap. This is reasonable up to a point. Since the focus is now on arresting force, not just strength, a test weight made of solid steel is preferred for more reproducible results.

Measuring instruments have a sensitivity represented in hertz (Hz). The force transducer, which is used to measure maximum arresting force (MAF), can register from 0.1 Hz to 10,000+ Hz. However, the fall equipment test rig may interfere with the test results obtained as low as 250 Hz and produce spurious values, unless these undesirable frequencies are filtered. In Britain, for many years, a 1,000-Hz sensitivity level was chosen. But the human body is a very much better shock absorber than a steel weight, and the exact reproducibility of a drop is a difficult task, so the mid-height of the wave was deemed to be the appropriate force level documented by the force transducer in a fall test.

Work done by Harry Crawford of the National Engineering Labs in Scotland for the British Standards Institute has shown that a sensitivity of 100 Hz is more than adequate for personal fall device force measurement.[7] Ulysse and Sulowski have shown that a steel test weight produces a force 20% to 50% higher than an anthropomorphic dummy does.[8] And Chen Wang estimated forces 50% to 100% higher than the human body.[9] OSHA has adopted a 1.4:1 force factor of a steel weight to the human body. In the U.S.A., a maximum sensitivity level of 100 Hz to 125 Hz has been proposed, based on a report to the ANSI Z359 Committee by Jim Brinkley of the Aerospace Medical Research Laboratory at Wright-Patterson Air Force Base. This recommendation is based on ejection studies, cadaver skull resonance, and related data.[10]

At 100 Hz or 125 Hz, the actual dynamic peak should be recorded when a fall system arrest force is charted.

FALL HAZARD ANALYSIS

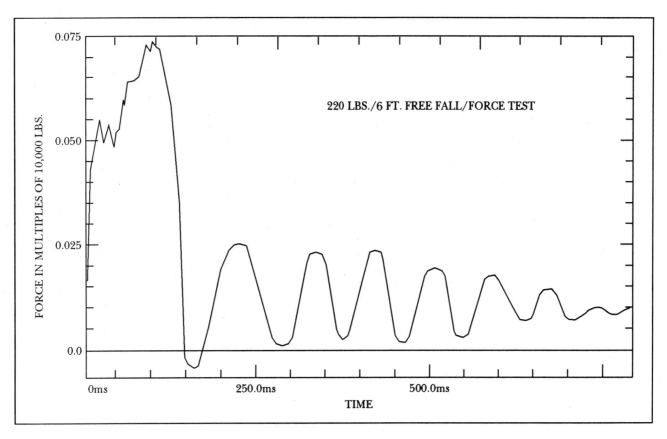

FIGURE 6.13
Fall force testing results, copyright 1990, Research and Trading Corporation.

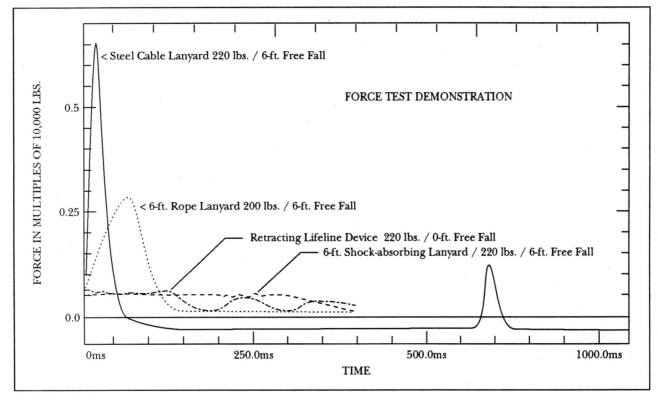

FIGURE 6.14
Force test demonstration results, copyright 1990, Research and Trading Coporation.

See the graphs in Figures 6.13 and 6.14 for the results of two force test demonstrations. All resonance due to the test rig and other unrelated peaks can then be eliminated or disregarded. OSHA has adopted the requirement that the test rig have a maximum deflection of 0.04 inches (1mm) when a 2,250-lb. static force is applied vertically[11].

Notes

1. Chapanis, Alphonse. "To Err is Human, To Forgive - Design." Speech given at the American Society of Safety Engineers, Nations Conference, New Orleans, LA, June 1986.

2. Proceedings of the U.S.A.F. Highwork Safety Conference. Air Force Inspection and Safety Command (AFISC). December 5-7, 1978.

3. *The Ironworker Magazine* (September 1986): 54.

4. Ibid.

5. Working Safety in High Places-A Study of U.S.A.F. Accidents 1970-77. Air Force Inspection and Safety Command (AFISC), Norton Air Force Base.

6. Hardesty, Charles, Charles Culver, and Fred Anderson. "Ironworkers Fatalities in Construction." *Occupational Hazards Magazine* (June 1993): 47-48.

7. Crawford, Harry. Letter to OSHA. National Engineering Laboratory. E. Kilbridge, Scotland. May 1986.

8. Ulysse, J.F. and A. C. Sulowski. "Fall Arresting Systems: Dynamic Load Test Conversion Factor Defined for Various Types of Test Mass." *Professional Safety* (May 1982): 32-36.

9. Wang, Chen H. "Free Fall Restraint Systems." *Professional Safety* (February 1977): 9-14.

10. Brinkley, James W., et al. *Evaluation of Fall Protection by Prolonged Motionless Suspension of Volunteers.* Harry G. Armstrong Aerospace Medical Research Laboratory, Wright-Patterson Air Force Base, 1986.

11. Federal Regulations 29 CFR 1910.66 App. C.

Review Questions

1. A rail car unloading procedure requires the operator to climb up the ladder at the rear of the car and walk along the tank to open the hatches. A worker falls off and suffers severe head injuries. What procedures do you recommend in the future?
   a. Tie off to the rail surrounding the hatch.
   b. Exercise greater caution when on top of rail cars.
   c. Use a combination of horizontal and vertical lifelines.
   d. Use a portable extension ladder to directly access the hatch.
   e. Build a scaffold next to the car with a fold-down ramp.

2. What is the quickest means of gathering information on elevated fall hazard exposures?
   a. Observation backed up by video of work methods.
   b. Interviews with workers and supervisors.
   c. Review of literature and available industry news.
   d. Accident analysis.
   e. Association meetings and seminars.

3. What criteria suggest that an elevated fall hazard has a high risk?
   a. Most frequent.
   b. Greatest elevation.
   c. Most severe.
   d. Most frequent and severe.
   e. Workers request fall protection.

4. How can elevated fall hazards be classified?
   a. By required mobility.
   b. By type of trade.
   c. By the capability of on-hand equipment.
   d. a and b only.
   e. By rescue time.

5. What is the overall purpose of analyzing fall hazards?
   a. To match equipment capabilities with required mobility.
   b. To identify exposures.
   c. To eliminate areas that are not significant.
   d. To determine those trades that should be exempt from the fall policy.
   e. To prevent reoccurrence of fall incidents.

WHICH FALL PROTECTION SYSTEM SHOULD BE USED?

With the right to choose
comes the responsibility
to choose wisely.

-INDIANA JONES IN *THE LAST CRUSADE*

❖ Part I: Hierarchy of Fall Protection Solutions

❖ Part II: Fall Arrest Equipment Capability

❖ Part III: Residual Hazards Associated with
the Use of Fall Arrest Equipment

❖ Part IV: Equipment Inspection and Maintenance

Knowing how to use fall arrest equipment is as essential as having it; using safety equipment improperly is the same as not having it at all.

This chapter is divided into four parts. Part I reviews the order in which fall protection solutions should be implemented. Part II discusses the various types of fall protection equipment available. Part III discusses the residual hazards associated with the use of fall arrest equipment. And Part IV provides guidance for equipment cleaning and maintenance.

Part I: Hierarchy of Fall Protection Solutions

☞ A person's balance should be backed up with a positive, effective means of fall protection. This means that administrative changes should seldom be used. Good fall protection control management calls for a priority system to tackle foreseeable fall hazards, as follows, in this order:

1. Eliminating fall hazards
2. Preventing fall hazards
3. Arresting falls
4. Administrative techniques

Eliminating fall hazards means finding a way to avoid the necessity of exposure to heights. For example, building a roof truss framework at ground level is better than assembling it in the air.

Preventing fall hazards is the provision of same-level barriers, such as floors, walls, covers, guardrails, handrails and perimeter cables.

WHAT IS FALL PROTECTION?

Continuous fall protection uses one or more of these means:

Fall Prevention
   Warning Lines at least 6 ft. from edge
   Barriers, Covers
   Guardrails
   Perimeter Cables

Fall Arrest:
   Safety Nets
   Walls, Fences
   Platforms, Buckets, Aerial Lifts
   Scaffolds, Planking
   Fall Arrest Equipment Systems

FIGURE 7.1
The means to achieving fall protection.

Arresting falls is the proper use of fall arrest equipment such as safety nets and personal protective equipment (fall arrestors), where there is sufficient clearance.

Administrative techniques are those procedures that deal with work methods to reduce fall hazards, such as specific routing to a certain elevated work area, or the correct way to set up a ladder. Where edge fall hazards occur, the use of warning lines set back from an edge is reasonable. Debatable methods include the qualified climber concept, safety monitoring close to roof edges, one-time-allowed exposures for inspection or job quotation, warning signs, and just plain old "being careful". The "qualified climber" is an attempt to rationalize training and frequency of climbing. However, the author believes this concept is convenient but futile. Perhaps it should be renamed the "lucky climber" concept. One mistake in a worker's career is all it takes to disprove this theory.

Figure 7.1 defines what means are used to achieve the end of continuous fall protection.

From this primary hierarchy of fall protection arises another hierarchy – that of work platforms and how workers access them. In order of desirability, they are:

1. Eliminate the need for access/fall protection
2. Engineered platforms
3. Aerial platforms
4. Scaffolds (temporary platforms)
5. Work positioning using belts/seats
6. Ladders and administrative techniques

Part II: Fall Arrest Equipment Capability

The purchaser has the important responsibility for choosing and using fall arrest equipment only for the application recommended in the literature, instructions and on the label. Companies should never allow the use of manufactured equipment in applications not recommended by its manufacturer.

For example, don't expect a saddle belt to be applicable for fall protection unless the manufacturer states that it is. Also, don't expect a snaphook to be functional when attached to an angle iron edge, bolt hole, or small D-ring. And don't expect a lineman's or tree trimmer's belt and strap lanyard to provide dynamic fall protection, other than static support around a pole above a step or brace in the first case, or where crotched and around an up-branch or leader in the second case.[1] The purchaser must match the fall protection or work positioning system with the application, and it must be used that way by the worker as a result of diligent training and work observation.

Only one fall arrest system per worker is required for proper protection. However, if the worker is

WHICH FALL PROTECTION SYSTEM SHOULD BE USED?

THE FOLLOWING IS A SUMMARY OF ANSI Z359.1 KEY REQUIREMENTS FOR FALL ARREST EQUIPMENT AND FALL ARREST SYSTEMS

Full body harnesses (FBH) are permitted for fall arrest.
Body belts are not permitted for fall arrest.
Horizontal lifelines are not addressed in this standard.

Fall arrester (FA) classification:
Type 1: Used on vertical lifelines (VLL)
Type 2: Used on horizontal lifelines (HLL)
Type 3: Used on a lifeline of any orientation

System Components	Min. Strength	Min. Side Load	Min. Gate Load	Proof Load
Snaphook	5000 lb.	350 lb.	220 lb.	3600 lb.
Carabiner	5000 lb.	350 lb.	220 lb.	3600 lb.
D-Ring	5000 lb.	N/A	N/A	3600 lb.
O-Ring	5000 lb.	N/A	N/A	3600 lb.
Buckle	4000 lb.	N/A	N/A	N/A
Lanyard Rope	8500 lb.			
Lanyard/EA	5000 lb.			
Straps	5000 lb.: 1 5/8 in. min. width			
Anchorage Connector	5000 lb.			
Harness, Static	5000 lb.: 1 in. max. slip through buckles			
Fall Arrestor	3600 lb.: Salt spray at 48 hrs.			
Synthetic Rope Lifeline	5600 lb.: Max. 22% elongation at 1800 lb.			
Wire Rope Lifeline	6000 lb.: Min. Diameter 0.3125 in. (8 mm)			
Vertical Lifeline Subsystem(VLSS) (YLLSS)	5000 lb.			
Self-retracting Lanyard (SRL)				
SRL - Static	3000 lb.			
SRL - Dynamic	1000 lb.: AFTER dynamic test			
SRL - Rope Line	4500 lb.			
SRL - Webbing	4500 lb.			
SRL - Wire Rope	3400 lb.			
SRL Retraction Force	1.25-25 lb. range			
Steel Test Weights	Dynamic Performance Test: 220 lb. ±2 lb. (Also test torso)		Dynamic Strength Test: 300 lb. ±2 lb.	
Wire Rope Termination	80% of wire rope			
Adjustable Lanyard	2000 lb. min. slip force			

Test Conducted	Min. Opening Force	Max. Elongation	Max. Arrest Force (MAF)
Lanyard (L) Dynamic Performance Test*		42 in.	1800 lbf.
Energy Absorber (EA)*	450 lb.	42 in.	900 lbf.
	Max. Arrest Distance	**Max. Arrest Force**	
SRL Dynamic Performance Test*	54 in.	1800 lbf.	

System Tested	Max. Lanyard Length	Max. Deceleration Distance	Max . Torso Angle	Max. Arrest Force
Full Body Harness + Lanyard	6 ft.	42 in.	30 deg.	1800 lbf.
Full Body Harness + Energy Absorber	6 ft.	42 in.	30 deg.	1800 lbf.
Full Body Harness + Energy Absorber + Lanyard	6 ft.	42 in.	30 deg.	1800 lbf.
Lanyard + Energy Absorber	N/A	42 in.	N/A	1800 lbf.

Continued on next page

FIGURE 7.2A

Summary of ANSI Z359.1 key requirements for fall arrest equipment and systems.

System Tested	Max. Arrest Distance	Max. Arrest Force
Fall Arrester Connecting Subsystem (FACSS)	54 in.	1800 lbf.
FACSS (Max. 3 ft. fall arrester to full body harness)	54 in.	1800 lbf. Min. strength after Dynamic Performance Test: 1000 lb.

System Tested:	Torso Weight	Free Fall	Feet First	Head First
Full Body Harness + Lanyard (integral)	220 lb.	6 ft.	one test	one test
Full Body Harness + Fall Arrester + Vertical Lifeline	220 lb.	6 ft.	one test	one test
Full Body Harness + Lanyard + Fall Arrester + Vertical Lifeline	220 lb.	6 ft.	one test	one test
Full Body Harness + Energy Absorber + Fall Arrester + Vertical Lifeline	220 lb.	6 ft.	one test	one test
Full Body Harness + Energy Absorber + Lanyard + Fall Arrester + Vertical Lifeline	220 lb.	6 ft.	one test	one test
Full Body Harness + Self-Retracting Lanyard	220 lb.	4 ft.	one test	one test
Full Body Harness + Energy Absorber + Self-Retracting Lanyard	220 lb.	4 ft.	one test	one test
Lanyard + Energy Absorber	220 lb. (Test wt.)	6 ft.	N/A	N/A

Qualification Tests**	Torso Weight	Test Weight	Free Fall
Full Body Harness + 4 ft. Test Lanyard	220 lb.		3.3 ft.
Lanyard		220 lb.	6 ft.
Energy Absorber		220 lb.	6 ft.
Self-Retracting Lanyard Dynamic Performance Test		220 lb.	0 ft.
Self-Retracting Lanyard Dynamic Strength Test		300 lb.	4 ft.
Fall Arrester + Vertical Lifeline Dynamic Performance Test	220 lb.		6 ft. or max. allowed by system
Fall Arrester + Vertical Lifeline Dynamic Stength Test	300 lb.		6 ft. or max. allowed by system

Anchorages
3600 lb. When certified
5000 lb. When not certified

---

* SRL + EA integral must meet same tests as SRL and not extend more than 24 inches beyond SRL.
Test instrumentation requirements: 1000 samples/sec. minimum sampling rate;
active response band up to 100 Hz (+1/2dB - 3dB).

** Environmental test preconditioning: Heat: 130 deg. C.
Cold: -40 deg. C.
Wet: Spray for 3 hrs.

NOTE: Careful reading of this standard in its entirety is required for proper understanding. In addition to Requirements and Qualification Testing summarized above in numerical context, the following parts are important to read:

Scope and definitions
Marking and instructions
User inspection maintenance and storage of equipment
Equipment selection, rigging, use and training
Acronym cross-reference
Illustrations

NOTE: *Snaphook* is referred to as snaphook in the Z359.1-1992 Standard and in OSHA 1910.269(g); as snap-hook in OSHA 1910.66 Appendix C; and as snap hook in older standards.

□

FIGURE 7.2A (continued from page 87)
Summary of ANSI Z359.1 key requirements for fall arrest equipment and systems.

permitted to use the fall arrest system as a tool, for example by transfering weight to it for support, then a second backup fall arrest system is required. The first line of protection against falls is the worker's balance. A fall arrest system is the backup.

The ANSI Z359.1 fall protection standard presents guidance for safety system components. Figure 7.2 summarizes this standard's key facts and requirements regarding fall arrest equipment. Figure 7.2-B offers the author's proposed equipment testing adaptations for better meeting these ANSI requirements.

Selecting Fall Arrest Equipment

A variety of equipment is available to help employers set up an effective fall protection program. Generally, this includes nets, body support mechanisms, climbing protection systems, vertical and horizontal lifeline systems, confined entry and retrieval systems and controlled descent-emergency escape systems.

The proper selection and purchase of safety equipment alone does not constitute a fall protection program. This is only one step. A complete, effective program ensures that:

SUGGESTED TESTING FALL ARREST EQUIPMENT FOR LIGHT AND HEAVY WORKERS

For non-standard conditions and for proper qualification of individuals to do work, the following is proposed:

1. **Fall Arrest Systems for workers over 310 lbs. up to 400 lbs.:** OSHA allows up to 310 lbs. including tools maximum weight for one person using a fall arrest system according to 1910.66 Appendix C.

For weights from 310 lbs. up to 400 lbs., the following is suggested:

Force Test:	Drop test weight 300 lbs.:	
	Free fall:	6 ft. free fall lanyard systems
		0 ft. for self-retracting lanyards/lifelines
Strength Test:	Drop test weight 425 lbs.:	
	Free fall:	7.5 ft. free fall for lanyard systems
		4 ft. for self-retracting lanyards/lifelines

Note:
Human weight 310 lbs. up to 400 lbs. including tools. Fall distances remain the same as current OSHA requirements 1910.66 Appendix C. Basis of testing is by ratio of weights and convenience in assembling torsos of appropriate weight. All systems shall incorporate shock/energy absorbers.

Results:
Force test 900 lbs. limit for harness.

2. **Fall Arrest Systems for workers over 90 lbs. but under 130 lbs.:** ANSI Z359.1-1992 limits workers to 130 lbs. including tools minimum weight for one person using a fall arrest system.

For weights from 90 lbs. to 130 lbs., the following is suggested:

Force test:	Drop test weight 100 lbs.
Strength test:	Drop test weight 300 lbs.

Note:
Human weight 90 lbs. up to 130 lbs. including tools. Same free fall as above and for regular OSHA tests. Basis of testing is weight test appropriate to weight range of users; upper limit allows for use by average range of workers. All systems shall incorporate shock/energy absorbers.

Results:
Force test 900 lbs. limit for harness.

Summary:
Each type fall arrest system should be labeled to reflect usage by the intended weight range. All other requirements of OSHA 1910.66 Appendix C/Z359.1 apply.

FIGURE 7.2.B
The author's suggested testing fall arrest equipment for light and heavy workers.

1. appropriate anchorage points are established by the employer;
2. proper inspection and maintenance procedures are developed and carried out according to manufacturer's instructions; and
3. workers are trained and supervised regularly in proper application and use.

Following is an overview of the principal types of fall protection and emergency escape systems.

Nets

Nets may not save all people who fall from a project under construction, but they can do their vital part. For example, the first major construction project reputed to have employed safety nets is the Golden Gate Bridge. Fifty years after the bridge was built, an article commenting on the builder, Joseph B. Strauss, noted that his insistence on using nets paid off. The nets, Strauss said, saved 19 persons during the construction period, limiting occupational fatalities to 11 lives.[2]

Nets are designed to provide passive fall protection under and around an elevated work area. That is, the worker is not directly involved by "wearing" fall protection equipment. Rather, the net is there to catch a falling worker before he or she hits the ground or an obstruction. There are two major types of nets, one for personnel and the other for debris. Often they are combined.

Personnel Nets

Personnel nets can be used where many workers are employed, such as in bridge construction or repair and long-term structural projects. They are also used where large open areas or long leading edges expose workers to height hazards (up to 25 ft. below the work surface by current OSHA rules), and the use of personal fall arrest equipment is deemed impractical or not feasible for the work method. On bridges, nets can provide interior and exterior protection.

On buildings under construction, nets can provide exterior protection. Internal nets are often used if interior falls can exceed 25 ft. or two stories, according to current OSHA Steel Erection rules such as Stair or Elevator Openings. If interior decking is done more rapidly, falls could be limited to one story internally, but even this fall distance may not be acceptable to safety professionals who can plan movement with fall protection limiting falls to 6 ft. or less.

Passive net fall arrest equipment, once installed, serves to arrest workers' falls without any active or conscious effort on their part. The advantage of nets is that individual worker training is not required. Once installed, nets are always in place and ready for use for the designated fall hazard. However, personal fall arrest protection must be provided during both net installation and removal.

One of the best systems to use is one where the net support cables and brackets are attached to trusses and girder sections before they leave ground or barge level. Then, with the load slightly raised, the net is fed under and snapped to cables on each side. The object is to provide a problem-solving session early on, to mate the fall protection plan and erection sequence together.

Personnel nets must be manufactured and tested in accordance with ANSI A10.11-1989 and OSHA 1926.105 requirements.[3,4] Mesh openings may not be greater than 6 in. x 6 in. Additionally, nets meeting these requirements must bear labels displaying the manufacturer's name and date of manufacture, together with testing data.

Nets should be as close to the work level as possible and must not be lower than 25 ft. (except with bridges, where the highest work level is considered the lowest part of the bridge by OSHA), and must extend outward 8 ft. from the structure. A National Bureau of Standards test report[5], however, proposes a 15-ft. extension. This is based on a worker's center of gravity projecting at least 7 1/2 ft. after falling 30 ft. According to ANSI A10.11-1989, nets must be tested in the field at successive 6-month intervals by withstanding a 400-lb. sandbag dropped from a 25 ft. height, without sustaining any broken strands. An engineer's evaluation report may be substituted.

OSHA has proposed new safety net extension standards for general industry (see Figure 7.3).

Debris Nets

Debris nets are designed to catch falling debris, such as tools, foreign objects, falling concrete and other construction debris, and to protect workers and pedestrians below. The strength and size of the mesh must be sufficient to sustain the impact, catch the size and sustain the weight of the objects that are likely to fall. Typical net sizes range from 1/4-in. to 3/4-in. mesh. To catch large and heavy objects as well as small and light objects, smaller mesh nets can be used in conjunction with larger mesh and stronger personnel nets.

Debris nets should project sufficiently beyond the perimeter of a building to catch falling construction materials or packaging from a given height. A single perimeter net system projecting 8 ft. beyond the exterior edge at the fourth floor level, for example, may not be adequate to catch objects dropping from the 20th.

Nets also can be used to catch both personnel and debris. In these cases, personnel nets must be used in conjunction with debris nets, and the nets must be cleared of debris on a regular basis to help ensure a

WHICH FALL PROTECTION SYSTEM SHOULD BE USED?

falling worker's protection. Use of pivoting brackets can help to keep the net from interfering with crane loads, and also simplify attachment of the net section to supporting cables.

Interior nets refer to personnel nets used on the interior of a structure.

Perimeter nets are installed along the outside perimeter of a structure where a worker could fall on the exterior. In this case, the personnel net should be placed under the debris net and the net always kept within 25 ft. of a potential fall.

Exterior perimeter netting vertical panels are frequently used in Japan and Europe to provide same-level debris containment. They can also provide a measure of personnel containment similar to using guardrails. These tightly-meshed nets are suspended close to each open-sided perimeter of a building under construction and are attached tightly to perimeter cables on each floor level. They often envelope the entire building. In 1987, New York City required this type of panel netting on buildings under construction with a 5-ft.-high installation on each floor.

A 42-in. perimeter cable meeting the 3-in. deflection rule and equipped with a vertical net panel attached firmly to the floor may substitute for a toeboard and midrail, according to OSHA (Lawrence Greenberg, Pearlweave. Personal correspondence to the author.)

☞ The installation of nets requires careful planning. Aerial lifts, manbaskets or personal fall arrest equipment is needed to protect workers exposed to a fall hazard while installing the nets, or when moving them. Nets and/or horizontal lifelines can provide many answers to fall hazards if they are planned, installed and used.

It should be noted that netting or tarpaulins or their equivalent, when used for wind or weather protection on scaffolds, require calculation to determine adequate stability against turning over or collapse.

Personal Fall Arrest System Components

All components comprising a personal fall arrest system must be used as part of a tested personal fall arrest system.

Body Supports

Body Belts
A body belt, sometimes known as a safety belt or waist belt, is a strap that workers secure around their waists and to which they attach lanyards or other devices.

☞ In practice, most belts are used (either by design or intermittently) for leaning, so that a worker's balance depends entirely on the belt and lanyard. When this is the case, a worker normally balanced on his or her feet has no backup fall protection. Therefore, harnesses have superseded belts in many areas of the world for fall arrest use.

Work positioning belts can still be used in addition to full body harness fall arrest systems to assist reaching a workstation. The ANSI Z359 Committee has not recognized body belts for fall arrest use. OSHA requires a 4-ft. freefall test for work positioning belts in its proposed 1910.130 standard. The author believes that belts may still be reasonable for fall arrest use if the total fall distance is less than 2 ft., reasonably enabling swift self-retrieval. (Suspension tests were conducted for OSHA at Wright-Patterson Air Force Base in 1986. These tests are discussed in the section on Potential Hazards: Body Belt Use for Significant Fall Arrest, later in this chapter.)

Safety managers may decide that harnesses are the correct general solution for a plant for all

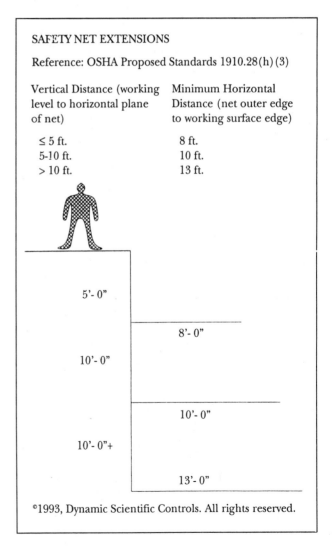

FIGURE 7.3
New safety net extensions from OSHA.

applications of fall arrest because the decision is easier to enforce.

Leather, which has been prohibited for body belts by ANSI A10.14 and OSHA 1910.66 Appendix C, has been replaced with more durable synthetic webbings, such as nylon and polyester. Belt widths typically range from 1 3/4 in. to 4 in. or more. The greater the width, the more support and comfort afforded to the worker's midsection during wear and before a fall arrest. The overall benefit is small, however, when the fall actually occurs, experience has shown. See Figure 7.4.

The configuration of the D-ring(s) to which a lanyard or device is attached depends on the type of protection needed. For example, a single D-ring at the center of the back would be for fall protection while working, whereas a front D-ring is designed for climbing with a fixed climbing protection system.

A modification of the body belt is the chest-waist harness, which also works for very limited falls. The higher position of the D-ring allows a more tolerable suspension after a fall. However, a proper fit around the waist is essential, and is something which workers may neglect because shoulder support can hold the harness in place. This means that a fall with a loose waist belt could have catastrophic consequences as a result of the worker falling out of the harness.

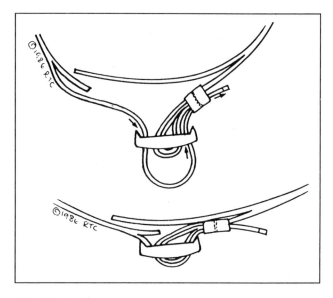

FIGURE 7.5
Example of a friction buckle, single pass design. Warning: single-pass and double-pass belts should never be mixed for work crew use, because doing so magnifies the unreliability of the double-pass belts to an unacceptable level.

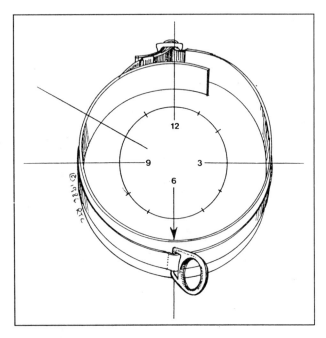

FIGURE 7.4
D-ring locations. Different D-ring locations serve different functions: Front D-ring (10 o'clock) is for climbing protection; Back D-ring (6 o'clock) is for fall arrest; and Side D-rings (3 o'clock and 9 o'clock) are for work positioning.

Body belts are designed to fit snugly around the waist between the rib cage and pelvic crest. Tongue-buckle body belts are effective only if the worker wears the correct size to ensure a snug fit. Under no circumstances should any user punch extra holes in the belt. Moreover, if the user can only pull the webbing through the buckle to the first grommet, then a larger belt should be requested.

Friction buckle body belts should only be worn by workers who have received instruction on how to properly use and adjust the buckle. A single pass friction buckle eliminates the extra pass back that a double-pass friction buckle needs to safely work, and that may be overlooked by a worker or become "too much trouble." For either, a minimum 5-in. webbing tab should always be maintained through the buckle for a secure attachment. Friction buckle belts can provide a proper snug fit for a broader range of users than tongue-buckle belts.

Many people ask which is stronger, a friction buckle or a tongue buckle? The answer is simple – when worn properly, both are strong enough to do the job. When pulled, both distort or creep well below the 5,000-lb. webbing strength. But both will support the worker if properly fitted and if the other parts of the lifeline system can absorb the shock. See Figure 7.5 and 7.6.

Note that friction buckles can loosen over time unless webbings are tightly held. Also, tongue buckles can come undone if excess webbing is not held securely due to snagging. In addition, tongue buckles can uncouple if they are loose (especially on harnesses).

WHICH FALL PROTECTION SYSTEM SHOULD BE USED?

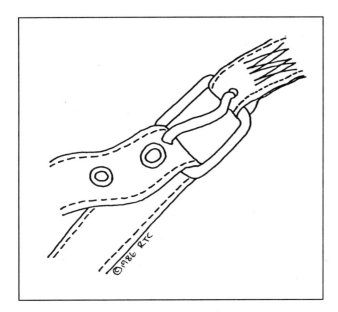

FIGURE 7.6
Example of a tongue buckle.

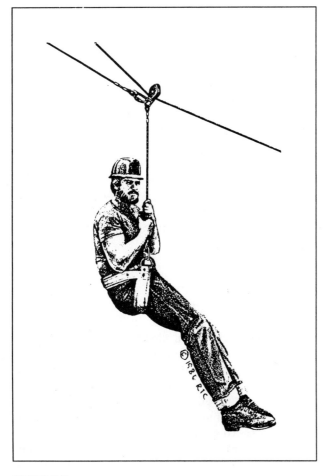

FIGURE 7.7
Example of a saddle belt being used for climbing and as well as for escape from oil rigs.

Work-positioning Belts and Harnesses

The saddle belt, also referred to as a tree-trimmer's or rigger's belt, is equipped with an extra subpelvic strap that is designed to provide support during climbing or positioning. The user is cradled in a relatively convenient sitting position for working for short periods or for suspension during emergency descent (Figure 7.7).

Other types of positioning belt systems are:

Lineman's belt and strap. This system is intended for positioning only. The equipment should meet a 4-ft. free-fall test of a 250-lb. bag of sand as well as the OSHA electrical resistance tests (the strap must withstand 25 kV/ft. ac for 3 minutes, dry, with no deterioration, and 3 kV over 1 ft. with a maximum leakage of 1 mA). If a lanyard is used in place of a pole strap, or vice-versa, OSHA requires a 6 ft. drop test.

Window cleaner belt system. This system should meet a 250-lb. steel weight fall test through 6 ft. (ANSI A39.1 and OSHA) because of the flexibility of movement required for this work. The A39.1 Standard calls for an anchor bolt strength of 6000 lb. minimum.

☞ Work positioning harnesses are becoming popular for form and rebar work. Employers must be careful when training workers to explain the proper use of each D-ring. The two side D-rings work together with a rebar chain/hook or lanyard for positioning, and the rear upper back D-ring is only for fall arrest. Some electric utilities have opted for separate components of work positioning (lineman's belt) and fall arrest (harness); others have combined them. It should be noted that if a belt/harness is used for work positioning, then fall arrest equipment also must be used if a fall hazard exists.

Full Body Harnesses

☞ Harnesses today are very different from the cumbersome heavy-duty designs of the past. They are light for almost all applications. A full body harness (sometimes still called a parachute harness) that can distribute arresting forces over the seat and shoulders as opposed to the soft, vulnerable midsection is preferred. A harness without a waist belt helps ensure unrestricted breathing, while an extra seat strap spreads the arresting forces on the most suitable part of the body, the buttocks, and provides additional support during suspension. (See Figure 7.8.) For female workers wearing harnesses, shoulder strap arrangements do not appear to be a hazard, although being suspended in them may cause some discomfort.

Chest straps between the shoulder strap should be worn above the breastline for both men and women, but below the collarbone, which limits any choking hazard after a fall. Once secured, this strap can be worn "loose" to avoid strap abrasion on the neck and chest (especially for women). Additionally, these designs typically are very painful under the arms during suspension, and the harness acts more as a belt during fall arrest.

☞ Color-coding harness top and bottom straps can help workers put the harness on easier, faster and with less frustration. Waist straps or rib straps which encircle the body give rise to harness sizes. Finally, a sliding back D-ring can help absorb force and position the body upright for optimal support during and after an arrest. This is particularly helpful for vertical retrieval through confined space openings. Full body harnesses with multiple D-rings that may allow fall arrest equipment to be inappropriately attached should be avoided, unless users are thoroughly trained. The Canadian CSA Z259.11 standard requires that each D-ring is given a prescribed letter to identify its purpose.

Harness D-ring attachment points typically are as follows:

1. Back D-ring on the upper back for fall arrest.
2. Side D-ring on each hip, usually with pelvic strap support for work positioning.
3. Shoulder D-rings on the shoulder for retrieval using a spreader bar.
4. Chest D-rings in the middle of the chest for ladder climbing systems and descent.
5. Shoulder Strap D-ring in the rib area for ladder climbing systems.

Because of potential misuse, the most simple harness with a back D-ring is recommended for most applications.

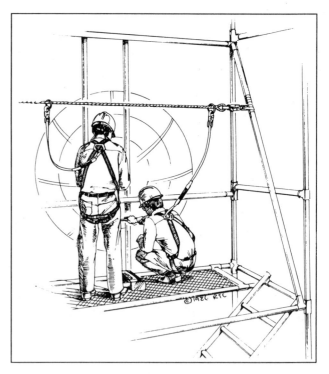

FIGURE 7.9
Example of a shock-absorbing lanyard in use. Note that anchorage strength requirements can be engineered down with specially designed fall arrest systems. (See Chapters 2 and 4 for details.)

As a special safety consideration, female workers with long hair should wear their hair "up" when on the job in order to avoid entanglement in sliding back D-rings. Wearing a ratchet-style hard hat helps.

It is important to note that harness designs should keep the back D-ring high on the back during use. Likewise, chest straps should remain high and above the breast line. D-rings lower than mid-back and chest straps lower than the solar plexus could result in fall-out if a head-first fall occurs.

Lanyards

A lanyard is a short, flexible rope or strap webbing connecting a worker's safety belt to the anchorage point or the grabbing device on a lifeline. OSHA requires at least 1/2-in. diameter synthetic rope for a lanyard[6] (5/8 in. minimum in Ontario). Some people recommend a 9/16-in. or 5/8-in. diameter lanyard rope to anticipate worker slack rope applications involving sharp-edge, wrap-around attachments, but this is not recommended in Canada. There is no limit to the length of a lanyard, but 2, 4 or 6 ft. are common lengths to help limit falling beyond a 6-ft. free fall maximum.

In cases where work task mobility can be limited to 6 ft. or less, for instance in bucket trucks, personnel lifts (such as in Figure 7.9) or outside of a guarded area,

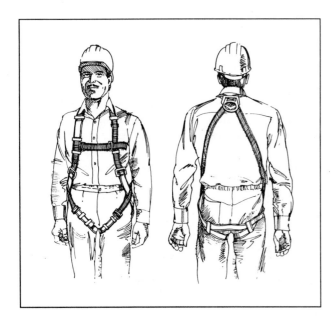

FIGURE 7.8
Example of a popular full body harness, with no waist strap. A subpelvic strap provides support after a fall.

WHICH FALL PROTECTION SYSTEM SHOULD BE USED?

lanyards can provide up to 6 ft. of protected mobility. Minimum attachment height should be at or above the level of the D-ring to ensure that any free-fall distance will be less than 6 ft. It is vital to have as little slack as possible in order to limit the free-fall distance to which a worker is exposed. Manually adjustable length lanyards should be used to take out slack where possible. In all cases, they must be connected so they allow no more than a 6 ft. vertical free-fall.

Unlike basic cable, web or rope lanyards, shock absorbing lanyards not only significantly reduce arresting forces on the body, but also provide a means to determine in-service loading. Typically, they include web-tearing or fiber stretch systems that activate during the fall arrest to absorb the energy developed. Shock absorbing lanyards usually have a warning label that is designed to appear after in-service or shock loading, in addition to the obvious deformation that clearly indicates that they have been stressed. This is a decided advantage over rope, web or cable lanyards; it is difficult, if not impossible, to tell if they have been in-service loaded. All loaded lanyards must be destroyed and replaced.

Shock absorbing lanyards offer the benefit of easy inspection and detection of use which should enable easier field inspection. Their primary benefit, however, is in reducing fall arrest forces.

With the use of shock absorbing lanyards, arresting forces should be limited to an average of 600 to 650 lbs. (be sure to request specific data from the manufacturer). This minimizes potential compounding injuries and also permits users to experience an actual fall arrest in training. Shock absorbing lanyards definitely should be used where longer free-falls are anticipated, or where steel cable lifelines and web lanyards are employed. A web shock absorbing lanyard tends to be stronger than rope when bent over edges and is easier to inspect than rope for wear and tear. Warning: Be sure to evaluate all edges over which lanyards may pass during a fall for catastrophic cutting potential.

Connecting Snaphooks

Locking snaphooks that require two separate forces to be opened can greatly reduce the potential for accidental disengagement or "roll-out".

Roll-out can theoretically occur when the fall arrest forces are transferred back through the lanyard or system with a twist, causing a single action snaphook to

---

CONSIDERATIONS IN THE SELECTION OF ANCHORAGE POINTS FOR LANYARDS AND LIFELINES

Members of the committee should be ready to consider the following points for lanyards and lifeline systems where workers must change from one anchorage point to another frequently.

1. Will you preselect the required anchorage points (tie-off points, installation points) for the predicted work area? Will you allow webbing or rope lanyards to be attached over sharp angled structures and then hooked back into the lanyards? Will you allow lifelines and lanyards to be wrapped around angle iron or each other and knotted?
2. Anchorage points should be 5400 pounds minimum strength for fall protection systems that allow free falls up to six feet, or alternatively, 3000 pounds for retracting lifelines that allow free falls of two feet or less. Since no worker can tell the true strength of a structural member, what should management do to increase fall safety reliability without exposing the worker to understrength anchorage points?
3. Can you designate each anchorage point location by painting it yellow or another bright color? Can you use specific bolt holes in I-beams or, perhaps, arrange overhead horizontal lifelines?
4. Can you make the anchorage rigid, and independent of the work station, or must you use cables? Have you calculated forces for falls from a horizontal lifeline to be sure the anchorages are strong enough?
5. Have you determined that the anchorage must be at least waist height to limit free fall from lanyard systems or, alternatively, have you determined the overhead height for reeling-type lifelines and escape systems?
6. How does the worker move from one work station to another, or climb up or down from a work station, without exposure to falls?
7. What will you have the worker hook up to when there is nothing above him/her but air?
8. Can you think of a safe method to install the fall devices so that the first worker up is not exposed to a fall hazard?
9. Can you think of a safe method to remove the fall device or lifeline from the anchorage so that the last worker is not exposed to a fall hazard?
10. Can you anticipate dangerous swing falls on lanyards or fall devices which call for additional anchorage considerations or horizontal lifeline installation?

Reprinted with permission of *Best's Safety Directory*.

FIGURE 7.10

Considerations in the selection of anchorage points for lanyards and lifelines.

ride up and around an anchorage, depressing the gate and suddenly disengaging the hook, potentially leading to a catastrophe.

Part III of this chapter contains guidelines for appropriate and compatible use of hooks when attaching to an anchor. Considering the practical level of field control, particularly when lanyards are wrapped around a structure and hooked back into themselves, it may be wise to use locking compatible (double-action) snaphooks across the board.

Other hardware, such as bolts, shackles, D-rings, and metal links, as well as snaphooks, are used to connect parts of a fall protection system together. OSHA currently requires 4000 lb. static tensile strength without permanent distortion.[7] ANSI A10.14-1991 required a 5000 lb. test without failure for positioning hooks only.[8]

D-rings must be proportioned in order to minimize accidental disengagement and help eliminate roll-out potential, as described in ANSI A10.14-1991.[9] Snaphooks must be attached to compatible hardware and never to each other to avoid unpredictable consequences. (See Figure 7.11.)

Knots: A Traditional Method of Connection

Not many supervisors are confidently knowledgeable about the different strengths and functions of the slide and lock type hitch knots that are sometimes used for attaching lanyards to lifelines. For those who have the knowledge, properly proportional triple hitch knots, assembled in tandem for extra security, are a highly reliable means of grabbing a lifeline. However, there are too many combinations that appear to work with just a manual tug but may not do so in a fall. Variabilities in knots are even greater for anchoring the lifeline itself.

The simplest bowline (a nonslipping bend knot) has traditionally been used for anchoring a 3-strand lay rope lifeline. It has been criticized because of its small bending radii, which can dramatically lower the tensile strength of the line.

The tracing, or follow through, figure eight knot for attachment around anchorage points has been recommended in at least one publication as a substitute for the bowline. The termination strength retention using the figure eight might be attributable to its construction, which bends more smoothly around two lines under stress, as opposed to the construction of a knot like the bowline, which bends sharply around and closely to one line. (See Appendix A-5 for more discussion on knots.)

The ease of tying, untying, and correctly tying the tracing figure eight are other reasons for favoring it over the bowline, double bowline (double bight) and other variations. However, the properly-tied bowline is reported to be much stronger than many hitch knots

---

CONSIDERATIONS FOR SNAPHOOK SAFETY

For Snaphook Attachment to Harnesses or Belts:
   The snaphook and belt or harness D-ring must be matched in a manner endorsed by the manufacturer.

For Snaphook Attachment to Anchorage Points:
   1. The snaphook must be matched to the eyebolt or other hardware as endorsed in writing by the manufacturer.
   2. No snaphook should be attached to any rope, cable, chain, or web lanyard unless endorsed by the manufacturer for specific applications.
   3. All snaphooks must be fully closed onto the matched anchorage point in a manner which does not stress the keeper or reduce the strength of the hook. Users should not rely on the sound of a hook closing; they should check it visually.
   4. Snaphooks that become ineffective because of lack of maintenance, dirt, wear and tear, or abuse, should be destroyed. "Ineffective" means bent, stressed, distorted, or exhibiting total or partial spring failure. Only snaphooks which operate in as-new condition should be used. Regular maintenance checks are required, as well as continued worker education, to make this effective.
   5. All possibilities for accidental disengagement ("roll-out") should be addressed by the Safety Director based on the normal type of work and work practice in the industry, particularly where the snaphook may receive a sudden load in an orientation where the hook must twist around the anchorage point.
   6. For applications where snaphooks do not have a history or demonstrated reliability, consider eliminating the snaphook entirely, or consider a forged shackle with a threaded bolt.
   7. Never attached a snaphook to an anchorage for horizontal lifeline use because of the additional dynamic load.

Reprinted with permission of *Best's Safety Directory*.

FIGURE 7.11
Considerations for snaphook safety.

WHICH FALL PROTECTION SYSTEM SHOULD BE USED?

and others that have one diameter rope bands and are subject to major stress.[10]

It is not unusual for workers and supervisors to clash over knot reliability because of their personal history and alleged experience, rather than established tested methods. There are several thousand knot variations and no one person has the skill to instantly know the characteristics of one type of knot on a specific diameter rope, nor can the knot be certified. Using mechanical grabs or other fall arresters is suggested, except perhaps for rescue squads and true emergencies with qualified personnel.

The spliced eye rope with 5 tucks, or kernmantle; a locking snaphook; and a properly-sized eyebolt remain the optimum choice for anchorage point termination hardware. Building owners need to equip roof areas with parapet or tie-back eyebolts for attaching safety lines and riggings for suspending scaffolds. Window cleaning contractors need to request these safety features when submitting bids to an owner. (Refer to Appendix A-5 for more information.)

Climbing Protection Systems

Climbing protection systems are distinguished from most lifeline systems by their inelasticity (a cable or rail rather than a rope, for example) and their ability to withstand long-term outdoor exposure. Protecting workers climbing on structures such as poles, ladders, towers, bridges, antennas, or rigs can be accomplished with taut cables or rigid rails running centrally or alongside the structure. The worker's body support is attached to the cable or rail by means of a climbing device that is designed to move freely up and down, but lock the instant a fall is sensed. OSHA does not permit ladders with negative inclines, with or without safety devices or cages.[11]

Basketcage protection consists of metal hoops installed around fixed ladders, according to an OSHA requirement (1910.27).[12] This arrangement offers the advantage of one-time installation, low maintenance and little or no training requirements. ANSI A14.3-1992 permits ladder safety systems to be used with cages for more safety.

OSHA requires protection for fixed ladders more than 20 ft. high or deep (if underground or in a confined space).[13] ANSI A14.3-1992 specifies 24 ft. but the author believes protection should be wherever practical, regardless of minimum height.

Ladder safety devices used in lieu of caging or wells require no offsetting landing platforms, and the ladder climbing safety system may extend the entire length of the ladder with rest platform breaks at 150 ft. maximum.

Since OSHA's standard on fixed ladders, in 1910

Subpart D, has been proposed for revision, OSHA Program Directive 100-57 makes ladder safety devices essentially an equal alternative to caging for all fixed ladders and not just those on chimneys, towers and water tanks.[14] Cages are recognized by safety professionals as failing to provide positive fall protection. They provide at best, perhaps, psychological comfort and "resting points." Therefore, climbing protection systems should be used in addition to cages for effective personnel protection. They are especially needed on tall ladders where workers become fatigued, if only for their economical advantages over cages in this application.

The psychological comfort or freedom from height vertigo experienced by climbers and others at heights is explained by the psychological response found in all normal persons to controlling the "falling over" illusion.[15] In 1978, Brandt, et. al. found that the retinal shift of visible stationary surroundings while the body is moving is the signal to activate sway correction. Quoting Brandt, "The visual detection of these surroundings causes increase in body sway when the distance increases. Beyond 45 ft., the perception of one's dangerous body shift is lost, saturating at 60 ft. distance. Presence of stationary objects within the peripheral visual field and maintenance of the head and body in the correct gravitational plane reduce this type of anxiety."[16]

Another type of height disorientation is alternobaric vertigo, caused by a rapid change in elevation, such as in an elevator in a tall building.

Experiencing one or more forms of vertigo can lead to an anticipated fear of heights, or acrophobia.

There are two main types of permanently attached climbing protection systems: a rigid rail carrier (Type I) and a flexible cable carrier (Type II). The rail or cable, called a carrier by ANSI A14.3-1992 and MIL-S-87966 (1980), runs the entire length of the ladder or tower and is a permanent fixture.[17]

For both types of systems, a sliding device or sleeve attaches the worker's body support to the carrier. The sleeve then travels up and down the carrier while the worker ascends and descends. Should a fall occur, the sleeve locks onto the carrier. Sleeves can be captive and remain on the carrier at all times, or removable to allow transport between many ladders and indoor storage.

Body support of choice is rapidly becoming the harness with a center or side frontal D-ring. A side frontal D-ring helps roll the body away from the ladder during a fall.

Belts should include a front D-ring (10 o'clock) if the rail or cable is in the center of the ladder. Side D-ring (3 and 9 o'clock) belts may be used if the rail or cable is on the side of the ladder. A close orientation between body support and sleeve is essential for the device to sense and arrest a fall quickly.

Cables

Vertical Cable Systems – A flexible cable-type climbing safety system is suitable for lower heights, such as illu-

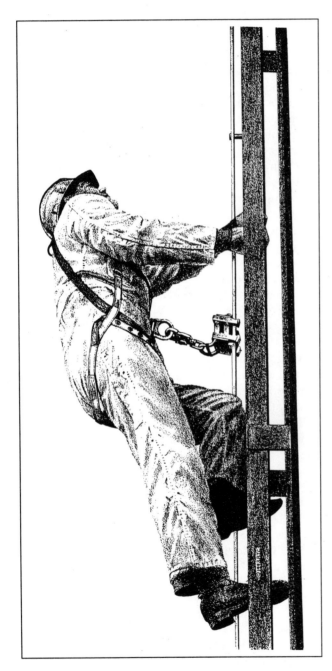

FIGURE 7.12.1
Example of a fixed rail climbing system. Note that this variation of the fixed rail climbing protection system incorporates the climbing structure itself into the rail. Specially-adapted "climbing boots" attach to horizontal bars which slide up and down each side of the rail, in addition to the center sleeve at waist-height. This can provide for more sure-footed climbing.

mination or communication poles and underground shafts, provided frequent inspections are conducted, preferably from an aerial lift. Cable devices are either captive or removable from the cable. Removable devices that involve the minimum of pins and parts are preferable, using one hand for installation if possible, and are ideal for use outdoors. For indoor applications, captive devices are always present and ready for use.

The advantages of cable-type systems are low cost and simple fixture to the brackets at the top and bottom of the climbing structure. Their disadvantages center around the weathering properties of steel cable outdoors, which may also affect the performance of sliding devices as well as the reliability of a single upper fixture point.

The cable should be kept taut by tightening devices to prevent damage caused by wind vibration. Cable guides should be positioned every 15 to 40 ft. to provide protection from wind whipping, and also to control bowing as the climber ascends or descends.

Cable guides that do not require manual manipulation to pass them are preferable. Weather resistant synthetic cables with long lifetimes in corrosive atmospheres are available. They offer the additional advantage of radio frequency transparency for antennas. Synthetic cables must be protected from wind abrasion with the structure by suitable clearance spacing.

Rails

Vertical Rail Systems – Rigid rail systems include shapes such as 1/4 in. x 2 in. bars, tubes (with or without notches), and various extruded channels and rails. These are usually available in steel, aluminum or fiberglass to suit the environment.

The advantages of rail-type systems are easy inspection, low-cost maintenance, and the fact that they allow several workers to climb at the same time. Structural attachments every few feet make these systems inherently more reliable and maintenance-free than cable-type climbing protection, which depends on a single upper fixture point. See Figures 7.12.1 and 7.12.2 for examples of fixed rail climbing systems.

Rail systems on tall towers or stack ladders can enable workers to use the sleeve to rest at any point they choose. However, since there is no backup when a worker leans back, a separate lanyard should always be used. Fall protection systems are for emergency use only.

Turntable systems in the rail can allow shift to horizontal movement mode in some designs (see the section on Permanent Systems in this chapter).

ANSI A14.3-1992, which only addresses fixed rails and cables, requires a 500-lb. weight drop test with 18 in. of freefall on climbing protection devices.[18] Note: The 500-lb. weight is a rationalization of an incapacitated climber of 250 lbs. being rescued piggyback style by a work buddy who also weighs 250 lbs., and both are 9 in. above the body support to climbing device connection.

The weight must be arrested. The test should be conducted at the weakest points of the system, such as at the top of or just below a rail splice. Fiberglass rails must be very carefully tested because of their sudden break characteristic under dynamic loads. According to this ANSI standard, an accidental fall should be arrested within a 6-in. sleeve movement.

Ladders that are not in use must be marked clearly or closed off with a suitable gate. The selected short connecting means must be long enough to avoid cramping the climbing style, and snaphooks should be useable with the heavy gloves associated with climbing ladders or those used in winter conditions.

For either system, a climbing extension above the dismount level ensures a protected transition and should be accompanied by tying off with a lanyard before the belt and safety sleeve are disconnected when on unguarded platforms. Climbing sleeves can also be prevented from unintentionally sliding off the top of the rail by using a "top stop," usually consisting of a protruding nut spacer and bolt. For underground or tank ladders with manhole covers, portable or retractable climbing extensions are recommended for protected access.

Rail is best for systems that may not be inspected with sufficient frequency.

Self-retracting Lanyards/Lifeline Devices

Automatic self-retracting lanyards/lifeline devices are finding increasingly practical applications for climbing protection on oil field rigs and during tank entry, as an alternative to ladder climbing devices. See the example in Figure 7.13. These retracting cable devices either lock to arrest a fall or lower one worker at an automatic rate following a fall, providing emergency descent.

Retracting cables are particularly helpful where a ladder angle of 10 degrees requires more body distance away from the ladder than is practical with climbing sleeves. Cables need to be kept free of dirt or salt deposits, and should be replaced if kinking occurs, interrupting normal use.

OSHA recommends a 250 lb./6 ft. drop test for fall

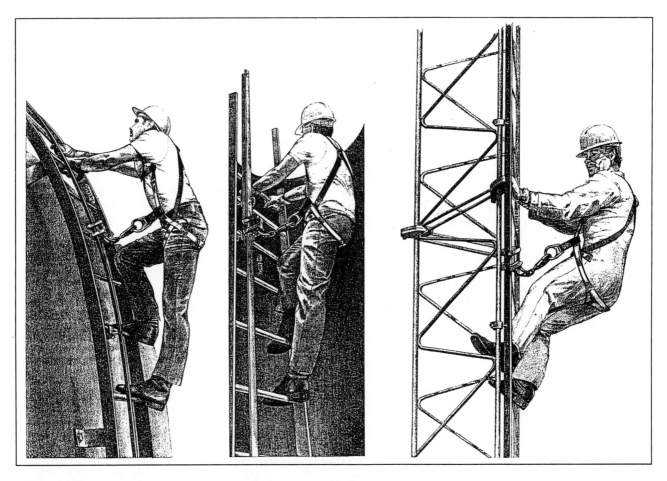

FIGURE 7.12.2
Three examples of rigid rail systems on fixed ladders. (Left) Curved ladder with rail system requires elevation of rail to handrail height near fineel ball. (Middle) Vertical rail system with side mount avoids frontal body impact. (Right) Guyed radio tower with rail mounted to side for climbing case and more foot space.

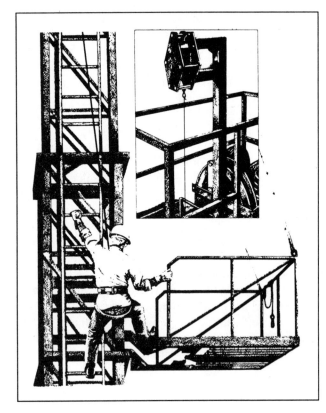

FIGURE 7.13
Workover rig climber transferring to tubing board with self-retracting lifeline protection.

arrest devices, and a 7 ft./sec. or less descent speed for lowering devices (1926.1053).

☞ Self-retracting lanyards/lifeline devices are suitable for outdoor climbing protection when they can be regularly inspected and maintained. Some applications in cold weather may require longer linkages and larger snaphook connectors to accommodate gloves and heavy clothing.

Climbing Assists

For long ladder climbs on structures such as drilling rigs or towers, a cable counterweight system, using a saddle belt, is often preferred as a "personal elevator," which reduces fatigue. The counterbalance weight should also permit a reasonable safe descent for emergency escape. Therefore, the weight should be carefully adjusted and tested to suit each user.

A device that can provide an automatically-controlled rate of descent, regardless of worker or counterbalance weight, can provide more reliability than simple pulley systems. This overspeed system combines climbing assist, fall protection and emergency escape, and is addressed in the proposed OSHA 1910.270 standard for oil and gas well drilling and servicing.[19]

First-Worker-Up Devices

When a company decides to make fall protection a mandatory requirement as of a certain date, a temporary system often must be used to achieve compliance where fall hazards occur before the permanent system is installed. Although this is sometimes burdensome in the short run, it can still be effective. A useful system for towers and ladders is a system which allows a telescopic reach to an anchorage point known to be adequate.

A first-worker-up portable climbing system consists of a shepherd hook on a pole, which incorporates a retracting lifeline or rope grab and can be pushed up to snag structural members. After climbing approximately 18 ft. to 20 ft., the climber belts off before pushing the pole further up the tower.

Portable systems can be used safely if they are practical and if the users avoid contacting conductors. Systems with dielectric properties should be tested by the user under his conditions of use.

Lifeline Systems

A lifeline is a vertical line that extends from an independent anchorage point, and to which a lanyard or body support is attached, using a grabbing device. This line should be at least 1/2 in.-diameter nylon or polyester (5/8 in. in Ontario). 5/8 in. polypropylene or 3/8 in.-diameter steel cable, all of which must have a minimum breaking strength of 5000 lbs.[20] Steel cable should be used only in spark or heat producing work operations, although it is popular for use with work at extreme heights such as chimney and bridge building and repair, where a limit on the lifeline elongation may be important. Ropes must always be protected from abrasive or cutting edges such as parapets.

Weather-protected nylon and polyester lifelines with neoprene jackets are available. Waxed polypropylene ropes are popular with electric utilities because of the low moisture absorption and high dielectric value. Ultraviolet (UV)-stabilized 5/8-in. or 3/4-in. polypropylene has become popular as a lifeline for many swinging scaffold operations because of its light weight and lower cost.

The proper light stabilization additives are critical in order for polypropylene to be as reliable as nylon and polyester, according to The Cordage Group. This is especially true in sunnier climates such as Florida, Hawaii, and southern California. The use of polypropylene containing a carbon black additive for lifeline applications seems very important in order to retard light degradation.[21]

Another lifeline design is the jacketed kernmantle. These tough lines resist dirt and prolong life, but are difficult to terminate effectively.

WHICH FALL PROTECTION SYSTEM SHOULD BE USED?

Contemporary lifeline systems are designed to go beyond the limitations of a belt and 6-ft. rope lanyard. They provide workers with protection from the time they leave the ground or grade level until they return, thus combining mobility with protection.

The two major types of lifeline systems, vertical and horizontal, can function independently or be integrated to provide two-dimensional fall protection. Lifeline systems should not be an excuse for not providing proper access or work platforms. For example, if a lifeline system is typically held by workers for balance, it is no longer being used as a lifeline. Similarly, if a lifeline is used to protect a worker in a silo who is trying to unblock a grain jam, the lifeline will be of little help in preventing asphyxiation if the grain shifts from underneath his or her feet.

Lifelines should be used for fall protection from suspended platform failure, overreaching, or edge exposures. The employer must correctly choose equipment for controlling specific job fall hazards. Be sure to account for long fall arrest distances typically found with rope grab lifeline systems.

Vertical Rope Grab Lifeline Systems

A rope grab is a device that connects the worker's body support or lanyard to a lifeline. It is designed to arrest a fall mechanically, bringing the worker to a full stop. Originally, this was a specific rope knot, called a hitch, tied by the worker to the lifeline. The Province of Ontario still recognizes the triple-hitch knot as a means of attachment to a lifeline.

However, with new or relatively untrained workers on the job, simple mechanical devices with predictable and tested locking features are preferred by safety

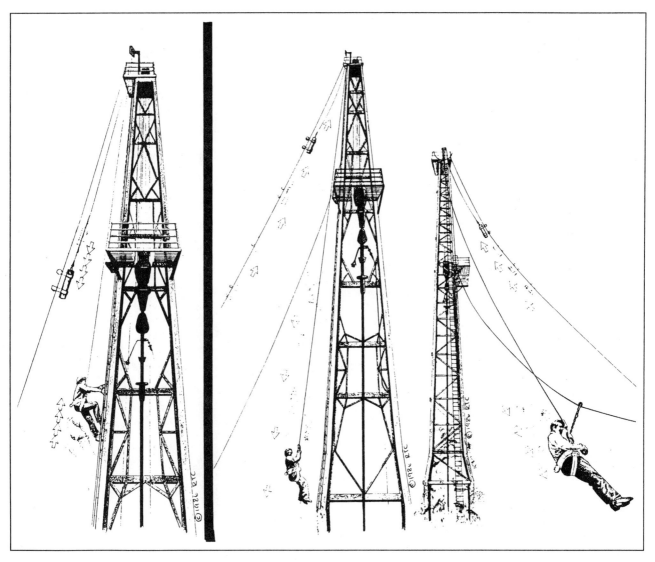

FIGURE 7.14
Left to right: Examples of climbing assist, fall protection and emergency escape.

directors and loss control managers to provide more reliable protection. In the event a fall incident occurs, mechanical rope grabs also provide a diagnostic tool for investigating what really happened, and whether the connection was ever made. Knots, however, might vanish after a fall incident.

Standard procedure with all fall injuries is to preserve the equipment in a safe place immediately after the incident, along with shoes, gloves and tools.

There are two types of cable or rope grabbing devices which can operate on wire cable or synthetic rope respectively: the manually operated grab and the mobile grab. Each must be compatible with its lifeline, and backed up by dynamic and operating tests for each line used, since no one can tell what may happen in a fall unless the drop test has been done.

Some grabs are captive, requiring the rope to be

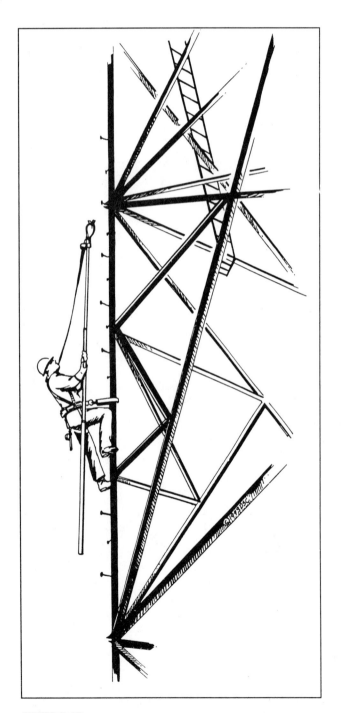

FIGURE 7.15
Pushing up a portable anchorage into position.

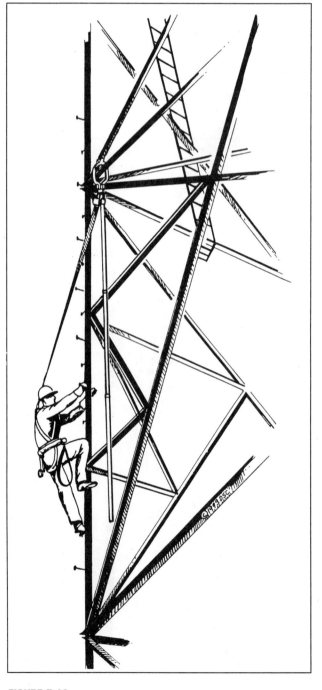

FIGURE 7.16
Climbing after the portable anchorage has been secured.

WHICH FALL PROTECTION SYSTEM SHOULD BE USED?

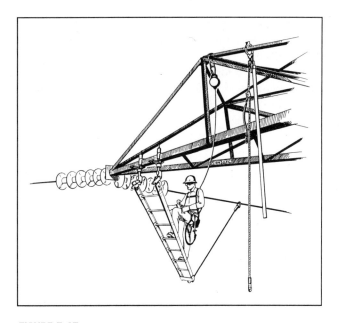

FIGURE 7.17
An example of 100% fall protection during an insulator change-out work procedure.

threaded; others are designed to fit onto the lifeline at any point. All ropes should be marked to demonstrate a system.

Manually Operated Grab – The worker moves this type of grab by hand, up or down the lifeline with relative ease. It is designed to be positioned above the work level when the worker is stationary.

The device actuates during a fall by squeezing the rope or tips in such a way to lock onto the lifeline by friction, thereby arresting the fall. A 6-ft. lanyard may be chosen to provide freedom of movement when the rope grab is positioned on the lifeline, but unless it is kept above foot height, this may lead to 12-ft. falls. The shortest lanyard should be used and the use of a 3-ft. lanyard can only produce a 6-ft. maximum free fall, the OSHA limit.

Shock absorption may be provided partly by slippage of the device down the rope during the arrest, or by the lanyard shock absorber.

Mobile Grab – This type of grabbing device travels freely on the lifeline, helping to provide "hands-free" move-

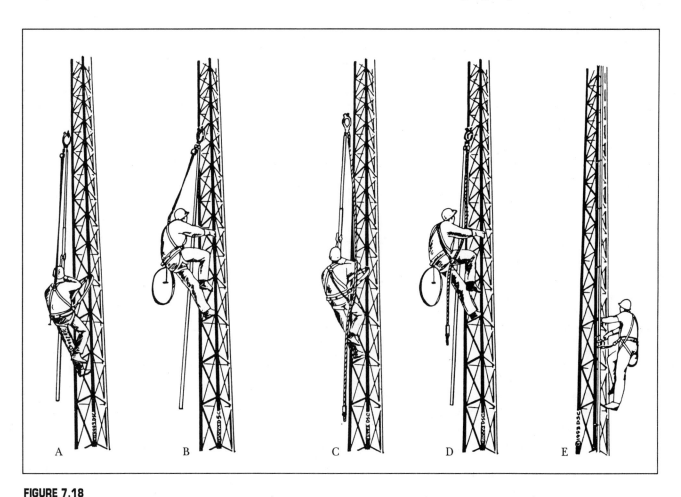

FIGURE 7.18
Left to right: A and B, first worker up, using a self-retracting lanyard/lifeline device; C and D, first worker up, using a rope grab system; and E, worker climbing in a permanently-installed rail system, the recommended method.

ment, but is designed to lock automatically when a fall occurs. Devices that roll freely along the rope without manual assistance can reduce worker frustration. They also avoid the potential of a worker holding a manual device open, with the consequences of a "death grip" during the panic of a fall. Only a 3-ft. lanyard should be used with such devices to avoid falls exceeding 6 ft.

In some systems, the device is activated by the inertial forces generated by a fall. The lock may consist of a ball cage and wedge or a balanced locking arm design. A short lanyard designed for the system is recommended but not always necessary. The body belt or harness

---

CONSIDERATIONS IN THE SELECTION OF A CLIMBING PROTECTION SYSTEM

A committee composed of civil engineers, site managers, and responsible climbers should carefully consider the following:

Performance Requirements
- Has the proposed climbing protection system been field tested by those who actually will do the climbing? Are written reports available describing personal experience?
- How many years do you expect the proposed system to be reliable?
- Is your ladder or climbing structure capable of sustaining dynamic loads, should a fall occur?
- Does the proposed climbing system allow sufficient flexibility to meet the needs of each climber, yet arrest the fall quickly and securely?
- Have you considered the effects of weather, corrosion, wind loading, and vibration? What about the tension of cables and expected problems with cable guides?
- How heavy is the sleeve? Are special belts required to use the proposed climbing system? How tiring will it be to use the system in long climbs?
- Will you allow parts of the system to be substituted? If so, which ones?
- Will the sleeve and the correct belt be available when the climb is made?
- Will the belt fit all sizes of workers, in all seasons?
- Does the climbing system meet the drop test and strength requirements of ANSI A14.3-1992? Will it do so when installed on your structure?
- How easy is the dismounting procedure? Is the worker still subject to a fall at the top?
- Will you allow the cable or rail to obstruct climbing in any way?
- How many persons will be using the same length of climbing carrier? Is this safe?
- What can go wrong? Can the sleeve be used with wrong-sized cables or rails? Will the system be ready for use in bad weather?

Installation Program
- Does the proposed climbing safety system interface with your structure in a manner acceptable to your engineering department?
- Are the correct materials being used to meet expected weather and corrosion problems? Can parts vibrate to cause damage? Who will inspect the installation?

Training Program
- Since installations usually are remote, will you be able to enlist the support of climbers to perfect each climbing system installation through careful field observations and constructive thoughts?
- How would you rescue a heart attack victim from the ladder above ground or below ground, if applicable?
- Can you actually demonstrate what will happen if a fall occurs?
- Are you capable of conducting semiannual meetings with climbers to show films and slides and discuss real or imaginary problems in detail?
- Are you checking to make sure that the system is used as intended? If not, why not?

Maintenance Program
- How often will you be able to check each climbing protection system? Will the parts be visually inspected along the entire length of the ladder or just from the ground? How thorough will the report be?
- Will your inspector be trained thoroughly to diagnose problems correctly? Can he/she correct problems in the field himself/herself, without a second visit?

Program Coordination
- Who will coordinate the climbing protection program, and who will maintain the appropriate records?

Reprinted with permission from *Best's Safety Directory*.

FIGURE 7.19
Considerations in the selection of a climbing protection system.

WHICH FALL PROTECTION SYSTEM SHOULD BE USED? 105

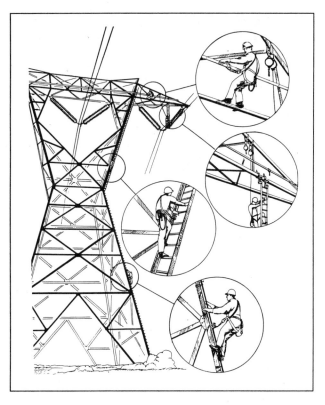

FIGURE 7.20
Examples of permanent fall arrest anchorages on a lattice-type transmission tower.

can be attached directly to the grabbing device, but a short lanyard up to 3 ft. in length may be helpful for all on swinging scaffolds.

While mobile grabs may be removable from the end of middle of the line, or held captive by design, an advantage of the captive mobile grab is that it cannot be removed or lost from the lifeline except possibly at the lower end. Mobile grab designs do not require worker manipulation on the lifeline while ascending, working or descending the lifeline by fixed ladder, single point or two point suspended scaffold, or during tower work.

"Hands-free" operation is particularly dangerous for workers operating suspension equipment, as well as for those needing both hands for climbing towers or other structures. A shock absorbing lanyard integrated with the device can provide mobility; a means of detecting in-service loading; and minimal arresting forces on the body and system.

A complete rope grab system is crucial for safety. The lanyard, if any, must be short and designed as part of the system when used. The rope grab and lanyard must be tested dynamically with its lifeline, and the results analyzed, before a particular combination is utilized for protection by any worker, to help avoid unforeseen failure of the system.

PROTECTION SYSTEM PREVENTS FALLS FROM METAL ROOF DECKS

A fall protection system has been devised by a contractor on an Alcoa Aluminum Co. project to protect the worker at the leading edge during metal roof deck installation.

The heart of the system is a 7 ft. (or shorter) gin pole and commercially manufactured retractable safety line, similar to the inertial reel restraint system on late model automobiles. The workers attach their regular safety belt lanyards to the retractable safety line devices, one worker per line, and a maximum of two lines per gin pole. The gin pole is firmly secured behind the leading edge to a roof purlin, not merely to the roof deck.

The device has 30 ft. of 9/16 in. nylon rope that is reeled out on demand but kept in mild tension by a spring in the unit, thus preventing the rope from becoming a tripping hazard. The inertial reel system dogs off immediately and positively whenever the rope reels out faster than a predetermined speed. The device is so effective that it will engage instantly by the worker simply walking at a rapid pace. The stopping mechanism will only release when forward tension is relieved; when relieved, the unit is again ready for service. In the event of a fall, forward motion is stopped immediately, minimizing the free fall.

This system has been used for a year. It has been well received by the contractor and workers alike. The system is also credited with saving the life of a journeyman sheet metal worker who fell when the unfastened piece of deck he stepped on slid out from under him. He sustained no injuries.

It must be emphasized that this system is experimental and that it has not received any formal approval or endorsement. It is being publicized as one approach to the serious problem of preventing roof edge falls, a longtime cause of construction falling accidents.

Karl L. Shipley
Aluminum Co. of America
Bettendorf, Iowa

Reprinted with permission from *Construction Newsletter*, National Safety Council, May-June 1981.

FIGURE 7.21
An example of new approaches to roof work safety.

Self-retracting Lanyard/Lifeline Devices (Locking)

Self-retracting lanyards/lifeline devices with locking features are designed to arrest free-falls in inches by eliminating the dangerous slack that can develop using fixed length lanyards. The line – either cable, rope, or webbing – extends or automatically retracts as the worker moves up and down. Overhead installation is critical for proper use in almost every situation.

Within the device, a centrifugal locking mechanism similar in effect to those in automobile seat belts is activated the moment a fall occurs, regardless of how much line is out of the unit. This limited free-fall distance, when coupled with an internal disc brake, can keep arresting forces to approximately 600 lbs. force.

Installed minimally above shoulder height at the highest point of climb, these devices can be accessed if necessary via a lightweight tag line, and workers can hook up at ground level for continuous protection. Units such as these, with lengths of up to approximately 200 ft., are extremely useful for helping to prevent the type of incident where a lanyard might not arrest a fall in time to prevent collision with an obstruction (see Figures 7.22 through 7.25). They must be installed overhead to avoid payout of the lifeline if a worker were to climb past the installation point, thereby producing a potentially long free fall. Similarly, when the worker moves horizontally, the device must either be high enough or move along with the worker in order to pre-

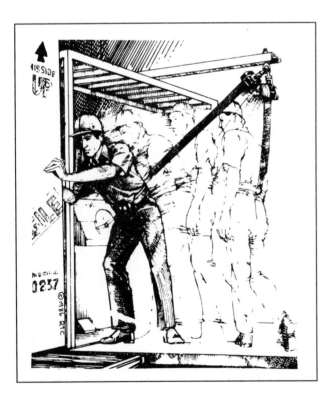

FIGURE 7.22
Example of a retracting web lanyard, used on a warehouse stockpicker. Note that swivels are sometimes necessary to counteract the tendency of some workers and work methods towards movement in a circular direction, which can twist the line. Employers should be especially careful to train these workers to use these devices as backup lifelines only, and not as lock and lean devices, which can substitute for repositioning the stockpicker. In the latter case, a second backup fall arrest system is required.

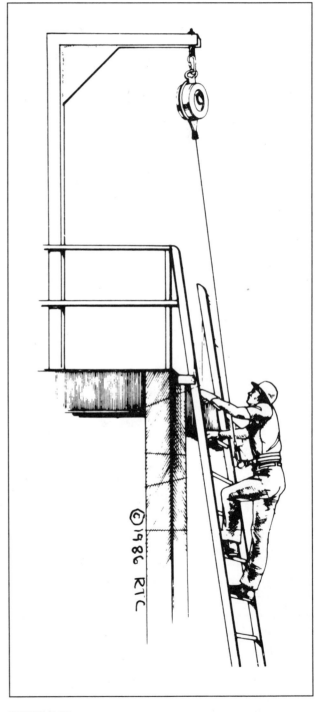

FIGURE 7.23
Example of a retracting cable lifeline, used on an angled ladder.

WHICH FALL PROTECTION SYSTEM SHOULD BE USED?

vent swing fall injury potential.

The sole objective of a locking retracting lifeline, when used properly, is to reduce falls to inches. Examples are shown for roof tiling and sheet metal decking, using suitable bracket installations posts.

Self-Retracting Lanyard/Lifeline Devices (Lowering)
Self-retracting lanyards/lifeline devices with a lowering feature are designed to arrest a free fall and simultaneously lower a worker at an automatic constant rate to grade level. Similar to the locking type, the cable extends and automatically retracts as the worker moves up and down. However, rather than arresting a fall and remaining locked until tension is relieved, the centrifugal braking mechanism provides an automatically

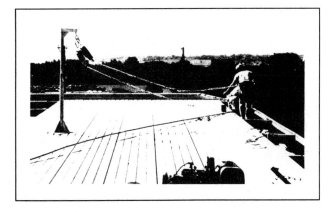

FIGURE 7.24
Roof deck workers attach safety belts to retractable lifelines, which lock when lines reel out above the predetermined rate.

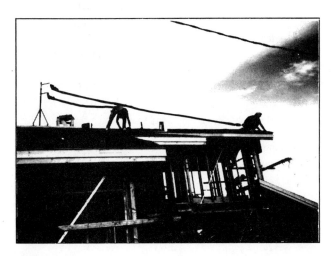

FIGURE 7.25
Roof workers using self-retracting lanyard/lifeline devices in California, 1986 (photo courtesy of Davey Roofing). Note that the entire fall protection system must be engineered in order to meet the 2:1 safety factor.

controlled descent. The worker essentially "floats" down at 4.5 ft./sec. (walking speed) or 9 ft./sec., depending on the model.

This automatic lowering feature can help eliminate costly and difficult high-level rescues and can control the fall hazard completely, rather than substituting a rescue problem. With cable lengths of up to 320 ft., workers inside a structure with a lower means of egress (such as a generating/recovery boiler) or outside a structure can have mobility with complete protection. See Figure 7.27.

Self-retracting lanyards/lifeline devices with an automatic, controlled descent feature also can provide the additional benefit of emergency escape, whether vertically or at an angle.

Horizontal Lifelines
Horizontal lifelines serve as anchoring lines that are rigged between fixed anchor points on the same level. These may be permanent, semi-permanent or temporary, depending on the length of the span, the number of workers and the duration of installation.

Horizontal lines are designed to help minimize the potential for dangerous "pendulum-like" swing falls that can result from moving laterally away from a fixed anchorage point. Swing falls can generate the same forces as falling through the same distance vertically, but with the additional hazard of striking an obstruction. See Part III of this chapter for further swing fall information. And see Figures 7.28 and 7.29 for examples of horizontal rail systems.

Horizontal lifelines should be installed without exposure to height hazards. They must be positioned above the waist-height of potential users.

Permanent Systems – Permanent horizontal lifeline systems should be designed to last as long as the structure to which they are attached. They can consist of a 1/4 in. x 2 in. rigid horizontal rail, or cable that allows a lightweight trolley to slide easily with the worker.

Since these systems are attached to the structure at regular intervals, they can accommodate several workers simultaneously (one trolley per worker). Special sections can allow the trolley to go continuously around corners so workers do not have to disconnect. The fixed rail trolley can be easily attached and detached at protected access/egress points. For crane runways, elevated catwalks and piperacks, permanent systems installed at waist height can provide continuous horizontal mobility with protection. For waist-height installations, a short shock absorbing lanyard is permanently attached to the trolley to limit arresting forces on the worker and system.

Some designs can be adapted from vertical climbing protection systems using a turntable to avoid disconnection hazards when switching from a vertical to horizontal movement. When the fixed rail system is installed overhead, it can be used in conjunction with a retracting lifeline for greater protected vertical mobility.

For piperacks in particular, regularly frequented areas can be more economically safeguarded when outfitted with a lightweight fiberglass accessway and rail system than with a full guarded walkway. Other areas may include cable trays, conveyors, vessels, tanks or loading docks.

The walking surface of this system is designed to help prevent slip falls through a skid-resistant surface and to control an elevated fall through the use of a low-friction

---

CONSIDERATIONS IN THE SELECTION OF A VERTICAL LIFELINE SYSTEM

The members of a committee consisting of the manager, an engineer, and users should be well-informed individually and ready to consider all the following factors.

Performance Requirements
- How far are you willing to allow your workers to fall? How will they recover or be recovered from a fallen position?
- What specific kinds of ropes or cables will you allow in your lifeline application and what kinds will you not allow?
- How far is the foreseeable vertical and horizontal movement?
- How much shock absorption is desirable?
- How long will the lifeline be left outdoors, and in what kind of weather?
- What component changes are you willing to accept without affecting the system's integrity?
- How many different applications are you trying to solve with one device? Is this safe? Have you listed each application and carefully considered the implications?
- What capability test has the proposed system met in the configuration of your application? What is the total distance to stop?
- Will you allow rope grab devices which are free-moving or those which must be moved manually?
- What can go wrong? Will parts of the system be replaced without authorization? Can the device be installed upside down? Will snaphooks accidentally become unfastened? Will the fall exceed system design? Will chemicals affect rope strength? Will harnesses be worn properly? Will the lifeline be used for other applications?

Installation
- Have you clearly identified the specific anchorage points of suitable design and strength? Will these be erected permanently for foreseeable scheduled workstations and work areas?
- Are you prepared to have engineering drawings made, showing the approved methods of installation?

Training Program
- How conscious are your workers of lifeline safety at this time? Will they follow your installation procedures? Are belts sized properly?
- Have workers had an opportunity to suspend in a belt and in a full body harness to determine which body support they prefer?
- Can your workers use the proposed system with little or no frustration?
- Do your workers really believe in fall protection? Are their work habits helping to cause damage to the system's integrity?
- Do you have films and slides geared to the usage of the lifeline in your application? How often will you show them to new and existing employees?

Maintenance
- Is your organization capable of supervising a visual inspection program which will quickly detect irregular performance of the system and damage to the parts? If so, do you have the capability to correct these defects quickly before system integrity is lost? How will you determine current break strength of the lifeline or whether it has been subjected to in-service loading?

Program Coordination
- Who will coordinate the lifeline program and who will maintain records?
- When will you meet again to evaluate progress?
- Did you answer these questions in sufficient details?

Reprinted with permission from *Best's Safety Directory*.

FIGURE 7.26

Considerations in the selection of a vertical lifeline system.

WHICH FALL PROTECTION SYSTEM SHOULD BE USED?

trolley with an integrated shock absorbing lanyard. The trolley rolls freely along the waist-high rail as the worker moves horizontally. Spans of up to 20 ft. are possible between structural supports, overhead, and 4 to 6 ft. at waist height.

A cable system employing specially designed supports approximately every 10 ft., and used in conjunction with a special pulley or slider design, can bypass supports to allow continuous unhindered travel horizontally. The larger cables (approximately 5/16 in. or 3/8 in.) may qualify for more permanent installation, based on corrosion potential and maintenance requirements. Some designs also may lend themselves for use on sloped working surfaces if they have additional locking features.

Semi-Permanent Systems – Semi-permanent lifeline systems are designed to provide service from months to several years. A lightweight synthetic cable can be tensioned in a near-horizontal plane to provide continuous protected mobility. Heavier aircraft cable or wire cable, however, requires careful engineering for proper installation, including the sag, tension and diameter of the cable relative to the length of the span and the number of users.

Synthetic cables with inherent elasticity can simplify

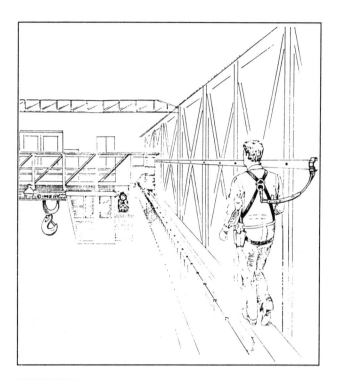

FIGURE 7.28
Example of a horizontal rail system.

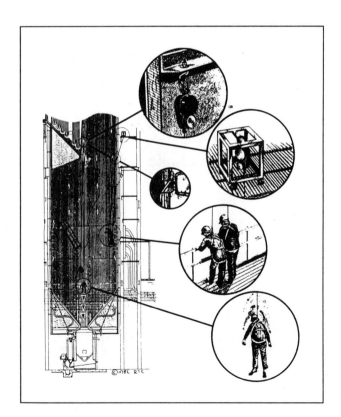

FIGURE 7.27
Example of a retracting cable lifeline with controlled descent used in utility boiler maintenance work.

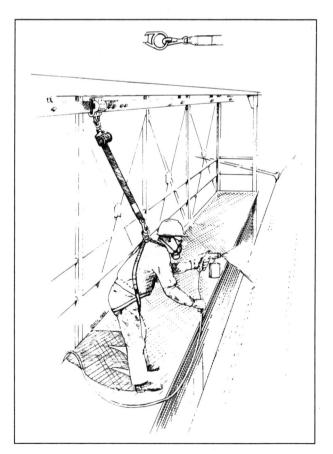

FIGURE 7-29
Example of a horizontal rail system with retracting web lanyard.

overhead installation. Moreover, they enable the connecting means, particularly fall arrester devices, to remain overhead when walking the entire span. Lengths of up to 200 ft. between supports are possible for up to three workers. Suitable areas include pipe-racks, roofs and railcar/tankcar loading and unloading.

☞ Where low clearances exist, dynamic sag must be small to avoid ground collisions. Lower spans and stiffer, tighter horizontal lines are called for with an engineered and documented solution. Trolleys on an I-beam are an alternative. For detailed discussion of these horizontal lifelines, see Appendix A-3.

Temporary Systems – Short-term horizontal lifeline systems are intended for a few days' to a few weeks' use. For example, these may be a horizontal rope lifeline and rope tensioner that can be installed with a wrench in minutes. Positioned between vertical support columns or fabricated end and mid-support posts, the system can provide protected horizontal mobility on roofs, tanks and in piperacks.

Synthetic rope systems are easily transported and do not take any longer to install than to do the job. Spans of 20 ft. between supports for use by two persons and 60 ft. for use by one person are possible with twisted rope designs. A system should be installed minimally at waist height for the attachment of lanyards, and overhead for use with devices. In both cases, the objective is to limit the free-fall distance as much as possible.

Wire rope systems (1/2-in. diameter seems adequate strength) should be considered where accidental collisions with crane suspended loads are foreseeable. Bypass of intermediate supports, using the split eyebolt concept, can be used in construction industry applications. Automatic roll-by or slide-by devices can be used in general industry applications.

Although double lanyard systems remain an obvious answer for moving horizontally on many present structures without the provision of horizontal lifelines, their use is cumbersome. An interesting variant used in

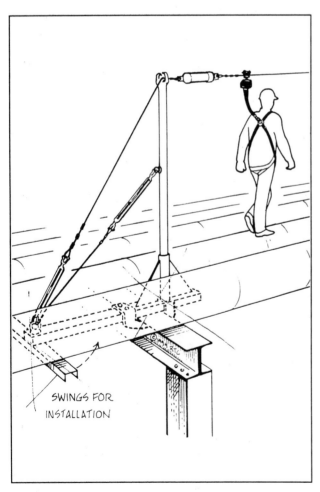

FIGURE 7.30
Example of a permanent horizontal lifeline accessway on a piperack.

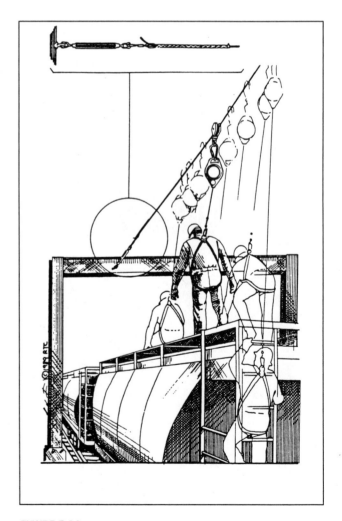

FIGURE 7.31
Example of a two-dimensional fall protection system. Notice the anchorage point structure (circled).

Japan allows a more simple system which includes a "key lock" attached to the worker's belt (See Figure 7.34). One lanyard key is inserted and remains attached until a second lanyard key is inserted in another opening. This action ejects the first lanyard key and can allow unhindered transfer past obstructions or supports and ensures continuous protection.

The railroad industry has adopted the "puppy-dog" system for unguarded bridge use where fall hazards exceed 12 ft. This consists of a rail slider at foot level and a lanyard attached to a worker's body support. Careful analysis is required to avoid falling more than 6 ft. and producing injurious collisions. Anchorage snaphooks must be carefully chosen to avoid damage to lanyard snaphooks when stressed by pulling or leaning, often when the "puppy dog" sticks or jams. A second "true" fall arrest system is called for in these applications with overhead anchorages.

Confined Space Entry and Retrieval

These four points form the foundation for any discussion and implementation of confined space entry and retrieval:

- The ANSI Z117.1-1989 standard stresses training.
- OSHA 1910.146, published in 1993, requires employers to designate whether the confined space is permit-required or nonpermit-required.
- Redesignation is required annually.
- Harnesses and mechanical winches are required for depths over 5 ft.

Entering confined spaces such as vessels, storage tanks, ship compartments, silos, pits, tunnels, vaults and pipelines often involves exposure to a fall hazard in addition to a potential need for emergency retrieval. By design, many confined spaces have limited openings for entry and egress. And, if potentially toxic conditions can be present, there is the added danger that rescue workers may be overcome and trapped as well. Venting and testing procedures are essential prior to entry as well as the proper personal protective equipment and rescue equipment.

☞ Many safety professionals agree that work crew extrication is an essential ingredient of confined space work training programs. Crew removal from the confined space is an ideal starting point for rescue teams.

Confined work space can be categorized by the degree of danger according to NIOSH Criteria Document 8-106.[22] These categories are summarized as follows:

- Class A is the most dangerous to life because of oxygen deficiency, or toxic or explosive atmospheres.
- Class B has the potential for causing injury and illness without any immediate threat to life.
- Class C confined space does not require special work procedures.

Rescue equipment is required for all classes according to this NIOSH document.

☞ The author believes that manholes and entrances of 18 in. diameter or less may be inherently hazardous and can trap or delay workers and rescuers regardless of training techniques. Internal baffles trays in pipe systems add to the danger of prolonged entrapment. Preferably, openings of 18 in. and less should not be entered by workers.

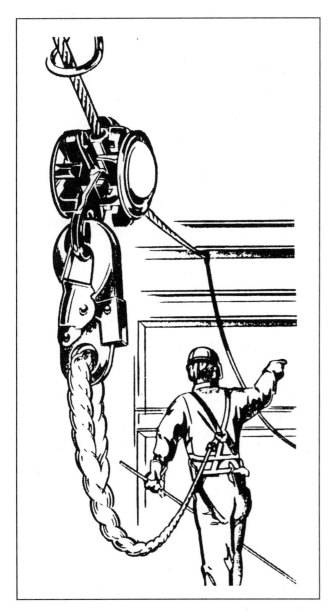

FIGURE 7.32
Horizontal lifeline intermediate support roll-by device. Courtesy of Fall Arrest System.

The more the danger, the greater the need for the medical certification of workers prior to entry and the need for a higher standard of preplanning and training. Besides receiving a thorough physical examination and X-rays of knees and lower back, the worker also should be tested for both acrophobic (fear of height) and claustrophobic (fear of enclosed places) tendencies.

☞ **Entry and Emergency Retrieval**

With confined entry and retrieval systems, all the additional dangers can be significantly minimized. A worker entering a space via a ladder or suspension equipment with a fall hazard or potentially toxic conditions (even after purging) should be hooked up to a lifeline first, which is also designed to be used for a rescue. Then, because the worker already has his or her lifeline

attached, a standby person or attendant outside of the space is able to retrieve the worker more easily should an emergency occur, without having to enter the space and also possibly becoming a victim. NIOSH Hazard Alert #86-110 (January 1986) points to approximately one-half of confined space victims being rescuers. It appears that many struggle to get out, yet fall from the ladder close to the opening. Thus, this lifeline procedure alone could save many lives.

For horizontal manway entrances and low ceiling vertical entries, winches must be rigged with pulley systems located for unobstructed pulling or lowering. Preplanning is essential.

Portable Tripods – An extension davit or other permanent means can provide suitable anchor points for retracting cable lifelines used for fall protection, and

---

CONSIDERATIONS IN THE SELECTION OF HORIZONTAL LIFELINES

Performance Requirements
1. Will you purchase a complete lifeline designed for horizontal use or construct it yourself?
2. What length of line do you envisage?
3. How many workers will use the line simultaneously?
4. What strength anchorage points do you need?
5. What sag in the line under dynamic load is tolerable?
6. Will you use lanyards or retracting lifelines attached to the line, and how will you attach them?
7. Is the line temporary, semi-permanent or permanent in nature?
8. Are you intending to use perimeter cables meant for restraint instead of fall protection, and are they strong enough for the intended application?
9. Do you need to construct anchorage posts if no supporting steel is available?
10. Can you move lanyards past anchorage posts without detaching the snaphook?
11. What can go wrong?
    a. Can all workers fall at one time? What will happen?
    b. Can lanyard snaphooks detach accidentally from the line?
    c. What happens if a crane load hits one of the anchorage points?
    d. Will the lanyard or retracting lifeline slide smoothly without causing a swing fall hazard?

Installation Program
1. Can you install the lines without exposure to falls, for example, at ground level, before hoisting?
2. How will you remove temporary lines without exposure to a fall hazard?
3. Has the degree of installation sag and sag following a fall been taken into account?

Training Program
1. Will the work procedure have to change when the lifeline is used? Why?
2. Do workers feel safe if they use the line as a handrail? Is the height and tension correct? Should you be using a horizontal safety rail or more intermediate posts for stability? Will other contractor personnel be required to use this line?

Maintenance Program
1. Will you use a colored flag to designate year of purchase and date of formal inspection?
2. Will the inspector actually observe each part of the system close up, or will he/she do so from the ground?

Program Coordination
1. Who will coordinate the material acquisition, installation, and maintenance programs?
2. Who will coordinate necessary changes in the system to speed work production, and how will that come about?

Reprinted with permission from *Best's Safety Directory*.

FIGURE 7.33
Considerations in the selection of horizontal lifelines.

WHICH FALL PROTECTION SYSTEM SHOULD BE USED?

some type of mechanical device designed to lift a victim vertically from vertical openings, such as a winch or block and tackle. Manual winches may be adequate to lift victims from about 50 ft. without exceeding a medically critical 3- to 4-minute time period (which is the predicted point of onset of permanent brain damage for respiratory or cardiac arrest victims).

At greater depths, power winches with a maximum lift of 1 ft./sec., and a 500 lb. slip clutch to avoid hangups (on ladder rungs, for example), are recommended, along with lifelines. All manual and powered winches should have manufacturer approval for use as a personal lifting device and a mechanical advantage of 4:1 minimal;[23] preferably 6:1 or even up to 8:1, and not 2:1 as proposed in one standard.[24] Radio communications can assist at depths exceeding 30 to 50 ft. or more, in case prompt action is needed in an emergency.

☞ *Access Systems* – Be careful to understand the differences between a winch or hoist and a backup lifeline system. The lifeline device must be passive until it operates automatically such as by arresting a free fall. A winch is a device that is used as a primary hoist to raise and lower personnel, and which must be backed up with a lifeline safety device, usually a retracting lifeline.

With the exception of elevators, very few hoists or winches are "man-rated" in the sense that they are of a sufficiently rugged design to be used to lower and raise workers reliably. Even those that are man-rated by a nationally recognized laboratory require a backup lifeline device when used for accessing workers up or down. Testing for access hoists should meet national requirements for such scaffolding equipment, or if no

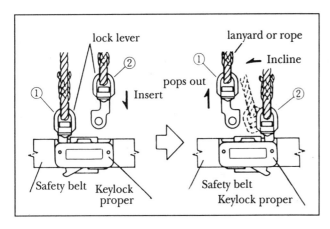

FIGURE 7.34
This is a general representation of how a key lock operates. Courtesy of Fujii Denko, Inc., Japan.

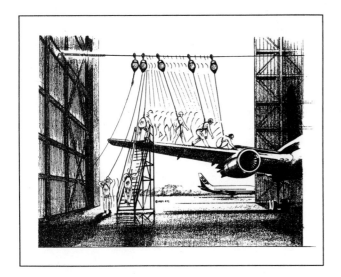

FIGURE 7.35
A fall arrest system for wing walking in a hangar.

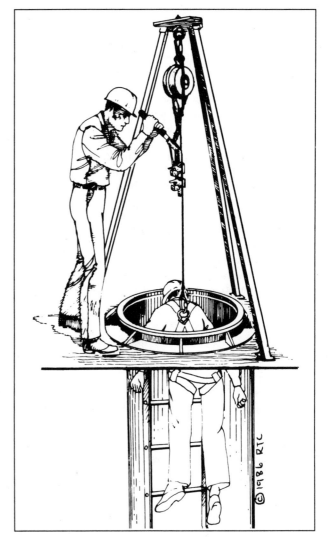

FIGURE 7-36
Example of a confined-space entry and retrieval system. Newer models incorporate the winch, providing greater head room.

requirements exist, then a 250 lb./4 ft. free-fall test should be conducted, as proposed in OSHA 1926.502 for positioning systems.

☞ Winches used for personnel should have an easy means of operation and be unable to "free-wheel" when the crank handle is released, unless an inertial lock is incorporated. Rescue devices, when used for emergency only, may be a single line. However, if training is done with them, then the backup lifeline must additionally be used, if the fall exceeds a nominal 10 ft. in the training process.

The mechanical advantage is based on a 220-lb. victim divided by the advantage of 4, which requires a 50-lb. force by the rescuer or attendant. (See Appendix A-5 for comments on one-man rescue lines.) A 50-ft. depth limit seems reasonable for a one-person mechanical winch rescue, because tests show rapid tiring occurs quickly at 20-ft. depths, regardless of the lifting ratio. Note that ratchet action by a 100-lb. rescuer could probably exert 50 lb., but not for a crank action winch where a 25-lb. limit to rotate seems more in order for lighter-weight attendants.

CONSIDERATIONS IN THE SELECTION OF A CONFINED SPACE LIFELINE AND RESCUE SYSTEM

Members of a committee consisting of a manager, an engineer, a hygienist, and users carefully should consider all of the following aspects of confined space:

Performance Requirements
- Agree on what a lifeline should do for a confined space worker.
- Agree on a time limit to complete a rescue of one or more workers.
- What is the type of work to be performed?
- Will the worker(s) be able to enter and exit easily using the proposed harness and will this be required to be worn at all times?
- Can the proposed belt or harness fit comfortably over protective clothing?
- What will happen to the worker after a fall has been arrested if he/she is not conscious?
- Will other workers be required to attach a rescue line to the worker to retrieve him/her and, if so, can this be done without endangering the lives of the rescuers?
- Will you allow your workers to enter manholes less than 24 inches in diameter, where they could become trapped?
- What are the qualifications of the proposed stand-by person?
- Will the proposed harness hold an unconscious worker sufficiently vertical to allow retrieval above the confined space? Could the victim be injured further by dragging him/her across baffles or in the direction of side exits?
- Will you consider a powered winching system for depths over 50 feet, instead of relying on manual winching?
- Does the proposed system for lifelines and rescue solve all reasonably predictable problems or just a single predictable problem, such as a fall or a breathing hazard?
- What can go wrong?
- Does the proposed winching system have manufacturer approval for lifting of personnel?
- Will a standby person holding a line be able to arrest a fall or raise a "dead-weight" reliably?
- Does the winch have a mechanical advantage of 4:1 minimally?

Installation
- Will you rely on portable installation points such as tripods, or a permanent overhead installation point above the entrance? Will a proposed tripod system be adequate for dynamic loads if a lifeline is attached?
- Will you have engineering drawings made showing the approved installation methods to meet your needs?

Training Program
- Do your workers understand their obligations to help develop a workable system which may save their lives?
- Do you plan to develop a slide presentation or film to demonstrate confined space lifeline and rescue procedure?
- Do workers know that, at depths of more than 5 feet, OSHA requires harnesses and a mechanical lifting device?

Maintenance
- Who will inspect the equipment regularly and report defects or damage?

Coordination of the Program
- Who will monitor the system, maintain records, and propose changes to help make the system more efficient?

Reprinted with permission from *Best's Safety Directory.*

FIGURE 7.37
Considerations in the selection of a confined space lifeline and rescue system.

WHICH FALL PROTECTION SYSTEM SHOULD BE USED?

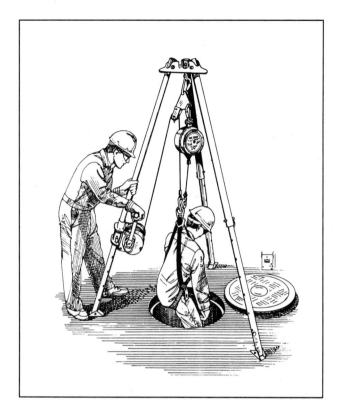

FIGURE 7.38
Example of a confined entry personnel access and retrieval system.

Again, if the confined space has a lower means of egress, a self-retracting lanyard/lifeline device with a controlled descent feature that automatically lowers a worker at a constant rate following a fall from a swinging scaffold may be preferable, in order to avoid rescue time for a suspended worker using the more common fall arrest systems.

☞ Alternatively, a self-retracting lanyard/lifeline device incorporating a retrieval winch can be selected, which winches downwards as well as upwards.

For deep confined spaces with several workers involved, all special-design collapsible scaffolds, boatswain's chairs, floating work surfaces, and other access systems and platforms should meet the performance requirements for scaffolds in other industry applications. Redundant backup winch systems are advisable for all primary hoist systems.

Lifelines and retrieval gear should preferably be combined into a single system for each worker to reduce the number of lines through tank entrances. Live training, under realistically simulated but reasonably safe conditions, is absolutely necessary before entry.

Emergency responders, including outside fire departments, should practice enough confined space rescue entry and retrieval scenarios to be sure they have optimally planned for most situations. Rescuers should also be protected from fall hazards, and have retrieval systems ready for speedy extractions in all foreseeable confined space rescues.

Other types of worksites present more questions. These are worksites that have many workers, or are tunnels or deep shafts. Answers can include refuge areas, respiratory protection systems and more advanced access systems that can provide more options for group rescue and can become a part of the organization's OSHA-required written emergency action plan.

Emergency Descent and Lowering Systems

The overall idea behind industrial egress is to provide every worker with a means of emergency escape from his or her workstation. Workers at heights, whose only means of access and exit are via fixed ladders or moving machinery, are subject to being trapped in an emergency. This can result, for example, from fire, gases and weather changes on chemical towers, or from fire, smoke and fumes around overhead crane operators. Sick or injured workers in high places present a similar challenge – getting them down safety and quickly.

The Life Safety Code sparingly addresses individual egress and relates to egress from fire situations.[25] The NIOSH Criteria Document on Emergency Egress from Elevated Workstations looks at the industrial egress problem in more detail, and recommends in its report to OSHA that the employer consider special means of escape to allow employees to evacuate elevated workstations quickly and safely when standard means of egress are impractical.[26] These special means of escape include approved controlled descent devices, slides and chutes. An appendix to subpart E of OSHA 29 CFR Part 1910 serves as a guideline for the development of employee emergency evacuation plans.[27] The 1910.38 regulation states that an Emergency Action Plan must be prepared in writing by every employer for each emergency and that Action Plan training also must take place.

☞ Unlike NFPA 101, or the building codes, OSHA 1910.35 has allowed the consideration of windows and similar wall openings for escape in addition to the concept of waiting for rescue, as explained in the Summary and Explanation of this final rule on September 12, 1980.

There are several points to consider before choosing an emergency descent system, as follows:

Anchorage Points for Descent Devices – Similar to fall protection issues (see Chapter 6), anchorage points for descent systems should not be left to chance or worker choice. One practical guide is that the anchorage point strength for descent devices should equal or exceed the line strength. Depending on application, minimum breaking strength in the direction of pull for the descent device line should be designated as follows:

- Working descent device
  (boatswain's chair)
  - single rope load line: 5000 lb.
  - self-contained cable winch: 3000 lb.
    and seat system
- Rope grab friction-type
  descent device lifeline
  (working from a boatswain's chair): 5000 lb.
- Retracting descent device
  lifeline (working a one or
  two point scaffold): 3000 lb.
- Emergency escape only, with
  limited initial free fall
  less than 2 ft.: 1800 lb.

☞ The operating principle is that any descent devices used as vertical fall arrest systems should minimally have the same line strength as a fall arrest device that is designed to stop the fall. However, when used for escape only, the minimum break strength should be as required by a nationally-recog-nized testing laboratory, for example UL Standard 1523, if no other national standard specifies such a limit.

Vertical Descent

Typical industrial applications for vertical descent devices include emergency escape from overhead cranes of all types, oil and chemical towers, cement silos, grain elevators, elevated work platforms and chimney worker cage hoists.

Descent devices are "systems designed to lower one or more persons by either a variable or an automatic constant speed method," according to an Industrial Safety Equipment Association definition (1977) prepared by the Descent Control and Controlled Descent Subcommittee of the Fall Protection Groups.[28] Both devices are mechanical and do not require the use of power or electricity.

There are two types of descent devices: automatically controlled descent devices, which are controlled with a maximum lowering speed inherent in the device, and manually operated lowering devices, which require user control at all times. Both types must have an overhead anchorage point.

CONTROLLED DESCENT DEVICES SPEED ANALYSIS APPLICATION GUIDE

Approximate Rate of Descent (100-300 lbs.)	Comments	Casualty Risk
Less than 2 ft./sec.	Too slow.	Only from slack cable and swing
2 to 4 ft./sec.	High confidence for first time users, and through witness eyes is very acceptable.	Cable gripping causes skin burns—stucco wall may cause slight abrasion to exposed arm or leg
4 to 6 ft./sec.	O.K. for trained industrial, commercial users. "Best speed" to these people.	Same as above. Training is reasonable with minimal risk of injury from low heights.
6 to 10 ft./sec.	O.K. for severe emergency such as oil blow-out.	Touchdown can be awkward for some people, and wall scrapes are possible. No problem with self-contained escape chutes.
10 to 16 ft./sec.	O.K. for angled descent escape along guide cable in an imminent danger escape application.	Touchdown vertically is usually on the seat for those weighing over 190 lbs.—may cause twisted ankle, unless angled descent employed.
More than 16 ft./sec.	Beyond user's control or reaction time relating to impact on touchdown.	Requires skilled landing techniques, such as parachute landing roll. (NAS 804: 21 ft./sec. descent rate maximum over final 100 ft.)

NOTE: Harold Steinberg, in his 1977 "Study of Fall Safety Equipment," addressed descent devices having a speed limit of 15 ft./sec. or less for an uninjured person and 10 ft./sec. or less for an injured person. Safety professionals now recommend 7 ft./sec. maximum rate with a tolerance of 2 ft./sec. The author's experience with various descent speeds and human behavior dates to 1970 and the speed analysis chart is based on his experience with hundreds of individuals.

FIGURE 7.39

Controlled descent devices speed analysis application guide.

WHICH FALL PROTECTION SYSTEM SHOULD BE USED?

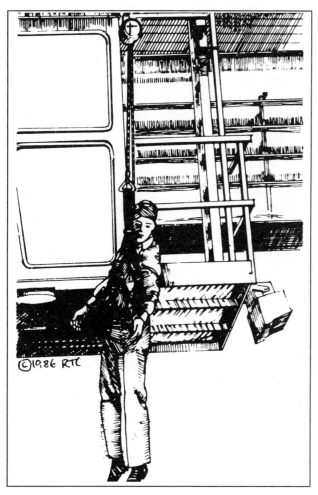

FIGURE 7.40
Example of an emergency controlled descent device from a crane cab used with quick-use escape belt.

☞ *Automatically Controlled Descent Devices* – This type of velocity-limiting descent device automatically controls the speed of the descent; one unit is factory pre-set for general use at a maximum descent rate of 3.5 ft./sec. ±10%. Various applications can call for speed limits up to approximately 12 ft./sec. (see Figure 7.39). This inherent speed control is designed to permit reliable descent under emergency or panic conditions without user presetting or manipulation.

The OSHA 1926.1053 ladder safety device requirements specify a speed limit not to exceed 7 ft./sec. U.S. Coast Guard requirements for offshore rig (artificial island) egress specify 7 ft./sec. to 12 ft./sec.

A typical controlled descent system incorporates a pulley mechanism equipped with a centrifugal brake. The escape belt is slipped over the head and under the arms and pulled tight to the chest with a buckle. The return cable is held initially during launch and provides the full control needed by the escapee to steady himself. A second escape belt at the opposite end of the cable returns automatically for the next user, providing continuous individual escapes without manual adjustment.

Another design has a retractable cable which returns the belt after the escape is complete; the lengths available are 35 to approximately 200 ft. With either device, the descent speed remains constant, regardless of the weight of the individual. The device typically stays attached to the installation point to ensure readiness. When purchasing this equipment, a test certificate should be required in addition to UL listing or the equivalent. Such documentation can promote user and management confidence.

☞ *Manually Operated Lowering Devices* – With this type of lowering device, the rate of descent is determined by a combination of the following three factors: 1) friction of a certain number of turns of the descent line around fixed parts of the device body, 2) the weight of the operator and 3) the conscious manual control of the operator. The device typically moves down the rope with the user/operator and is used with a boatswain's chair for work positioning access. (See Figure 7.40.)

One such unit incorporates a spring locking mechanism. Descent continues only while there is positive, downward pressure on the control unit handle. The mechanism is designed to lock automatically if the worker releases his grip on the handle. Descent then can be resumed under the conscious control of either the worker or a coworker standing below.

Another device can be utilized with a boatswain's chair and "locked off" by looping the line over the descent mechanism. This stopping option encourages use of these units for work positioning such as inspection, window cleaning, painting and riveting work, similar to a single point scaffold, so an additional lifeline is required. When the device is used as an independent lifeline, the system provides a means by which a conscious worker may lower himself after a fall or equipment failure, when he can reach the length of his lanyard and when the line has been 'locked-off' to provide fall arrest.

Some suppliers provide two lines with one device offering work positioning and lifeline as one unit. Check with local OSHA officials on their views for that region on these type devices.

It should be emphasized that there is no inherent speed limit with user-controlled devices. Many have to be preset manually before each use, necessitating careful regular checks for continued or emergency reliability, as a function of rope and device wear and tear.

Lever and push-pull devices that allow a "sweet spot" to permit descent, but jam when pushed or pulled too hard, provide more security.

An overspeed device fitted to one model activates at a certain rate of descent to lock the rope movement. For all safety equipment, and especially emergency safety equipment, "forgiving" designs make the difference between a convenient tool and a true safety device. A true safety device has a performance that can be tested. The supplier should provide a certificate with each device showing compliance.

Again: for all safety equipment, and especially emergency safety equipment, "forgiving" designs make the difference between a convenient tool and a true safety device. Independent lifelines are required with the use of all manually-operated lowering devices.

Angled Descent

Where there is sudden danger from fire below the escape point or from the effect of blast, angled escape away from the structure via an angled guide cable or chute affords more personal protection than does a vertical descent system. (See Figure 7.41.)

Vertical descent devices, however, can be hooked up to these angled cables. Steady descent speeds of 10 to 12 ft./sec. are preferred for angled descent, and automatic speed-limiting descent systems provide the necessary predictable performance for a reliable touchdown that enables the escapee to continue to move away. Manually-operated descent devices and cable slide devices also have been in use for many years, but these devices require the conscious control of the worker and appropriate anchorage at each end to ensure safe escape. (See Figure 7.42 for selection considerations.)

Proposed OSHA Standard 1910.270 for oil and gas well drilling and servicing addresses angled escape on rigs, and either limits controlled descent speeds to 15 ft./sec. at touchdown or requires manual system guide cables to enable the device to come to a stop before it reaches the ground anchor.[29]

Group Evacuation – Where group protection is required, safety concepts include means of fire and smoke detection, smoke barriers, alarm systems, extinguishing systems, refuge areas and means of escape to reasonably meet the OSHA required emergency action plan.

Self-contained emergency escape chutes capable of evacuating 30 to 40 persons per minute await adoption in the USA for building and industrial use. Japan and Europe are current users of these systems. The Japanese fire code includes the use of escape chutes. These can be utilized vertically, or at an angle if supervised. Vertical chutes have an internal spiral design to slow descent to a comfortable rate. Escape chutes should provide inherent descent speed control up to approximately 10 ft./sec. and reasonably ensure a continuous descent to a soft touchdown at the bottom.

Offshore platform escape provisions for groups of 20 or 30 at a time, for instance, require suitable automatic controlled systems to give reliable access to water level. For cold-water emergency use on rigs and platforms, self-contained controlled descent capsules, which also serve as navigable escape craft, are available. Personal controlled descent devices or approved means of abandonment (U.S. Coast Guard) are needed for stragglers on offshore platforms.

Emergency Escape Training

Training is the key to the successful use of any emergency egress procedure or device. Comprehensive and frequently repeated training sessions without exposure to height under 10 ft., for example, help to overcome the panic that may confuse or even paralyze workers in an emergency situation. Equipment must be reliable, visible, simple to operate and thoroughly familiar to the workers whose lives may depend on it. Some equipment manufacturers have prepared manuals and consulting services to assist with employee training programs.

Personal Rescue Systems

Competent rescue teams develop techniques for the recovery of workers who may be injured or trapped in difficult positions. It is important to remember that when rescuing an injured or sick worker from his or

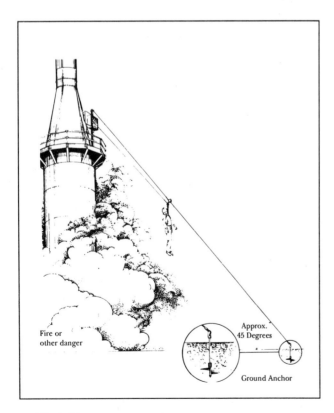

FIGURE 7.41
Example of an angled emergency escape system with controlled descent.

WHICH FALL PROTECTION SYSTEM SHOULD BE USED?

CONSIDERATION IN THE SELECTION OF A PERSONAL EMERGENCY DESCENT SYSTEM

A committee comprising all levels of management and workers should carefully consider all the following factors:

Performance Requirements
- Have all the committee members experienced the feeling of descent on the escape system through actual personal demonstration? This should be mandatory.
- What do you foresee to be the needs of your workers in an emergency? How much time will they have? Will the means of escape be available when needed?
- What is the maximum descent speed that you will tolerate?
- How quickly must the workers be able to reach the ground? How many workers are there altogether?
- How many features or applications are you trying to combine in one device? Can this be done safely?
- What limitations does the escape system have?
- Does the proposed escape system have written approval for usage in the specific application from your corporate safety officer and from a nationally recognized testing laboratory? Is each device factory tested and serially numbered?
- What kind of weather, corrosion, fire and electrical problems and abuse factors will you face? Will the escape device need special protection?
- What can go wrong? Will the system always be ready for use? Does it work equally well for all workers, whether they are conscious or unconscious? What kind of misuse or lack of attention can you expect? Will this create flaws in the required performance?

Installation
- Have approved installation points been documented on your company engineering drawings?

Training Program
- Are you willing to conduct frequent training, either quarterly or semiannually?
- Are you willing to develop a formal training program which will expose workers to heights and yet provide sufficient reliability for your workers so that accidents will be avoided?
- Is a film or slide presentation available to show workers how the system works? Will it be a job training requirement for all new workers?
- Will the trainer be prepared to answer fully all questions from workers?

Maintenance Program
- Are you able to inspect the escape system visually in a detailed manner and at least semiannually?
- Are you willing to consider annual recertification of the escape system to check its worthiness and reliability?

Program Coordination
- Who will be responsible for coordinating training and maintenance programs on an on-going basis?
- When will the committee meet next to review the overall escape program?

Reprinted with permission from *Best's Safety Directory*.

FIGURE 7.42
Considerations in the selection of a personal emergency descent system.

her workstation, time is critical. The first few minutes for a heart attack victim, for example, can be vital.

Many lives can be saved if employers build rescue techniques into their workplace operations techniques that require less skill and training than those used by highly trained rescue squads.

If safety lines such as ropes and cables are used for manual hand-over-hand or block and tackle rescue, they should have a minimum braking strength of 2,650 lbs., according to OSHA. Chafing over sharp edges should be avoided in order to avoid weakening the system.

If space permits, a stretcher or basket should be used to support the victim, but in tanks with small manhole entrances, wristlets in combination with body

harnesses and suitable D-ring locations can be used to hold the worker in a vertical position during the retrieval process. A safety feature should be incorporated to prevent falling back into the manhole.

Rescue from Above-Ground Level
Descent devices permanently installed or immediately available at such workstations as overhead crane cabs, grain elevator workhouses and elevated platforms on towers or vessels can be used effectively for lowering an injured member of the crew quickly and safely to ground level.

Devices with no inherent speed control require the presence of a trained rescue team or trained coworkers

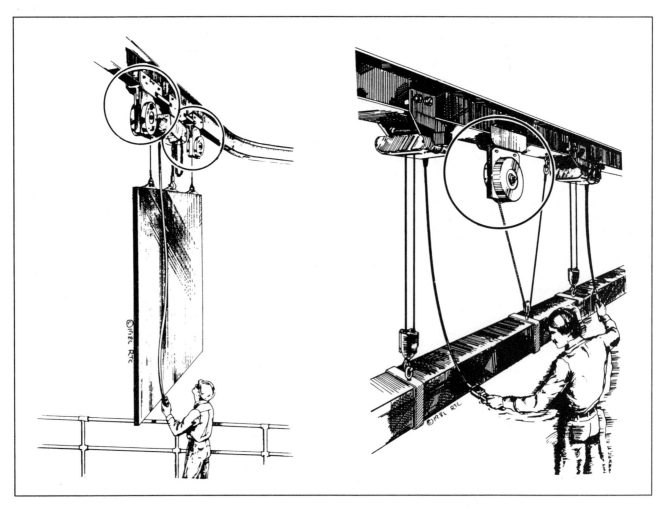

FIGURE 7.43
Quick-acting load arresters (circled) offer worker protection from falling loads, for example, a portable gate section from an underwater nuclear reactor rod storage area (left) and a length of steel at an automotive plant (right).

to supervise the rescue operation. Automatic speed-limiting (controlled) descent devices reduce or eliminate the need for trained rescue personnel – the machine itself controls the rate of descent of the injured worker.

Rescue cradles are an alternative to stretchers, provided that neck or back injury is not suspected. They are useful for small, cramped spaces in crane cabs and towers, but rigid stretchers should be available for victims with suspected broken bones or internal injuries, to be sure that the injury is not compounded.

Aside from helicopters, multiple person rescue from heights can include the optional use of permanent or temporarily-installed chutes for vertical descent.

Load Arresting Systems

For work tasks or manufacturing operations that require personnel to move beneath suspended loads, a backup load arresting system must be used. For instance, custom molds, utility turbines and automobile bodies could cause substantial personal injury and property loss if the hoisting mechanism suddenly fails. A retracting cable unit with a suitable load limit can serve to arrest a fall of a suspended load within a prescribed distance (see Figure 7.43).

Part III: Residual Hazards Associated with the Use of Fall Arrest Equipment

☞ No personal fall arrest equipment system can guarantee that workers will not sustain any injury if a fall occurs. The best that can be expected is a substantial reduction in the likelihood of injury. What is certain is that the improper use of equipment will vastly increase the chance of serious or fatal injury, because misuse builds false security. In particular, safety belt use, swing

WHICH FALL PROTECTION SYSTEM SHOULD BE USED?

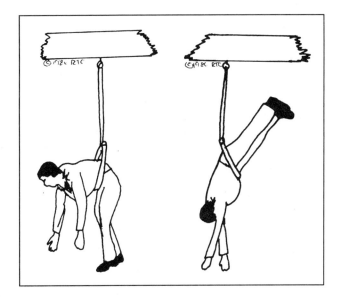

FIGURE 7.44
Examples of falling out of a body belt.

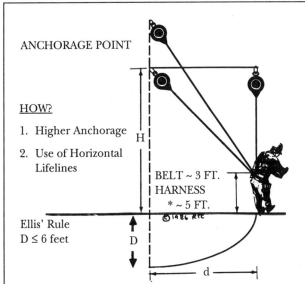

Minimize vertical free-fall distance and swing hazards. If D is chosen as 4 ft., then:

Maximum d (ft.)	Minimum *H (ft.)
5	6
10	15
20	53
50	316

Note: This table addresses vertical fall distance, but obstructions may still be a hazard and must be avoided.

FIGURE 7.45
How to address the problem of swing fall hazard.
Copyright 1986, RTC.

falls, roll-out, equipment originally intended for mountaineering use, home or shop-made equipment and mixing-and-matching equipment designs all can be associated with the misuse or misapplication of equipment for its intended purpose.

☞ The author invites medical directors to read Part III, especially the section dealing with the use of body belts. Some hazards relating to equipment use are described in the following sections.

Note that this is not an exhaustive list of hazards to be expected while using fall protection without adequate forethought of the consequences. It serves only as a guideline for further thought.

Hazard: Body Belt Use for Significant Fall Arrest

The following potential problems should be evaluated.

1. Falling out of a belt.
2. The worker's vulnerable midsection.
3. Prolonged suspension.

1. Falling out of a safety belt poses a serious threat during a fall arrest.[30] Safety belts are sometimes worn loosely and, quite often, are slung down over one hip like a western gun belt. The position of the belt on the body at the beginning of the arrest influences the victim's center of gravity. Should the center of gravity tip the legs downward, the belt might slip up and catch under the arms. On the other hand, if the head and trunk tip forward, the victim can slip headfirst out of the belt and fall to grade level. This is of particular concern with workers who are overweight because it is more difficult to get proper initial fit, and, in addition, the body shape is "top heavy". Belt security depends on catching the rib cage for a feet-first fall, and the hip crest for a head-first fall.

2. The energy generated from free falling can be dramatic. During a fall arrest, forces are transferred to the body and distributed over the body support device. The combination of a narrow belt around the soft, vulnerable midsection and a long free fall is almost certain to result in serious internal injury.[31]

3. Prolonged suspension in a body belt following a fall arrest, in one case, has led to technical asphyxiation.[32] Construction of the diaphragm and other internal organs significantly limits a victim's ability to survive until rescued, especially if unconscious.

A study conducted for OSHA at Wright-Patterson Air Force Base (1986) found that participants were able to hang suspended in a jack-knife position for an average of 1 minute and 38 seconds. Subjects reported abdominal pressure and breathing difficulty. In comparison, the mean suspension time in a full body harness was 30 minutes and 7 seconds.[33] The report concludes that those wearing belts presenting circulatory problems are at greater risk.

What are the alternatives?

- A full body harness, which can distribute arresting forces over more appropriate areas of the body, such as up under the buttocks and, to some extent, over the thighs, shoulders and chest. A harness with a sliding back D-ring can also provide proper upright support, both during and after a fall arrest. An absence of a waist belt enables unrestricted breathing. Rigid discipline on anchorage point designation is required, since the harness D-ring is at least 1 ft. higher than the belt D-ring. Therefore, the anchorages need to be above shoulder height, as opposed to waist height for belt use.
- Limited use of body belts, to free falls less than 2 ft. and to situations where workers can foreseeably recover their position within a few seconds.
- Body belts with a front D-ring, which should only be used with fixed climbing protection systems to help ensure that the device quickly senses a fall and activates fall arrest.
- Workers' choice of body support, which should be available after seeing a videotape of an articulated dummy falling in different types of body supports[34] and after personally experiencing a few seconds of suspension in both a belt and harness.
- Live fall arrest training to simulate field use. This should only be conducted with properly designed and fitted full body harnesses.

Hazard: Swing Falls

☞ Potentially dangerous "pendulum-like" swing falls can result when a worker moves horizontally away from a fixed anchor point and falls. The danger of such a fall is that the arc of the swing produces just as much energy as a vertical free-fall through the same distance. In addition, the hazard of swinging into an obstruction is a major factor. Swing falls are of particular concern with self-retracting lanyards/lifeline devices, because of the longer cable lengths and the worker's ability to move freely.

What are the alternatives? Figures 7.45 and 7.46 illustrate the author's recommendations. "Ellis' Rule for Planning" is that the vertical distance (D) of an arc drop, or the maximum allowed by the agency having jurisdiction, should be less than 6 ft.

Swing falls can be controlled in at least two ways. First, using an appropriate horizontal lifeline can help maintain the attachment point overhead, thereby allowing the fall arrest to occur in a vertical plane. Secondly, raising the height of the anchor point can reduce the angle of the arc and the force of the swing.

On steep angle residential roofs, tests conducted with self-retracting lanyards/lifeline devices by the author indicate swing falls over wood eaves edges were not a serious problem provided the cable would snag within a few feet, and also provided that there was no obstruction immediately below the eave line into which a worker could swing. Central ridge mounting of these retracting devices on a post can also minimize the hazard from roof side falls. Higher post systems are required if tiles are used to avoid obstructions.

For planning purposes, try to to design the system so that D is 2 ft. or less (see Figure 7.45).

Hazard: Roll-out

☞ *Dynamic roll-out* – This can occur when a non-locking single action (originally called single-locking) snaphook is seemingly harmlessly but improperly mated to an attachment point (such as a small eyebolt shape); to another snaphook; to certain D-rings, or to another

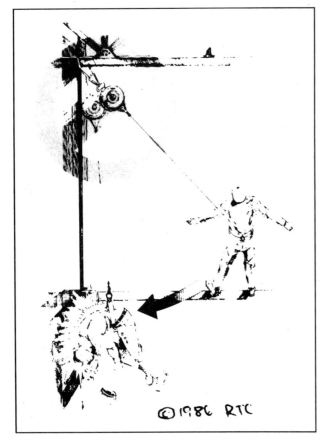

FIGURE 7.46

Example of a swing fall hazard caused by obstructions. Copyright 1986, RTC.

WHICH FALL PROTECTION SYSTEM SHOULD BE USED?

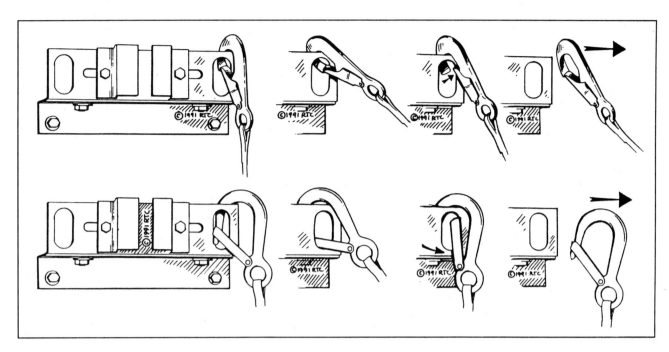

FIGURE 7.47
In a slotted fixture, examples of (top) dynamic roll-out and (bottom) static roll-out.

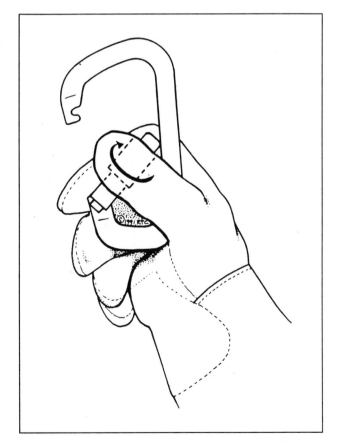

FIGURE 7.48
Field use of a carabiner locking snaphook.

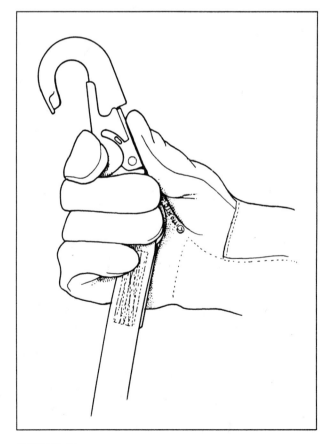

FIGURE 7.49
Equipment section use of a locking snaphook.

shape. For example, accidental disengagement or roll out can result when the force of a fall arrest rebounds back up through the lanyard/lifeline constructed of twisted rope lanyard/lifeline, driving the hook up and around the attachment, depressing the gate, and allowing the snaphook to pop loose or "roll out". This appears to be possible in just a few milliseconds.

A gate strength of several hundred pounds using a positive locking snaphook is sufficient to divert rotational unlocking forces and prevent roll-out; however, a simple self-closing gate snaphook requires only 2 lbs. (approximately) of force to open it. (Information is provided here according to the views of the late Don Beck, D.J. Assoc.)[35]

Static roll-out – This can occur when low forces of just a few pounds are applied in a twisting action between the snaphook and its attachment, so that the gate unlatches and disconnects the two components.

Snaphook roll-out is an accident theory which can be easily demonstrated but hard to prove when alleged.

For example, unknowledgeable workers sometimes erroneously decide the answer to the need for a longer lifeline is to add two lines together, perhaps by connecting the snaphooks of each. Also, they might attach a lanyard snaphook to the wrong-sized structural member (small eyebolt, bolt hole, etc.). Or they might snap onto a horizontal line or around a member back onto their own lanyard. All are conditions which can conceivably result in snaphook roll-out during a fall.[36] However, a more probable disconnection theory is more likely to be the result of no hook up initially.

Roll-out is also possible when a lanyard or lifeline is wrapped around a structure and hooked back onto itself. The twisting and turning of the line under sudden stress against the gate can cause the snaphook to open, releasing the attachment very suddenly and potentially catastrophically.

☞ There are precautions to take against roll-out. When a non-locking single action snaphook is used, strict adherence to the guidelines below should be a minimum safety policy, and indeed is required by OSHA 1910.66 Appendix C.

1. Never attach two snaphooks together.
2. Never attach a snaphook back onto its own lanyard.
3. Never attach a snaphook directly to a horizontal lifeline.

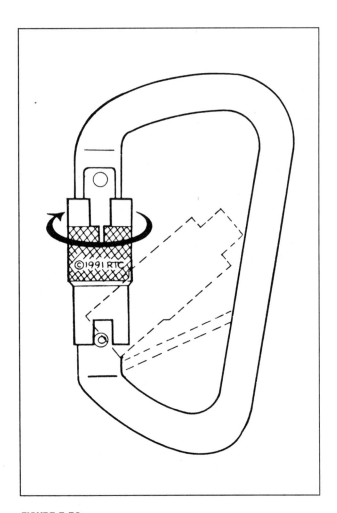

FIGURE 7.50
Function of a type of locking snaphook.

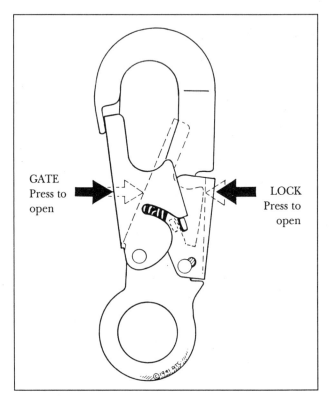

FIGURE 7.51
Function of a type of locking snaphook.

WHICH FALL PROTECTION SYSTEM SHOULD BE USED?

4. Never attach two or more snaphooks to one D-ring.
5. Never attach a snaphook to a webbing loop or webbing lanyard.
6. Never attach a snaphook to a D-ring, eyebolt, rebar or other attachment point that has improper dimensions in relation to the snaphook dimensions.

Locking (originally called double-locking) snaphooks that require two separate forces to open the gate can significantly reduce the potential for accidental disengagement or roll-out. If the hook is twisted momentarily against its attachment point during a fall, the gate keeper is designed to keep the gate locked, thus deflecting the load from the gate to the main strength-beams hook components.

It should be noted that roll-out allegations or capability increases as the snaphook size increases. For example, ladder hooks with approximately 2 in. openings can have more misuse potential than the smaller lanyard-type hook with an approximate 5/8 in. opening.

Attachments to girder bolt holes and angles and flanges are good examples. The need for the locking designs is paramount, in the author's opinion, because sufficient warnings cannot fit onto slender hook designs.

Since there is such a great variability in currently available anchor points at worksites, and because workers may only be able to hook lanyards and lifelines around the anchor and back onto the line, particularly when field supervision is limited, the use of functionally suitable fall arrest snaphook connectors is a vitally important safety consideration for management to address.

Hazard: Mixing and Matching Equipment

☞ A personal fall protection equipment system should be designed, tested and supplied as a complete system. When purchasing any fall protection or emergency escape equipment, it is best to purchase a complete system from a reputable manufacturer or authorized dealer. A complete system should minimally include not only the device and all accessories, but also service, repair and comprehensive instructions required for proper use.

☞ Both the employer and employee should realize that components of a system may not be interchangeable. For instance, if a commodity grade rope is used for a lifeline, it must meet certain manufacturing standards and performance requirements to be considered of a sufficient diameter and strength for use with a specific rope grab device on a prolonged basis.

☞ No component of a fall arrest system should be substituted or changed unless fully evaluated and tested by a competent person or the equipment manufacturer. Large corporations with fall protection audit committees should make it a priority to have on board a competent person familiar with the technical details of mixing and matching equipment. Not only should standards such as ANSI Z359.1-1992 be followed, but also individual components must be tested in house for reasonably expected methods of use.

Hazard: Equipment Misuse

☞ Poor work habits, lack of supervision, and a desire by many workers to declare themselves experienced with rigging lifeline arrangements can lead to uses that are not safe or recommended by the equipment manufacturer.

Considering the use of mountaineering snaphooks and harnesses in an industrial fall arrest system is a lure few industry people can resist, because of usually attractive, lightweight, low-cost designs. However, it is potentially dangerous to consider equipment components which have not been designed into an industrial fall equipment system and approved as such by a competent fall arrest device supplier. Let's discuss this trap for the unwary.

The buyer and user of nearly all mountaineering equipment hardware, harnesses and rope is one and

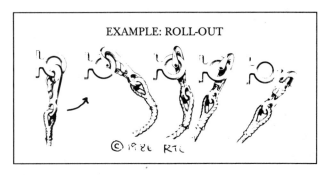

FIGURE 7.52.1
An example of roll-out.

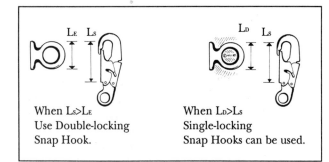

FIGURE 7.52.2
How to determine the proper snaphook.

the same person. The responsibility for equipment use is clearly the user's, and this equipment is for a sports activity, not a work occupation. Hence, for example, a snap with no safety lock or manual screw lock may be a reasonable design.

In industry, workers are often reluctant to use fall arrest equipment unless they have been trained – the responsibility rests with management for equipment use and maintenance. Furthermore, equipment abuse in industry, lack of maintenance, and especially the opportunity for dirty conditions are not foreseeable in mountaineering equipment design.

The best approach here is to stay away from this type of equipment and to request industrial-grade models certified to meet OSHA requirements and ANSI standards. Indeed, industrial grade self-locking carabiners are not a popular alternative to the traditional safety snaphook, but they must be carefully selected and inspected regularly.

Hazard: Electrical

Electric utilities need to provide standards for the use of fall arrest equipment, including the following issues.

☞ Transmission and distribution live-line work calls for fall protection and arrest equipment systems to meet electrical resistance requirements, similar to those of hand, arm, foot and climbing gear. Ontario Hydro has proposed testing be on wet lines and should not exceed a flow of 1 mA when 30 kV are applied over 1 ft.

Static electricity build-up and potential discharge to create a spark creates the need in mines, refineries, etc., for grounding and for minimizing frictional static build up caused by lines rubbing.

Spark discharge from sudden contact between two metal surfaces is conceivable with fall arrest equipment use. Plastic, grounded shells for fall arrest equipment and their synthetic lines, such as a self-retracting lanyard/lifeline device, should provide protection against exterior collisions.

Centrifugal locking pawl action in a self-retracting lanyard/lifeline device is a sudden contact, but within the enclosed device. For protection of snaphooks, D-rings and buckles, a fresh wrap of insulating tape has been recommended by the US Air Force (AFISC/Air Force Inspection and Safety Command). Plastic-coated hardware could become a problem at wear points in a short period of time.

Note that the ignition risks of ordinary flashlights (PSD2212) and ordinary telephones (PSD2213) in Class I, Group D vapors has been studied by the American Petroleum Institute.[37] The reports indicate there is no basis for considering these devices as ignition sources.

Hazard: Heat

☞ Ropes and webs in lifelines can be cut very quickly by inadvertent torch handling or from a welding rod laid down on the steel next to the synthetic material. And steel cable lifelines can ground out welding equipment by inadvertently burning wires. Protection from these heat hazards, as well as from welding flash, is provided with a section of slit air hose or a leather cover. Kevlar® or Nomex®[38] sleeves can be valuable aids to deflecting slag on all types of lanyard and lifelines, if specified by the employer.

Hazard: Cutting Edges

☞ The sharp edges often found on plate glass window panes, angle irons, and fabricated steel shapes can cut web or ropes instantly and disastrously.

Parapets can abrade rope lifelines.

And nip points on swinging scaffold platforms can snag or cut the lifeline.

These various cutting hazards must be carefully analyzed by the employer, and where such cutting edges are found to be a realistic possibility, the lifeline must be protected, or changed, or the hazard eliminated.

Conversely, steel cable lifelines may themselves be a cutting agent for glass-lined tanks or leading and trailing edges of aircraft wings. A synthetic lifeline could answer this potential problem.

Hazard: Intense Cold

☞ Metal may embrittle at temperatures approaching 40° F., which is not uncommon from the Central Plains to the Canadian Arctic.

Snaphooks and eyebolts should be cooled in a dry ice bucket and then impacted with a heavy hammer to obtain qualitative testing results. 4140 steel has been widely used for added security.

Hazard: Corrosion and Dirt

☞ Unless the metal has a large enough cross section, every steel part should be coated with zinc to protect it from salt, air or other common corrosion and to prolong its useful service life. Aluminum parts should be anodized if the parts may come into contact with steel.

Stainless steel cables, springs, and other critical parts are favored over regular steel parts, but many zinc-

WHICH FALL PROTECTION SYSTEM SHOULD BE USED?

MAINTENANCE AND INSPECTION GUIDE FOR FALL ARREST AND WORK POSITIONING EQUIPMENT

Components	Lifetime (yrs) Service	Shelf	System Rating*	Check at 3-6 mo. intervals
Webbings (Belts, harnesses, lanyards)	2-3	7	5000 lb. OSHA – static 900 lb. OSHA for belts – dynamic 1800 lb. OSHA for harnesses – dynamic 600-800 lb. shock absorber – dynamic	• Cuts, wear, burns; pull one unit sample. • Owner self-certifies every 6 months maximum.
Ropes (Lifelines, lanyards)	1-2	5	5000 lb. OSHA – static	• **Synthetic:** cut in strand, paint, worn, dirt inside of rope. For strength: pull end sample. • **Cable:** Kink, broken wire, terminations. Owner self-certifies every 6 months maximum.
Hardware				
Hooks	3		5000 lb. OSHA – static	• Cracks, distortion, wear points, corrosion.
D-rings	5		5000 lb. OSHA – static	• Low temperature service impact reliability.
Fall Devices - Locking				
Rope grabs	1-3		1000 lb. before slip	• Recertification**
Self-retracting lanyard/lifeline	1-2		3000 lb. OSHA, static pull at drum	• Distortion, wear.
Climbing protection device	5		350-450 lb. before slip 1000 lb. proof load – static	• Cleaning difficulty. • Compatible parts. • Operates manually as intended.
Personal Lowering Devices				
Self-retracting lanyard/lifeline	1-2		4-9 ft./sec., † 3000 lb. line strength	• Recertification**
Controlled descent device	5		3-6 ft./sec., † 1800 lb. line strength (UL)	• Distortion, wear.
Descent control device	1-2		Overspeed limit, 5000 lb. line strength	• Controlled payout, equipment readiness for emergency. • Operates manually as intended.

* System Rating: Minimum break strength, maximum arrest force range.
** Recertification: manufacturers offer reconditioning and inspection services.
† Descent speed at 310 lbs. load.
Note 1: Metal goods should have no limit on shelf life expectation as long as they meet the current standards for use. **Check date stamp on each piece of hardware** before requesting information.
Note 2: **Warning!** Any broken stitches must be the signal to remove any webbing product from service because failure could occur at any time with subsequent stresses.
Note 3: Old or obsolete models may not meet current industry specifications and should be replaced.
Note 4: UL means Underwriters' Laboratories.

FIGURE 7.53

Maintenance and inspection guide for fall arrest and work positioning equipment.

aluminum alloys also can work. The ASTM B117 Salt Spray Test on Hardware (exposures to industry norms) is a useful pre-test for fall arrest equipment.

Dirt is a pervasive problem. It has a similar effect and produces the same consequences as corrosion does, namely, making moving parts stick so that the device or system becomes nonfunctional. A preventive maintenance program is required in almost every application of fall arrest and escape equipment to keep systems working properly.

Polymer-filled cables help keep cables flexible in dirty and salt air environments. Watch for corrosion at the lower end of self-retracting lanyards/lifeline devices that are exposed to weather.

Part IV: Equipment Inspection and Maintenance

☞ All equipment manufacturers' instructions need to be incorporated into a corporate and plant inspection and preventative maintenance procedure.[39] This periodic inspection program should be conducted by a competent person.

☞ In addition, all workers need to be trained to manually inspect their equipment. They should be trained in the basics of static loading of fall equipment for test purposes and also in how to look for equipment damage before each usage.

☞ All fall arrest components should be bar-coded by employers to keep track of inspection.

Figure 7.53 presents a recommended maintenance and inspection guide for fall arrest and work positioning equipment. It is very important to note that it is not intended as a complete reference, but only to serve as a guide for employers in establishing and administering their equipment inspection and maintenance programs.

Special situations such as radiation, electrical conductivity, spark generation, chemicals, etc., all must be considered. The recommendations shown in Figure 7.53 should not be regarded as an industry consensus but rather the author's recommended considerations for safety in company procedures.

Cleaning

Synthetic Ropes, Belts and Harnesses
For removing loose debris from these items, washing in soapy water is best, followed by rinsing with fresh water. Drying in a cool area away from UV light is recommended. Always make sure that labels are still legible after cleaning.

Do not use industrial solvents on synthetic materials. These can degrade the product by leaching out oils used in the manufacturing process which provide strength in the final product.

Fall Arrester Devices
Again, washing with soapy water is best for removing loose debris. Alternatively, for caked materials and paint overspray, solvents such as wood alcohol or 1.1.1 tricholoroethane should be used for metal parts. Always make sure that labels are still legible after cleaning.

Do not oil moving parts unless instructed by the manufacturer. For some parts, such as rollers or bearings, which are subject to heavy use or dirt, such lubrication may be reasonable. On the other hand, oil could interfere with descent device brake efficiency, which is unacceptable. However, any lubrication should only be with the manufacturer's approval. Many manufacturers offer reconditioning programs and retesting documentation to aid the equipment owner with device maintenance.

Storage

Keep synthetic materials away from bright light and UV light during storage, and maintain them in a cool dry place. The fading of dyed synthetic color is an indicator to signify UV exposure, which may be unfavorable and call for regular testing or replacement.[40, 41]

Notes

1. ANSI Z133.1-1982 Requirements for Tree Care Operations. New York: American National Standards Institute, 1982.

2. "Golden Anniversary." Time Magazine (May 25, 1987).

3. ANSI A10.11-1989 Requirements for Safety Nets. New York: American National Standards Institute, 1989.

4. Occupational Safety and Health Administration. OSHA 1926.105 Requirements for Safety Nets. Washington, DC.: Department of Labor.

5. Yancey, C.W.C., et al. Perimeter Safety Net Projection Requirements. NBSIR 85-3271.

6. Occupational Safety and Health Administration. OSHA 1926.104 Requirements for Safety Belts, Lifelines and Lanyards. Washington, DC.: Department of Labor.

7. Ibid.

8. ANSI A10.14-1991 Requirements for Safety Belts, Harnesses, Lanyards, Lifelines and Droplines for Construction and Industrial Use. New York: American National Standards Institute, 1991.

9. Ibid.

10. Longerich, Randy, New England Ropes. Personal communication with the author.

11. Occupational Safety and Health Administration. OSHA 1910.27(d) Requirements for Personal Protective Equipment. Washington, DC.: Department of Labor.

12. Ibid.

13. Ibid.

14. Occupational Safety and Health Administration. OSHA Program Directive 100-57. Washington, DC.: U.S. Department of Labor.

15. "Fixed Ladders and Climbing Devices. NSC Data Sheet 1-606, Rev. 83." National Safety News (April 1983): pp. 58-61.

16. Brandt, T., W. Bles, F. Arnold, and T. Kopteyn. "The

Psycholophysics and Posturography of Visual Destabilization at Free Stance." Barany Society Ordinary Meeting Abstracts (June 1978): pp. 25-26.

17. ANSI A14.3-1992 Requirements for Fixed Ladders. New York: American National Standards Institute, 1992.

18. Ibid.

19. "OSHA 1910.270 Proposed Rule for Oil and Gas Well Drilling and Servicing." Federal Register (December 28, 1983).

20. Occupational Safety and Health Administration. OSHA 1926.104 Requirements for Safety Belts, Lifelines and Lanyards. Washington, DC.: Department of Labor.

21. Haas, Frank J., cordage consultant. Correspondence with the author, 1983.

22. National Institute for Occupational Safety and Health. NIOSH Criteria Document 80-106. NIOSH 76-128 Emergency Egress, 1975. Cincinnati, OH.

23. ANSI Z117 Standard for Confined Spaces. New York: American National Standards Institute, 1987.

24. Occupational Safety and Health Administration. OSHA 1910.272 Final Rule for Grain Handling and Storage. Washington, DC.: Department of Labor.

25. National Fire Protection Association. NFPA 101-A39.2.2 (1980) Life Safety Code. Escape Chutes and Controlled Descent Devices. Quincy, MA: National Fire Protection Association, 1980.

26. NIOSH Criteria Document 76-128. Egress from Elevated Workstations. National Institute of Occupational Safety and Health, 1975. Cincinnati, OH.

27. Occupational Safety and Health Administration. OSHA 1910 Subpart E. Requirements for Means of Egress. Washington, DC.: Department of Labor.

28. Subcommittee on Descent Control and Controlled Descent. ISEA Definition on Descent Devices. Industrial Safety Equipment Association, 1977.

29. "OSHA 1910.270 Proposed Rule for Oil and Gas Well Drilling and Servicing." Federal Register (December 28, 1983).

30. Sulowski, Andrew C. "The Safety Belt Question." National Safety News (February 1985): pp. 44-46.

31. Ibid.

32. Ullyse, J. INRS. Personal communication with author, June 27, 1986.

33. Harry G. Armstrong Aerospace Medical Research Laboratory. Evaluation of Fall Protection by Prolonged Motionless Suspension of Volunteers. Wright-Patterson Air Force Base: 1986. U.S. Government.

34. National Engineering Laboratory. Drop Comparison of Safety Belts and Harnesses. Glasgow, Scotland, 1975.

35. Beck, Donald. Guide to Load Bearing Parachute Harness Hardware. U.S. Forgecraft. 1975.

36. Sylvester, Len. "Reduce the Chance of Roll-Out Occurring." National Safety Council Construction Newsletter (November-December 1986): p. 6.

37. American Petroleum Institute. "Preparation of Equipment for Safe Entry and Work," Chapter 5, Guide for Inspection of Oil Refinery Equipment. Washington, DC (1878).

38. Registered trademarks of DuPont Co., Wilmington, DE.

39. "Use Fall-Protection Devices Safely-Follow Instructions." National Safety Council Construction Newsletter (November-December 1986): p. 6.

40. The Cordage Group. "Environmental Degradation of Rope." Product Bulletin-R-5. April 1978.

41. Madigan, Doris L. "Sunlight Degradation of Rope. National Safety News (March 1984): pp. 54-56.

Review Questions

1. What is the main difference between a vertical lifeline and a lanyard?
   a. They are both flexible lines, but the lanyard is stronger.
   b. The lanyard is a shorter flexible line than a lifeline.
   c. A lifeline is longer than a lanyard.
   d. They are the same.
   e. A lifeline is used to extend an anchorage point while a lanyard is used to absorb energy.

2. What is a shock absorber in a fall protection system?
   a. A device which absorbs energy in a fall.
   b. A belt which absorbs shock.
   c. A nylon lanyard.
   d. A bungee cord.
   e. Stretch.

3. You have been purchasing rope grabs from a supplier for years but not the rope lifeline, which comes from your construction warehouse. What potential problem do you face?
   a. An accident from an untested subsystem.
   b. No problem. It's the equipment manufacturer's problem.
   c. No control over the usage.
   d. Workers may object to using the equipment.
   e. OSHA may find something wrong.

4. Other than the fall itself, what additional hazards are possible when experiencing a fall arrest in a loose body belt?
   a. Neck injury.
   b. Collision with an obstruction.
   c. Asphyxiation.
   d. Fall out of belt.
   e. All of the above.

5. What might occur if a worker moves away from the anchorage point of a fall protection system?
   a. The fall device may not work or or it may lock up.
   b. A swing fall can occur.
   c. The fall distance is increased.
   d. The g-force becomes less.
   e. The fall device may not be long enough.

ANCHORAGE POINTS

The quality of a fall arrest anchorage is a benchmark for a fall protection program.

❖ Anchorage planning: the key to fall protection

❖ Elevated falls kill workers

❖ Tools for safety

❖ Elimination of hazards

❖ Employing competent persons

❖ Tying it all together

8

Anchorage Planning: The Key to Fall Protection

☞ Every anchorage point must pass each of the following nine tests for safe usage.[1]

1. Height

- Does the anchor-point height reduce free fall to the shortest distance possible?
- Is the anchor point away from possible collisions with the body or the head?
- Is the anchor point unaffected by the local environment, or contamination such as paint overspray?

2. Location

- Is swing fall reduced to a reasonably safe minimum in order to reduce the potential for collision injury and to allow for self-recovery?
- Is the anchor point continuous by design (to accomplish the task without intermittent fall hazards)?
- Is the anchorage reachable, to permit connection without a hazard?

3. Shape

- Is the anchorage point compatible with the attachment method of the deceleration device? Many shapes are not attachable with snaphooks, including certain eyebolt shapes.
- Will the likely method of attachment cause damage or failure to the deceleration device? Looping a lanyard around an angle iron could cut the lanyard in a fall.
- Will the likely method of attachment be to a bolt hole? Snap hooks can detach from slotted bolt holes with as little as 2 lb. of steady force.
- Can the attachment method allow sliding-down falls or permit cutting the line?
- Will the attachment method of a lanyard to a flange edge without closure of the snaphook gate be prohibited? This is a formula for disaster, even for a few seconds.

4. Strength

- Has the anchor point been recognized as part of a group of engineered anchorpoints, or has a civil or structural engineer certified that specific point for its intended use?

- Is the anchor point reliable if it has long been exposed to the elements, such as salt air, for example?
- Will a tie-back point prevent any additional free fall if a primary anchor point fails?

5. Usage

- How many workers can be safely attached to the same common anchor point? This is an engineering question if the answer is more than one worker.
- Are the load-bearing suspension line and the lifeline attached to separate support systems?
- Is tying knots prohibited for providing anchor point attachments? Knots aren't reliable without a strict worker training system and a single method of tying them.
- Has wrapping a line around a typical structural member such as a I-beam been tested by the company for sufficient strength?
- Is it prohibited to attach snaphooks to each other or to a lifeline or lanyard? Doing so results in hazards such as roll-out and loss of strength.
- Will the snaphook be used for attaching to the structure or for pulling loads? Enormous forces develop in mechanical equipment that will damage fall protection equipment.
- Will the method of use force workers to disconnect themselves at heights because they can't reach their task?

6. Stability

- Has attachment to the lip of an I-beam flange been prohibited? A snaphook may slip off with an angled pull and cause system failure.
- Has attaching a lifeline to a projection been prohibited? The lifeline can detach by movement off the end.

7. Independence

- Are the anchor points independent? The independence of each anchor point from the main work-positioning anchor support is an important principle. Where tripods or the building or structure itself are concerned, the question to address is, what kind of failure would likely produce an injury? Anchor point design should address all predictable scenarios.
- Is the fall protection system engineered? An engineered system may permit the lifelines to be combined for several workers, as long as they are separate from the main work positioning support.

ANCHORAGE POINTS 133

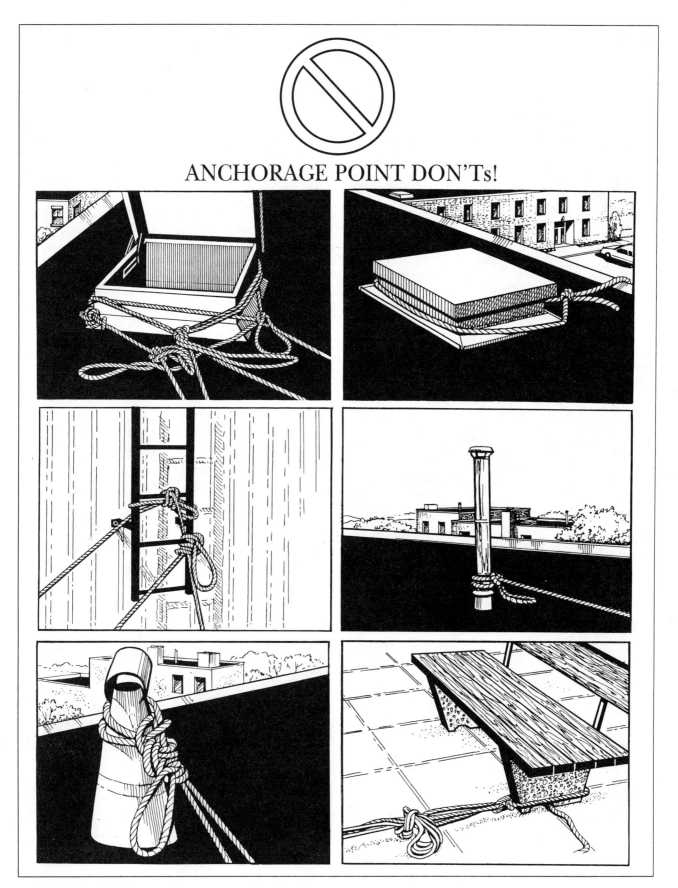

FIGURE 8.1
Anchorage Point Don'ts

ANCHORAGE POINT DOs!

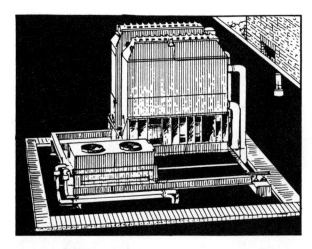
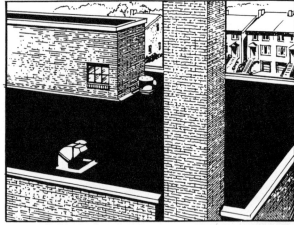
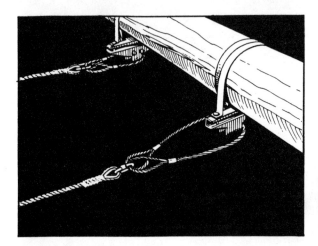
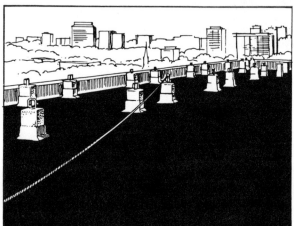
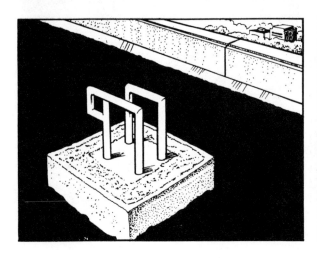
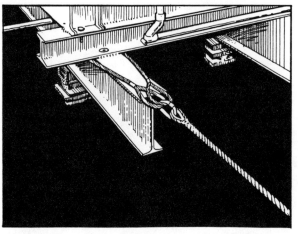

FIGURE 8.2
Anchorage Point Dos

ANCHORAGE POINTS

8. Protection While Moving

- If horizontal lifelines are used to allow protected movement, have they been engineered for this purpose? A horizontal line may be intended as a hand line or perimeter cable. Termination of lines or butting them with mechanical clips can be dangerous under dynamic conditions.
- Do the horizontal lines allow enough sag under the dynamic conditions of a fall to permit the

---

CRITERIA FOR TESTING, LABELING AND RECERTIFYING ANCHORAGE POINTS

Anchorage point choice:
- Non-engineered: 5000 lb. (5400 lb. in 1926.104)
- Retracting lifelines only, non-engineered: 3000 lb.
- Engineered system: twice the maximum arrest force of the fall system, minimum

Permanent anchorage point details

1. Labeling –
   ☞ The following informational content is suggested for a tag:
   - Color
   - Certified to x lb. static load
   - For Fall Arrest use only
   - Approved fall arrest equipment required
   - Warning: Not for any other use
   - Drawing #
   - Call 1-800-xxx-yyyy
   - Last date inspected: dd/dd/dd
   - Must be inspected every y years
   This should be designed as a permanent tag, but replaced every three to five years, or when the tag has deteriorated.

2. Testing Anchorage Points at the Time of Installation –
   Proof load to one half of rated load, statically in the direction of the foreseeable fall.
   The preferred method of anchor bolt installation is through bolting, with a backup distribution plate on the inner wall, or structurally fastening or welding to the structural steel framing of the building or structure.
   Adhesive installations should be tested for an axial strength of 4000 lb.

3. Recertification of Permanent Anchorage Points –
   Test to one half of the certified load capacity, statically in the direction of the foreseeable fall or worst case.
   Any permanent deformation is a signal to reject the anchorage point.
   Stamp the date on the permanent tag.
   Test frequency: group into 1 year, 2 years, 3 years, and grade accordingly.
   - 1 year – frequent use of the area by user trade or other trades
   - 2 years – moderate use of the area by people
   - 3 years – infrequent visits by various people

4. Recertification of Permanent Horizontal Lifelines Attached to Permanent Anchorage Points –
   Inspect annually for any degradation, and if necessary, replace damaged or worn parts. Check torque on any bolts against specification.
   A Professional Engineer should certify, in writing, that the horizontal lifeline assembly is fit for use.
   Stamp the date on permanent tag after inspection.

5. Temporary Anchorage Points –
   Temporary anchorage points should be modeled and approved by a registered Professional Engineer.
   Railings should not be used as anchor points without engineering verification.
   Lifelines should not be attached to parapet wall clamps unless tied back to an acceptable anchorage point.
   Lifelines with or without parapet wall clamps should be in line with the point of suspension when practical, but not more than 10 ft. horizontally, or more than 25 degrees offset.
   Every static and horizontal lifeline that is rigged between anchor points, and to which lifelines or primary support lines are directly attached, shall be used as a Professional Engineer suggests. (This last sentence has been taken from the Ontario Ministry of Labour's Guidelines for Roof Anchorage for Fall Arrest Systems.)

FIGURE 8.3
Criteria for testing, labeling and recertifying anchorage points.

worker to avoid colliding with an obstruction or the ground? Careful analysis is required here for a designed system.

9. Labeling

- Can the anchor point be marked for future recognition and limited specific use? Can anyone claim to recognize a 5,400-lb. anchor point, let alone the other criteria to avoid a predictable system failure in the long run? Of course not. Many managers simply shrug their shoulders — putting a belt and rope lanyard in the hands of the worker, and administering an admonition to tie off, have long been the alibi with these managers for fall protection planning.

The samples shown in Figure 8-1 illustrate six poor choices for anchorage points, based on application of the criteria discussed above. The samples in Figure 8-2, on the other hand, illustrate six good anchorage choices. For a detailed discussion of testing, labeling, and recertification criteria, see Figure 8-3.

Roof Anchors

The following 18 points address design and installation considerations for roof anchors as recommended by the Ontario Ministry of Labour in its Guidelines: *Roof Anchorages for Fall Arrest Systems*, published in September 1991. The recommendations quoted here appear on pages 8 and 9 of the Ministry's Regulation for Window Cleaning, Ontario Regulation 527/88.

"1. Anchors for lifelines, equipment tie back and direct attachment of primary lines for suspended equipment should be designed to resist without fracture and/or pullout a force of 22.5 KN (5000 LBF), applied in the most adverse direction. Equipment tie backs and lifelines shall not be attached to the same anchor. The anchor welding shall confirm to CAN/CSA W59 and carried out by companies certified in accordance with CAN/CSA W47.1. All manufactured window cleaning anchors shall be capable of withstanding the following tests:
   A. A force of 22 KN (5000 LBF) without fracture applied in the direction in which the anchor will be required to withstand tension in service when a worker falls.
   B. A drop test with a 100 kg (220 lb.) rigid mass falling a distance of 1.2 m (4 ft.) without fracture. The test lanyard shall consist of a wire rope 1.8 m (6 ft.) long and 9 mm (3/8 in.) diameter, having an independent wire rope core.

   The above tests shall be witnessed and certified by a professional engineer.

2. For swing stage use, davit bases can be used as a lifeline anchor if it can be demonstrated by a professional engineer that they have been designed or analyzed for the worst loading condition, meet the requirements of Item 1, and are considered a component of the permanent structure. Additional anchors (minimum two) for lifeline attachments shall be provided if davit bases spacing exceeds 7.3 metres (24 ft.). These anchors shall be spaced at 1/3 point of the davit base spacing. If boatswain chair is used, the rigging shall conform to Item 12 of the Guidelines.

3. A continuous rail can be substituted for a series of separate anchors. It is acceptable to tie both equipment tieback and lifelines to the rail or beam provided the system is designed by a professional engineer for all loads likely to be applied as if it were an extension of the roof structure, and installed in accordance with the design. The design loads should be consistent with Item 1 of the Guidelines.

4. The preferred method of anchor bolt installation is through bolting with a back-up or force distribution plate on the side of the wall opposite the connecting "eye" or structurally fastened or welded to the structural steel framing of the building.

5. If through bolting is impractical, only adhesive inserts are acceptable. Adhesive installations shall incorporate a minimum of three adhesive inserts per anchor. If three inserts are incorporated, each insert shall have a minimum diameter of 20 mm (3/4 in.); if four or more inserts are used, each insert shall have a minimum diameter of 16 mm (5/8 in.). All adhesive inserts shall be stainless or corrosion-resistant material. These installations shall be designed and installed under the direction of a professional engineer.

6. Adhesive installations shall be field tested for an axial capacity of 18 KN (4000 lbs.). As an absolute minimum, 25% of the inserts must be tested with a minimum of one insert in every anchor assembly. The tests shall be witnessed and the results documented by a professional engineer who shall give an opinion in writing that the anchorage system is acceptable for window cleaning operations. More stringent testing or rejection of all or some anchors shall be at the discretion of the professional engineer.

7. Static or horizontal lines that are rigged between anchor points for window cleaning operations are not recommended unless Section 29 and Section 10(6) of Ontario Regulations 527/88 is complied with.
    29.(1) Every static or horizontal line that is rigged between anchor points and to which lifelines or primary support lines

are directly attached shall be used as a professional engineer directs, and the professional engineer shall certify the maximum load to be applied to the static or horizontal line.

(2) The support capability of an anchor point shall exceed the total breaking strength of all support lines attached to it.

10.(6) c A lifeline used in a fall arrest system, shall be suspended separately and independently from any suspended scaffold, boatswain's chair or similar single-point suspension equipment.

8. Precast concrete and cast in place concrete parapet walls designed as part of original wall design are acceptable for installation of anchors for window cleaning purposes and/or the support of parapet wall clamps, provided the parapet wall is approved by a professional engineer who is aware of loads to be placed on the wall.

9. Brick parapet walls or brick face parapet walls (with concrete block back-up courses) are not considered to be capable of maintaining the integrity required for anchor installation over a period of time.

10. If a parapet wall is less than 900 mm (3 ft.) in height (i.e. serves as guardrail), fall arrest protection must be provided whenever the worker approaches within approximately 2 metres (6.5 ft.) of the roof edge.

11. If a boatswain's chair or similar single point suspension equipment is used having the primary support lines directly attached to anchors, the horizontal portion of the descent line (that portion of the support lines from the anchor to the roof edge) should be in a plane at right angle to the face of the building at the drop.

12. Life-line anchors and tie-back anchors for outrigger beams and parapet wall clamp should be located in line with the point of suspension whenever practical, but shall not be offset more than 3 m (10 ft.) measured horizontally from running at right angle to the building face at the point of suspension. The angle created by the offset distance shall not exceed 25 degrees.

13. Anchors shall be manufactured from corrosion resistant material or of mild steel that is properly hot-dipped galvanized for the application.

14. The roof sketch shall include the layout and details of the anchor bolt installation and a cross section through the parapet wall. Spacing dimensions of the anchors and the window locations shall also be indicated.

15. The roof sketch shall be reviewed by a professional engineer acting on behalf of the owner of the building(s) and the installation of anchors be inspected and reviewed by a professional engineer.

16. The lifeline of a worker's fall arrest system shall not be tied to a parapet wall clamp.

17. Suspended stages used for window cleaning must have a full front guardrail.

18. Where applicable, it is recommended that rope guides or line stops designed for all loads and forces they may be subject to, be installed at the roof or parapet to prevent the swing and impact of a worker on a building side in a fall arrest situation."

The above 18 roof anchorage recommendations are courtesy of the Ontario Ministry of Labour.

Elevated Falls Kill Workers

On December 12, 1990, window cleaner Jeffrey Suchanec fell 400 ft. to his death from the Academy House condominium building in downtown Philadelphia. All of his equipment, ropes, lowering device and lifeline immediately followed him to the street below.

Suchanec was wearing a harness, and his rope grab was attached to the lifeline, but he was not as safe as he looked.

☞ It is in situations such as this one that the older fall protection methods break down. Who can guarantee that any worker can select any of the criteria listed above to best suit a particular kind of work or work method? Personal choice is not what elevated fall protection is all about.

Fall hazards at the same level, on steps, and on stairs are an engineering subject having to do with visibility, wear and tear, friction in wet and dry conditions, behavior, and inclement weather such as snow. Spills, oversprays and mists such as paint, oils or greases add to the considerations. Timely housekeeping can control the variables, and a plan for material placement can limit trip falls on construction sites.

Fall hazards at heights should be engineered out if possible. Those hazards remaining deserve a backup system for when the worker forgets or momentarily loses control. Why? Because these hazards are so lethal. Eventually, conditions will combine to produce the scene for a disastrous fall, one which is entirely preventable in almost every case if workers follow proper procedures.

If this perspective fails to impress the old guard who responds, "You can't provide protection from every hazard!" or "You can't guarantee safety!", read on to see what can be done.

Tools for Safety

Railings, perimeter cables, scaffolds, and aerial platforms are the first choice for fall prevention.

In general, however, there are two types of equipment used at heights – work positioning equipment and fall arrest equipment.

If the worker's weight is actively and steadily applied to the equipment to help the worker do the job, then that is work positioning equipment. For example, a lineman typically leans on a belt and strap system.

Fall arrest equipment, however, is passive. The only force you see, other than the weight of the equipment itself, is dynamic force during an accidental fall.

We can plan safety at heights and we can train employees in better work methods, but too many company supervisors still leave the entire choice of work method and safety provisions to the worker. "After all, he chose this line of work and has the job experience, so he should know best," goes the reasoning, along with "I can't be with the worker and do her job for her."

However, the actual tools for safety too often have not been provided to the worker. The critical safety knowledge needed to deal with heights safely is not inherent in the minds of most managers. It needs to be learned. Tolerating fall hazards has become an unconsciously accepted practice many managers develop early in their careers. They unfortunately think workers who fall weren't careful enough, or simply were unlucky.

Elimination of Hazards

It's true that all hazards can't be eliminated from a particular situation. However, by addressing the known hazards we can predict how most of them can be eliminated, or reasonably controlled, before workers are exposed to them. A simple checklist is often all that's needed, because it forces visualization of how the work is supposed to be done.

Aren't Fall Hazards Obvious?

Isn't it obvious to any person (who may someday sit on a jury) that height hazards are a known severe injury producer, if not a reasonably certain fatality producer? Then why don't employers address this hazard exposure as one which can be reasonably eliminated or controlled? Why is such a severe and foreseeable hazard left for the worker to solve alone? And why do so many employers and managers think they are immune from responsibility as a result of the workers'-compensation system?

A casual reading of a 1984 Bureau of Labor Statistics report on falls in the workplace confirms that permanently disabling falls can occur from a height of 10 ft. or lower. They don't have to be from 100 ft. or 200 ft., where a fatality admittedly is more certain.

The key word should be thoroughness, not simply awareness, when it comes to providing proper fall protection. Notice use of the word provide, not ensure. Beyond training lies a failure to follow procedures. How do you prove what really happened, for proper accident analysis, if you've let workers randomly select their own anchorages?

The Pandora's Box of assumptions in fall protection practice starts with management and leads directly to the worker. Permitting guesswork automatically implies worker negligence; this must be replaced by provable sequential facts if fall protection is to be applied in a reasonably scientific manner.

Important Anchorage Factors

Anchorage point engineering may have to take advantage of the OSHA 2:1 factor of safety to provide anchorages for such items as railings, tubular-frame scaffold members, antenna parts, ladder rungs, and wooden structures.

Should anchorages be strength or dynamic tested? The answer is, strength-tested, but not necessarily on an individual basis. Classes of anchorages can be addressed on engineering drawings with written directions to workers to be applied in training courses.

A short fall allows a reasonable self-recovery to a walking/working surface. Free falls should not exceed 2 ft. Anchorage point height must be above the D-ring (fall arrest attachment point) and next to the worker at all times, even within a changing work area such as a construction site. Scenarios for potentially serious line abrasion and collisions during a fall are part of the employer's analysis required in each special application.

Employing Competent Persons

Now is the time for employers with recurring fall-hazard exposures to appoint a competent person to evaluate fall hazards, as required by OSHA. This individual should be familiar with fall protection methods and their limitations, and should be authorized to abate the foreseeable hazard.

Also required now is the appointment of a qualified person, a representative of the civil or structural branch of engineering, to assist in eliminating or controlling fall hazards at the design and planning stages of each new construction and maintenance project.

Who Creates Fall Hazards?

Designers, engineering consultants, design-builders, architect/engineers, suppliers, construction managers, superintendents and knowledgeable owners must realize that they create the work environment and thus its fall hazards. They, more than anyone else, need to apply the proper knowledge and training to the project to address fall hazards. It's time that a formal fall protection plan accompanied each project, with awareness by the designer of how fall hazards can be dealt with.

Potentially qualified individuals should upgrade their qualifications to support field experience, to which proper fall protection has never been previously applied. Qualifications include becoming a board-certified Safety Professional or a Professional or Registered Engineer. These designations afford the professional application of practical people safety skills and simple mechanical engineering calculations to each potential fall hazard situation. And they afford personal commitment to the subject of fall protection and to the needed control measures.

Tying It All Together

Down-to-earth facts show that fall protection provisions can reasonably be made at the job-planning stage. Since we know where the workers must go and what they must do, let's plan for them to do it safely.

Too many owners and managers lump slip, trip and fall hazards into one category, and thus think in simple terms for solution — "Watch your step," "Be careful," and "Take your time and don't take chances." These managers are from the awareness school. But worker awareness on the job is like much like bananas on the kitchen table — a quickly perishable commodity.

☞ Work can't be done efficiently and productively without the proper tools. Likewise, elevated fall protection can't be accomplished without the proper tools. But selling the attitude of practical fall safety has never been simple, and the job is never finished. Anchorage-point planning and documentation is the trail by which our efforts will be measured.

Notes

1. Ellis, J. Nigel. "Anchorage Planning: The Key to Fall Protection". National Safety Council. *Safety and Health*, September 1991: 66-70.

Review Questions

1. A railing traditionally has been used as an anchorage point for many years, during shutdown maintenance on a flare stack while moving from a manbasket to a permanent platform at a height of 300 ft. A structural engineer who is asked to calculate the strength of the top rail determines that the upper strength capacity (to yield) in new condition would be 2000 lbs. You, as safety professional, must decide what to do as follows:
   a. Tell the contractor the strength limit.
   b. Instruct the contractor to use shock-absorbing lanyards.
   c. Review the contractor's fall protection program and either accept or reject it.
   d. Tell the contractor that he or she cannot use the railings.

2. A 20-ft. scaffold is to be built on the outside of a vessel up to a manway starting 45 ft. above ground. After thorough training, what fall protection would you expect to see planned for use for each worker during erection?
   a. Lanyard and belt.
   b. Two lanyards and harness.
   c. Retractable lanyard and harness.
   d. Horizontal lifelines, rope grab and belt.

3. A scaffold is to be built starting at the 250-ft. platform level of a three-legged flare stack up to the 295-ft. level under a platform which is to be extended. What should be used for an anchorage point during erection?
   a. Rope grabs with lifelines attached to each of the three tower legs (20 ft. apart).
   b. Two lanyards and harness per worker attached to scaffold legs.
   c. Retractable lifelines attached to flare stack flange lugs.
   d. Horizontal lifelines between scaffold members.

4. A vessel is to be scaffolded, but there is no convenient anchorage point above the manway to be reached. What is required for use of the scaffold as an anchor point?
   a. Two lanyards.
   b. Railings.
   c. Tie-in of the scaffold and minimum two to one safety factor for scaffold members.
   d. Tie-in of the scaffold and 5000 lb. strength requirement.

5. A 10-ft.-wide piperack has a cabletray running parallel over the same supports in a petrochemical plant and which seems to have the highest frequency of travel in the plant. Your fall arrest

manufacturer salesperson says he will be happy to provide you with one lifeline. You stop to consider:

a. Anchorage point locations.
b. Clearance distances.
c. Sufficiency for two persons.
d. The various ways of access that may be made.

6. In a heavily trussed production building, a roof project involves changing out concrete roof that has a history of not supporting human weight reliably as it has aged. The workers have caulked translucent panels regularly and have been told to walk only on the purlins to which the panels are attached. Your horizontal lifeline solutions are installed, but workers are afraid that they will swing back through the opening into the building ceiling obstructions. What to do?

a. Provide a cover for the opening before it is created.
b. Use a second lifeline attached to each person.
c. Re-roof the building with a reliable sealer.
d. Put the roof off-limits.

7. A contractor is building a warehouse extension which will bring the building to 200 ft. long and 150 ft. wide. The ridge is only 3 ft. elevation above the eaves. Even though the contractor indicated that fall protection was 100% and had workers who appeared to be tied off, a worker falls to the concrete floor from the ridge opening at 28 ft. and is severely injured. The contractor proposes to attach the crane hooks of two mobile cranes together over the roof to which workers will attach lanyards for protection. What is your response?

a. Ask for an engineering assessment.
b. Deny the request based on crane manufacturer's literature.
c. Permit use if the strength is sufficient.
d. Permit use if shock absorbing lanyards are used.

APPLICATIONS

No fall protection system can make up for a poor work method.

❖ Roofing work

❖ Swing/suspended scaffolds

❖ Scaffolds

❖ Lifts and aerial platforms

❖ Ladders

❖ Confined spaces

Guide for Roofing Work

A vast number of work methods exist that foresee movement on roofs. This vast number gives both construction and maintenance a very complex set of options for fall protection. There are two types of fall hazards: those through the roof or floor, and those off the edge or perimeter.

Falling Through

A major problem with roofs is that workers can fall through a skylight, skylight opening, air duct opening, or other various openings, even if the openings are small. To the author's knowledge, there have been catastrophic falls through openings of 14" x 53" and 21" x 23". Sealing holes and openings the moment they are created – or guarding them effectively – is the only reasonable solution.

The most dangerous fall hazard is a sudden collapse. Renovating buildings with suspect floors or roofs calls for an engineer's plan for demolition, such as described in OSHA 1926.850 (a), before contractors or employees are permitted to use them for access. Spreading the load with plywood boards for anticipated access may be a reasonable solution.

Falling Off the Edge

OSHA's fall protection for slopes less than 4 in 12 is based on guarding low–pitched roof perimeters during the built–up work phase (OSHA 1926.500 (g). The options for fall protection at sides and edges over 16 ft. eave height are as follows:

1. Motion–stopping systems. Motion–stopping systems include scaffolds or platforms with guardrails, safety nets and fall arrest systems.
2. Warning lines. A warning line is a flagged cable, rope or chain between 34 in. and 39 in. high, set back 6 ft. or more from the edge. Stanchions must support a 16 lb. tipping force at 30 in., and the line must be 500 lb. minimum tensile strength.
3. Safety monitoring systems. The safety monitoring system cannot be used when mechanical equipment is on the roof.

Although OSHA does not provide for a hierarchy of protection, the author believes that protection can reasonably be provided with motion–stopping systems and warning lines. A safety–monitoring system may not be effective, based on the following analysis.

A safety–monitoring system is defined in OSHA 1926.502(p)(8) as follows:

A safety system in which a competent person monitors the safety of all employees in a roofing crew, and warns them when it appears to the monitor that they are unaware of the hazard or are acting in an unsafe manner.

The safety monitor must be on the same roof as, and within visual sighting distance of, the employees, and must be close enough to verbally communicate with the employees.

A safety monitor system is usable on roofs 50 ft. or less in width, where mechanical equipment is not being used or stored (1926.500 (g) (1) (iii)).[1]

In the roofing trade workers frequently work backwards. This raises the probability of falls, because workers are unable to directly or peripherally observe some stepping or elevated hazards.

Can trained and hazard–knowledgeable monitors provide effective fall protection? See Figure 9.1 and consider the following:

- According to University of Michigan research in the 1970s, and the author's own tests, workers can fall from a standing position over an edge within 6 ft. by tripping, slipping, stubbing their toe, or other loss of balance. In such situations, the monitor can't react effectively to stop the fall over the edge by voice contact alone, once the fall has started in that direction.
- How far from the edge should an employee be before being warned about stepping over the edge? The minimum distance to warn an employee who may trip is 6 ft., which is the basis of the

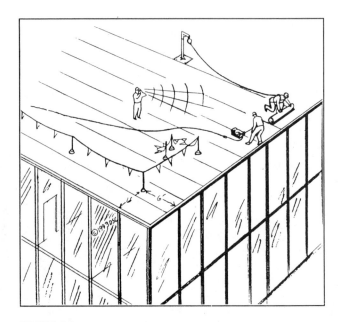

FIGURE 9.1

Safety monitoring versus positive fall protection. A shout may be the last thing a worker hears as he or she hurtles to the ground.

warning line distance rule. Since work inside this 6 ft. limit is the basis of the safety monitor role, if the trip or slip occurs, the monitor is powerless to stop the fall.

- The monitor may become inattentive over a period of time. It is not reasonable to expect continued focused attention on one or more workers near a roof edge. Each worker requires separate monitoring for predicting a dangerous step toward the edge. A monitor's attention may easily be diverted for several seconds, which is enough time to permit a worker to step over the edge. An analogy may be a lifeguard who has to watch many swimmers, but has difficulty tracking even one. Yet the lifeguard has only a few seconds to react and reach a potential victim.
- The monitor may be distracted by noise and other environmental conditions over an eight–hour day. Equipment and machinery noise in the area could obscure warning sounds. If work is started early or finishes late, the light may diminish and reduce visibility. Artificial lighting provides shadows, which permit some fall hazards to go unnoticed.
- The monitor must warn the worker while the worker still retains control over his or her balance and before he or she inadvertently steps over an edge. This is at least one step, or 3 ft., away from the edge while moving backwards, before an attentive monitor can be convinced that a fall is imminent. Yet 50% of the time inside the warning line may be within the 3 ft. limit from a roof edge. A step occurs at the rate of 3 ft./sec., and one or two steps to the edge take only one or two seconds. (See Figure 9.1.)
- A warning must be heard by the worker. He or she could be deaf on that side, have ears obscured by head coverings, or could have a head cold. Also, the worker could be startled by a machine starting up or be unaware of a warning because of background noise.
- A warning from 50 ft. is much less effective than one from 10 ft. More time is required to give and receive warnings at longer distances.
- Some roofing felts may extend over the edge without being tacked or wrapped. This could lead to both the worker and monitor being unaware of unstable footing. This results in a step close to the edge and an immediate fall over the edge. Even if both monitor and worker are aware of this, it's an easy fact to forget momentarily. The eye can be deceived when attention is diverted, even briefly.
- A worker's reaction to spilled hot roofing liquids may cause him or her to step quickly to the side and possibly off the roof. This has occurred in the author's experience with the accident investigation of a fatality.
- Raising material to the roof by well wheel pulley requires a worker to be at the roof's edge, looking down and communicating with a ground person, and also to bring loads onto the roof. If the load is upset or the pulley system tips, then the worker can be pulled over the edge by the equipment.
- A worker can lose balance due to any of many possible events, such as the following: stepping onto a slight depression or elevation in the roof, backing into an obstacle behind the knee, experiencing a trick knee, turning an ankle, spilling hot liquid roofing material, fumes, vibration, pushing a wrench, looking up momentarily into bright sunlight, or watching a bird or plane overhead. Problems such as dizziness, sickness, getting up suddenly, rapidly bending down then up, and losing grip on a load or object, among others, may cause a fall, and are probably beyond the control of a monitor.

Flat Roofs

For flat roofs with slopes less than 4 in 12, catastrophic falls are predictable within 6 ft. of a roof edge, and are best stopped by fall protection, physical barriers and lifelines. These devices, when properly installed and maintained, can act automatically to stop such a fall. A monitor who has to react, warn, be heard and then heeded, involves too much time and uncertainty for a catastrophic fall hazard potential.

A situation where a monitor might be effective is when a roof is close to water, into which it is reasonably safe to fall and then be rescued. In some situations, a reasonable fall height is up to approximately 20 ft. Other surfaces, besides water, might offer an equal or better cushion for a fall without injury under normal conditions. It should be noted that the Federal Railroad Administration has reduced the maximum fall hazard from 20 ft. to 12 ft. from railroad bridges.[2]

It takes a minimum of 3/4 second to react to a road hazard, according to many state driver's manuals.[3] And in that 3/4 second, a worker can walk approximately 3 ft. – one full step – before the monitor is even able to raise an alert call. (According to a U.S. Army report, average walking speed is 4 to 4.5 ft. per second.)

According to the present standard, OSHA 1926.500(d)(4), any mechanical equipment used or stored on the roof (which may obscure visibility, produce smoke or fumes, or provide a noise distraction) must have a warning line 10 ft. from an edge or motion–stopping system close to that edge.

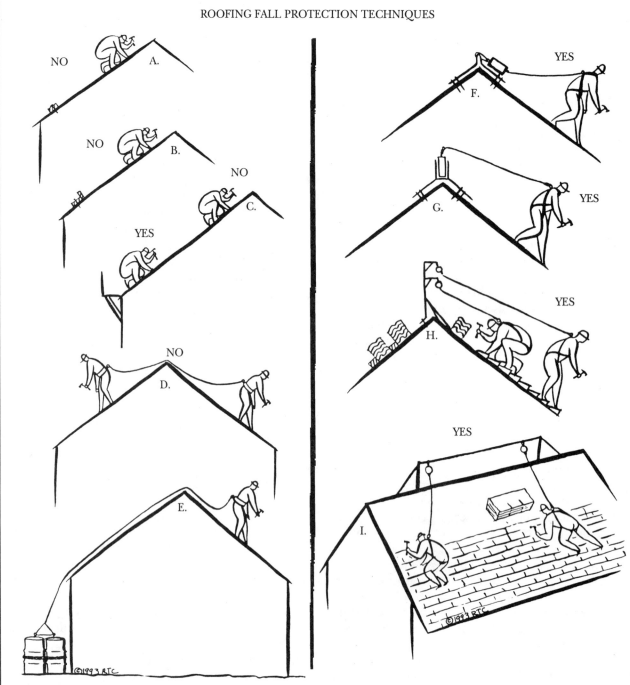

A. NO. Work practice of a "2-by-4" used for a slide stop or a hand grasp – rejected.
B. NO. Offered as an improvement to "A" above, to an Administrative Law Judge (Nicholas v. Secretary, OSHRC Docket #89-500) – rejected.
C. 10-ft. vertical height is the Washington State limit. It is also used for placing trusses.
D. NO. Human counterweight is sometimes used, but it is often impractical or even improperly applied.
E. 5400-lb. anchorage, with lifeline secured above the point of operation. Requires strict rules for proper usage.
F. Practical for securing upper boards in sheeting operation; also for planning shingles and shakes.
G. Alternative installation technique to "F" above.
H. Higher anchorage for tile operations used by two workers.
I. For use on commercial roofs with heavy-duty trusses or ridge beams.

FIGURE 9.2
This illustration of roofing fall protection techniques does not address gable fall protection techniques.

APPLICATIONS

145

Planning Safe Roof Work

It is the author's experience, after investigating many roof edge falls, that even skilled, knowledgeable roofers cannot maintain a constant awareness of site fall hazards while also concentrating on the roof work at hand for an indefinite period of time.

Thus, effective roof work planning must take into account many factors, including the following:

1. The nature of the work to be done, and the workers' physical fitness.
2. Access fall hazards, including ladder use and stability.
3. Through–the–roof fall hazards (e.g. openings, skylights, deteriorated structures).
4. Material handling access fall hazards.
5. Freedom to move without tangling lifelines.
6. Unusual stresses from proposed lifting procedures, and movement of materials to and from secure areas with fall–free access.
7. Emergency action plan OSHA 1910.38.
8. Training to meet OSHA roofing requirements, and routine testing for safety knowledge.
9. Positive fall protection options to suit the specific work.

Effective roof work fall protection techniques protect roofing workers while affording them the mobility and comfort they need to accomplish their work. See Figure 9.2 for an illustrated discussion of techniques.

Construction or Repair of Steep Roofs

Steep roofs with slopes of 4 in 12 or greater are addressed by OSHA 1926.451(u)(3), which calls for a catch platform when the eave height exceeds 16 ft. The catch platform must be 2 ft. wide, with guardrails, and with a toeboard. Catch platforms are effective only for workers close to the eave, so fall arrest systems are the systems of choice for most situations on steep roofs. (Several anchor point systems for various roof designs are shown in this book.)

Fall arrest systems for the gable edges of steep roofs should be planned so as not to permit dangerous swing falls. (OSHA regulations relating to gables are not specific, but 1926.500(d)(1) may apply.)

Roof construction, especially for residential roofing in North America, involves setting trusses, sheeting, and finally roofing with a water–resistant material. Present methods of construction bring trusses to the top floor by crane or forklift, where they are spread and nailed together with "2-by-4" pieces. This spacing and nailing typically exposes carpenters to both exterior and interior fall hazard from narrow lumber edges. Designers should consider a plywood floor where sup-

port exists, and firmly hook on railed platforms, to provide a reasonable walking surface for installing each truss sufficiently, from a central point.

A worker standing on plywood boards placed on the lower truss member can attach a waist–high "2-by-4" around the perimeter. Then the first two rows of sheeting can be positioned and nail–gunned from the interior to the exterior position before any access to the sheeting is permitted. A lifeline already attached to a center truss top point can be used for backup protection. On steeper roofs, a positioning system will also be needed.

Roof Maintenance Operations

Wherever routine work on an existing roof occurs, the same fall protection requirements will apply for general industry as for construction. Repairs and occasional work will usually fall under construction regulations.

Window cleaners who are letting down lines or hauling them up must be protected within 6 ft. of an edge; they should take advantage of the lifeline attached to its anchor point. The rope grabbing device can be moved along the lifeline until the worker is in position at the roof edge.[4]

Note that proposed OSHA standards intend to address heights over 6 ft.

Exterior Building Maintenance Safety Procedures for Elevated Work

Rules for elevated work are in addition to the rules for protecting the public below any area being worked. Examples of public protection rules are roping off ground areas and providing warning signs adequately placed to keep pedestrians away from the immediate area.

The proposed procedures that follow relate to elevated work and personal protection safeguards. Rules should be dated and given in card form to each worker, and explained in a meeting. Workers must be trained frequently on the rules, using slides or videos to emphasize points and to demonstrate techniques. Each rule should be the subject of a weekly safety meeting. Workplace safety problems should be fully discussed in these meetings.

Audits must be done continuously to maintain high standards of compliance. For these rules to be effective, the violation of any OSHA rule should be documented in a worker's personnel file with a warning. Workers should be allowed one warning only and then be dismissed for any further violations. Working foremen and workers are to be reminded that safety is not obvious or common sense in any way. Proper procedures must be followed according to company policy and rules. They should be reminded that the company supports this fully, with appropriate engineering support when necessary, especially for unusual conditions.

Building owners' specifications for anchorage points must meet OSHA requirements before the work is started. Do not use railings unless they have been proven to support 5,000 lbs. or other load as a part of an engineered system.

1. Two Workers Minimum

There must be at least two workers on a building. One worker is designated the safety person, who stays on the roof or the ground. Preferably, there is one person at both locations while any descent is being made. This person should safeguard the installation and ensure that visitors to the roof don't interfere. The safety person should remain on the roof until the descent is completed, and stay in radio communication with the company and the descending person(s).

If both workers must work on the side of the building, then there must be adequate provisions for safeguarding the roof area.

The rig should be effectively labeled with warnings to reasonably ensure that visitors to the roof don't interfere with the rig inadvertently.

2. Safety Checks By Workers

Each person on the roof doublechecks the other for safety before the one goes over (or both in case of a double drop). This check is a component check, including a lifeline anchorage system for each person. The lifeline system must be separate in its entirety from the load line and without any links or connections to the seat/chair or any of its related hardware. The harness must be worn properly, with straps correctly positioned and snugly fitted, and must be directly connected to the rope grab via a lanyard without being part of the load line system or seat support.

3. Maximum Free Fall Distance

No person should be able to fall more than 6 ft. in free fall at any time, at any position, because of the method of hook up to the fall protection system or because of lanyard length.

4. Fall Protection Near Edges

A fall protection system should be in continuous use when close to an exposed edge. An exposed edge is any one of the following:

- Any unprotected side (with a barrier such as a railing or parapet zero to 30 in. in height).
- Any unprotected side with a barrier incapable of taking a downward load of 200 lbs.

- Any unprotected side, where the height of a vertical barrier at least 30 in. high plus the depth of the barrier's top edge is less than 48 in. in total distance.
- Any barrier over which the worker's elbow may reasonably project in conducting work.
- Any unprotected side with a roof slope of 1 in 4 or greater.

Note: Buildings should have warning lines minimally 6 ft. from an edge as a permanent installation. If pulling mechanical equipment toward an edge, 10 ft. is required for a warning line, according to OSHA. The warning line needs to be 6 ft. from an edge normally to provide a "tactile" warning of the edge's approach.

5. Anchorage Point Checks

Each anchorage point should be capable of supporting a rated load and be labeled as such (see Chapter 8 for detailed anchor point discussion).

Each person, or the safety person, checks the other person's anchorage point and method of attachment on each building. A file should be maintained on each building, keeping a record of which anchorage points were used for which descent, for future use or to document how cables were attached.

Cable systems used for anchorages around buildings or structures on the roof should be stainless steel with fittings attached according to the wire rope manufacturer's instructions or standard rigging handbooks.

All temporary and permanent rope terminations, including wire cable, should be demonstrated to meet the minimum OSHA standards strength requirements by publishing diagrams for workers that illustrate the method of construction of the termination and verify the proper setting or torque. No deviations should be permitted without the express written approval of an officer of the contractor on a one–by–one project application basis. Such approvals expire within 30 days. This avoids the exceptions becoming the norm over time, and must be rigorously maintained.

6. Attention To Detail

Never take anything for granted! Each drop should be treated like a space shot, with great attention to detail. Remember that what worked yesterday or this morning may not be satisfactory this afternoon. There must be a backup for any reasonable predicted failure of any part of the descent system, in addition to human failure. Training, inspection and maintenance need to be applied to each building regarding anchorages, anchorage connectors, horizontal lifelines, rope grabs, lanyards and harnesses.

7. Horizontal Lifelines

All horizontal lifelines or lines to which vertical load lines or vertical lifelines are attached should be carefully engineered, and should be documented, with a report on file which can be used as a model for similar situations.

This type of lifeline system should not be used by more than one person at a time. This means that there should be no common parts, lines, hooks, tiebacks or anything except the building itself which would link the individual lifelines of two or more persons, unless the lifeline is engineered by a registered professional engineer who is knowledgeable in fall protection and building exterior maintenance work methods.

9. Descent Devices

Work positioning descent devices should have a dead man lever, in order to prevent inadvertent failure from lack of human operator control at some point in the lifetime of the descent device, regardless of the efficiency of any lifeline system. A lifeline system is designed only for unforeseen failures, not predictable failures, no matter how long it takes for a catastrophic event to occur.

10. Snaphooks

All snaphooks must be of self–locking design. Screw–gates are not effective. Never use a snaphook if it does not operate in perfect condition or even if it is without any apparent damage or visible stress. All snaphooks must meet OSHA requirements. Inspect all of them before each use. Refer to Chapter 7 for detailed inspection criteria and checklists.

11. Owner/Contractor Relationship Regarding Roof Anchors

Responsibility for new building roof anchors – The owner/building manager must be told that he or she is responsible for providing anchorage points suitable for foreseeable exterior suspended work. And there should be no exception for new buildings when the exact locations for tie–backs and anchors can be laid out based upon the contractor's experience and proposed work method.

Responsibility for existing building roof anchors – All building managers must be told in advance of the job that exterior work can be done more safely with properly–positioned roof eyebolts. The contractor can send a standardized proposal to the building manager after each contract is won, proposing that the eyebolt installation work be done at the same time as the maintenance contract for more economical results and more safety in the future.

Roof anchor design criteria – Eyebolts or fixtures for roof anchors must be engineered into the roof:

- Eyebolts must permit attachment of 5/8–in. or 3/4–in. opening snaphooks. The size of the eyebolt's "eye" must be compatible with snaphook design to prevent accidental disengagement, known as roll–out. Each eyebolt must be able to support a minimum of 5,000 lb. static loading for a personal lifeline anchorage support in the direction of foreseeable dynamic loading. Check load line support requirements with the scaffold or boatswain's chair system manufacturer or with the jurisdictional authority.
- Fixtures are desirable when retracting lifelines are expected to be used for approaching a building edge within 6 ft. without protection. They allow such a device to be suspended without contacting the surface of the roof, which can cause abrasion and premature locking. (For a survey of possible designs, see the September 1991 issue of *Safety & Health* magazine.)

Eyebolts and fixtures for roof anchors must be permanently labeled, tested for capacity and periodic testing records kept by the building owner/manager.[5]

Guide for Contractors Who Use Swinging/Suspended Scaffolds

All contractors who do elevated work should have a well–defined safety policy, detailed procedures and ongoing training for high work. This section addresses some aspects of a fall safety program. When there is a need for fall protection beyond the scope of these recommendations, further advice must be sought.

The standards in this field, including fall protection requirements, are noted in Figure 9.3.

Use of suspended work platforms, including boatswain's chairs, always requires fall protection. The OSHA 1910.66 requirements and the very similar 1926 subparts L and M are helpful revisions proposed and published in the Federal Register.

One exception to an independent lifeline requirement for each worker can be where each suspension rope is supplemented with a separate line equipped with an automatic locking device. In this case, attachment to a sufficiently strong scaffold structural member could be adequate, after an engineering review. Horizontal lines across the back of the scaffold and sliding attachments for short lanyards assist mobility while protecting against falls over the side.

When used on two–point scaffolds, a one–end failure results in a swing problem, which most probably will

Standards Addressing Fall Protection for Scaffolds and Elevated Platforms

General Industry

OSHA 1910.66	Powered Platforms for Exterior Building Maintenance
OSHA 1910.28	Safety Requirements for Scaffolding
ANSI A39.1-1987	Window Cleaning
ANSI A120-1992	Safety Requirements for Powered Platforms for Building Maintenance

Construction

OSHA 1926.451	Scaffolding
OSHA 1926.500	Floor and Wall Openings
OSHA 1926. 1050-53	Stairways and Ladders
ANSI Z10.8-1988	Floors and Wall Openings

Note: Several states have special requirements and some states permit approved fall protection equipment.

FIGURE 9.3
Standards applicable to scaffolds and elevated platforms.

cause severe impact injuries for the worker. The worker also will suffer an extremely long fall, even if the sliding device is a locking design. In addition, when close to the ground, swinging into the ground could cause severe injuries that might be avoided with an independent lifeline.

Independent lifeline systems can be of two types. Both types allow freedom to move vertically and, within limits, horizontally, and can sense a free fall and lock to arrest that fall.

Rope Grab Systems – Rope grab systems should be designed for industrial use; ascender devices designed only for mountaineering use should not be used. The three principle types of rope grab systems are cam, friction and inertial. The key is to move freely along the line with little or no friction, yet grab when a fall occurs. The component parts are the lifeline, the grab, the lanyard, the body support, and the anchorage point.

These parts must be connected with the appropriate connecting hardware, and more importantly, must be connected correctly. There should be no common element with the positioning lowering system or boatswain's chair itself, so that the independent lifeline system is kept independent. This also means that the designated lifeline rope should not pass through the lowering device, which would then become a common element.

Additionally, the fall arrest cushioning should not depend on lifeline rope stretch, but rather on grab deceleration and lanyard shock absorption. These are more predictable, regardless of the length of the lifeline. The rope grab should move with as little manual manipulation as possible to help avoid failure due to a panic grip during a fall.

Retracting Lifelines – The retracting lifeline's component parts are the retracting lifeline itself, the body support, the anchorage point and the connecting hardware. This system eliminates nearly all the problems with rope grab component attachments.

The maximum length of a retracting lifeline is presently 200 ft. to 300 ft. This device should be positioned above and removed from any dirty work. Note that all fall arrest systems must automatically bring the user to a halt. A variance would be required for applications where controlled descent is required to forestall difficult or lengthy rescue, or, for example, when time exposure to radiation is hazardous.

Fall Arrest System Components

Following is a discussion of the main components of a fall arrest system, in particular, a rope grab system.

The Anchorage

The universal problem for all suspended scaffolding window cleaning contractors is the lack of predesignated tie–backs for scaffold and independent lifelines on building roofs. One contractor in Wilmington, Delaware, manages a regional exterior building maintenance firm and installs roof–top wall eyebolts for this purpose upon request of the building manager. This particular contractor feels that the professional anchorage system, when it is available, assists with the safety performance of his maintenance crews.[6]

Using air–conditioning equipment, exhaust or piping systems for rigging tie–backs and lifeline anchorage points is not realistic for safe contractor work on buildings. Tie–back points should be permanently installed as soon as possible on contractor–maintained buildings. They should be painted yellow or other bright color for high visibility, and tagged with their purpose.

As an example, one enterprising contractor in New Hampshire created a counterweight bracket to hold his 100–ft. retracting lifeline 1 ft. to 2 ft. over and above the parapet to provide for proper suspension as well as the necessary tie–back.

The Lifeline

There are several safety points relating to lifeline use with rope grabs. Perhaps the most important point is that the rope grab and lifeline must be compatible and coordinated.[7] Other points are:

- ☞ *Approved rope lifeline.* The rope grab manufacturer has tested certain ropes with its device, but not all ropes. Only ropes the manufacturer has drop–tested with a 300–lb. weight attached to the lanyard and grab, according to proposed OSHA Standards, should be used with the rope grab, unless such tests can responsibly conducted with a different rope. Never rely on static holding of a worker's weight to prove the efficiency of the rope in a dynamic fall. Lifelines should be continuous in length. Two short lifelines should never be joined to create a longer lifeline. Preshrunk lifelines keep rope swelling problems in wet weather to a minimum to help reduce worker frustration.
- *Polypropylene rope lifeline.* This should be black in color to indicate the presence of a carbon UV inhibitor. Samples should be strength–tested at a local laboratory regularly, especially in bright sunny regions, to determine the effect of the sun's ultraviolet rays. Black 5/8–in. polypropylene (carbon UV–stabilized) rope degrades at about the same rate as the same size nylon and polyester rope — approximately 15% strength loss per year in the first year, according to one leading rope manufacturer. The author has recorded less than 5% strength loss in 5/8–in. black polypropylene rope, due to sunlight and environmental exposure, during the first year used in the Philadelphia area. Proper rope testing should follow the requirements of ASTM D4268–83 or the latest revision, for repeatability.[8]
- *Rope strength.* Only approved synthetic ropes should be used with rope grabs, because natural fibers rot too quickly, and strength loss below 5,400 lb. in any rope is not obvious. As a guide, pull–test end samples of your lifelines regularly. In the Philadelphia area, the author has found 1/2–in. nylon twisted ropes degrade by 50% in two years due to handling and dirt, although 5/8–in. ropes degrade more slowly.
- ☞ *Rope stretch.* A 100–ft. nylon rope will stretch elastically several feet in a fall, so that a fall within 15 ft. of grade could produce an injurious impact with the ground. Polyester has one-third of the rope stretch of nylon, and has better UV resistance.
- *Rope abrasion.* Taking care to use carpet or split hose to lower or raise rope over the side of the building is an important step. Polypropylene seems to react better to mild abrasion over a parapet than nylon and polyester, with less effect on the grab running freely due to "fluffing" of the rope.

- *Suspending scaffold weight on the lifeline.* When scaffold operators leave the scaffold, they frequently wrap the rope grab lanyard around the railing and lower the scaffold to tauten the lines to secure in case of wind conditions. This is not recommended because of rope wear over the parapet. Additionally, no lifeline in service should be stressed for any reason other than an accidental fall. If the rope has been stressed because of accidental fall, it should then be withdrawn from service and not used again for personal protection. Lifelines should be redeployed before each use as a sound work practice.
- *Rope weights on lifelines.* Weighted lines are very important to keep lifeline slack from developing as the scaffold moves up from grade. However, in some windy conditions, rope weights could damage the building, especially windows. Physically securing the bottom of the line could be the answer in this case. In addition, proper termination of a rope can prevent unraveling of the strands.
- *Catch points on the scaffold for the lifeline.* Be careful to eliminate nip points where the line can catch and snag if the scaffold were to fall. Be careful to avoid the grab catching on a railing during a descent and putting explosive dynamic stress on the line, which could spring dangerously into the face of the operator.
- *Attachment to anchorages if tiebacks are not available.* Web or steel slings should be attached around a substantial structure, capable of supporting 6,000 lbs. Steel snaphooks with locking design should be used to link the lifeline to the sling. Lifelines should be terminated in a splice. Various length lifelines should be available for different height buildings.

The Lanyard

☞ Lanyards should not exceed 3 ft. in length. Many operators will erroneously use a 6–ft. lanyard, meaning that a 12–ft. fall could occur. If the jurisdiction having authority has a maximum free fall of 5 ft., like New York State, then the lanyard should only be 2 1/2 ft. Boatswain's chair work may call for lifeline placement 18 in. to 24 in. away from the suspension line, between which the user must climb over the parapet. Mobility on a scaffold is achieved by correct placement of the lifeline, one quarter to one–third of the way across the scaffold. In this way, the pull on the lifeline is small as the operator moves along the scaffold. A smooth back rail, along which the lifeline can easily slide, is a big asset, especially at the lower levels of a building, to provide easier cross scaffold mobility.

Lanyards should be the shock–absorbing type, and preferably integrally–attached to the rope grab. This helps avoid the attachment of nonapproved and incorrect lanyards, and diminishes or eliminates the opportunity of roll–out. Cleaning instructions for hardware and lanyards should be available from the manufacturer. Solvents other than water should not be used to clean synthetic materials. A replacement lanyard program for integral grab-lanyards is available from some manufacturers.

Shock–absorbing lanyards offer several benefits to users. They can:

- Reduce shock load to a comfortable level.
- Reduce damage to the lifeline by the grab.
- Indicate when a fall has occurred.

The Body Support

Many scaffold operators and users have independently come to their own conclusion that full body harnesses are the only right way to go. Live training proves this is true. Full body harnesses allow the worker to withstand rescue time while suspended following an accident.

Chest waist harnesses are more painful during suspension than full body harnesses, and some users have failed to make a tight enough cinch around the waist, resulting in the worker pulling out of the body support during a disastrous fall. Lightweight full body harnesses are recommended over the body belt or other harness designs. A D–ring in the back of the body support should always be used for proper fall protection and subsequent support. The D–ring should be a circle design and proportioned to help avoid the possibility of roll–out.

The Connecting Hardware

The choice of snaphooks to link rope grab system components is a vital safety matter. Only the rope grab manufacturer's instructions should be followed to help ensure the hardware is compatible. No other snaphooks should be used to help avoid potential roll–out. Other parts of this book address the problems of mixing and matching, and misuse. All snaphooks should be of locking design, and they should be kept in as–new operating condition or discarded if they're jammed or damaged.

Testing

When an operator purchases a rope grab system or retracting lifeline, he or she should ask for documentation that the system being purchased meets proposed OSHA 1910.66 or 1926 Subpart L and M test requirements, and that it meets the strict force limits imposed by the standard. The distributor may be able to provide limited training for operators.

Other Considerations

Boatswain's Chair Systems – OSHA considers boatswain's chair systems to be single point adjustable suspended scaffolds. Contractors are directed to the OSHA proposed standards 1926 Subpart L and M. The lowering device should meet the overspeed brake requirements of this standard (1926.450(b)(31)). An additional separate feature of emergency descent (paragraph(b)3) can be provided.

Building Perimeters at Roof Level – Where a low–perimeter (less than 42 in.) or no-parapet wall exists, fall protection must always be planned for approaching within 6 ft. of an edge. Access to scaffolds from the roof must always be made with the lifeline system fully hooked up and operational.

Summary

1. Always wear and attach fall arrest equipment before exposure to any fall hazard. This especially applies to roof–stored scaffolding.
2. Window cleaners who use window anchors should follow the fall protection requirements of ANSI A39.1–1987. Single point suspended scaffolding should be designed so that an overhead guard or suspension bracket does not prevent safe use of an independent lifeline. Some users have tried to attach the lifeline to the gooseneck frame designs, but fall arrest requirements are now increased for the worker's weight and tools to 500 lb. or 600 lb., including the weight of the scaffold, and still the operator is not independently protected.
3. Steel lifeline devices, including retracting steel lifelines, are an alternative in heat–producing applications that are protected from grounding by a section of split hose, and are ideal for welding work.
4. Only use lifelines authorized by a reputable fall arrester manufacturer.
5. Separate emergency descent devices are required on scaffolds where power failure is anticipated, for example, on an air–powered scaffold with air–powered breathing equipment used for painting a water tower. Failure could expose the workers to asphyxiation from paint solvent fumes unless an emergency escape controlled descent device is ready for use.
6. Self-retracting lanyards/lifeline devices, which provide controlled descent from scaffolds, are useful for confined space work in boilers or when radiation exposure, for example, creates undue time pressure on rescuers.
7. Each contractor should have a written safety program outlining the policy and training and maintenance procedures. All equipment should be live tested under controlled conditions to realistically simulate foreseeable problems.
8. ☞ All positioning and all fall arrest equipment must be periodically reconditioned. Body sup-

APPLICATIONS

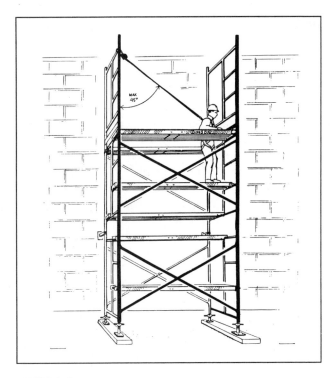

FIGURE 9.4
Scaffold erection with fall protection.

ports, lanyards, grabs and ropes should be discarded when signs of wear appear. Contaminants, such as oversprayed chemicals, acids, paint, gunite and dust, should be considered carefully before equipment choice is made. For example, fully diluted acid concrete cleaner can reduce nylon web lanyard strength by 80% in only one week's exposure, whereas under similar conditions, polyester web lanyards can maintain full strength. More details can be found in other sections of this book.

Scaffolds

Scaffolds can be stick–built or can be assembled from frames to elevate their structure for access and work.

Scaffolds in the USA are required to meet OSHA 1926.451 Construction or 1910.28 General Industry standards. A revision of the scaffold construction regulations was proposed in 1986, but had not yet been finalized at press time. ANSI A10.8 addresses scaffolding safety requirements in construction.

Suspension scaffolds (also called swinging scaffolds or stages) are addressed in other sections of this book.

Early in the 1980s, it was discovered that meeting standard fall protection requirements when erecting a scaffold requires a need to carefully plan and model.

It should be a standard rule that any scaffold started from any position above the ground, or where existing fall hazard occurs, must have a fall protection plan drawn up that protects workers 100% of the time for the foreseeable method of building and when using the scaffold.

For example, a project to replace a platform on a flare stack 250 ft. above the ground might require building a scaffold under the old platform from the structural attachments on the stack at the 200–ft. level or next level down. A fall protection plan is essential before work starts.

An evaluation is required to classify the scaffold design for fall protection for scaffold builders. The first step is to ask whether the location above a site for a scaffold can serve as an effective anchorage point. If the answer is yes, this is the first category of scaffold design. For example, a system scaffold is to be built up to a manway 50 ft. above grade on a distillation column. The other side of the column has an offset ladder and platform system up to the top of the tower. A projected secure anchorage using a small I–beam or channel can be used to reach directly over the scaffold.

Note: A structural engineer should provide guidance for such a design and method of reliable securing to the platform.

The next step is to evaluate the structural design of the scaffold itself as an anchor point. This is the second category of scaffold design.

A video has been prepared[9] showing scaffold erection and dismantling, including fall protection, on a single tower using 6 ft. 6 in. tie–ins at the ground or first level for stability assurance. The video shows pinning each frame leg securely, keeping to the center of the scaffold while erecting, and providing suitable anchors on the frames themselves, permitting workable techniques of scaffold erection with fall protection. The key is to provide a high enough anchorage to reduce the free fall distance and keep the swing fall angle as low as possible to limit potential swing injuries. Walk–through frames are a special challenge to provide platforms at an intermediate level and still permit a through–the–middle–access route until the scaffold is complete.

Figure 9.4 shows an erection worker attaching cross–braces to scaffolding. The angle of the worker's line should be kept less than 45 degrees to the vertical to minimize swing fall injuries should a fall occur.

Tube and coupler and system scaffolds can be erected with fall protection in much the same way, because the vertical posts provide the opportunity for a stable anchorage.

For long row scaffolds, such as masonry or stucco types, a fall hazard may exist after erection because of openings for material access and openings close to the building. In these cases, a horizontal lifeline can be designed to run part or all the length, where guardrails and/or planks and picks do not provide suitable protection from falls.

Following assembly, a longer self–retracting lifeline can be installed above the landing to provide access and exit protection while moving between the ground and the platform.

In summary, there is a hierarchy of scaffold fall protection as follows:

- Elimination of the need, or use of alternative access means.
- Anchor point above and on nearby structure.
- Anchor points on scaffold.
- Administrative instruction.

Workers must be properly trained to recognize fall hazards and learn the limitations of fall protection from railing and fall arrest equipment. Anchorage for fall arrest equipment must meet the 5,000 lb., 3,000 lb. or 2:1 safety factor alternatives explained in OSHA standard 1910.66 Appendix C. Scaffold manufacturers should provide sketches of models that have been tested with fall arrest equipment meeting OSHA 1910.66 Appendix C and ANSI Z359.1 requirements.

Aerial Lift Fall Protection

Why are workers required to wear fall arrest equipment while working in manlift equipment? What are the specific hazards?

The term *manlift* can be defined as an aerial lift used for one or more personnel. Different aerial lift equipment may have greater or lesser need for fall protection, depending on the application.

Aerial lifts are mobile work platforms used for personnel access and work at heights. The work is typically done over the side of platforms because it is easiest to work at waist to chest level, rather than overhead. Frequently, the work involves pulling, stretching and leaning over the edge.

Sometimes workers see the need to access onto a machine, fan, motor or other equipment. These operations lend themselves to falls out of the platform over the rails or sides. The very real possibiliity of the worker stabilizing the platform by pushing it under an object to hold it steady from swaying can release energy waiting to spring the platform loose under some uncontrolled condition. This released energy force may propel the worker from the lift platform in the same way that vehicular impact may eject a passenger. Or, alternatively, this force may collapse one wheel or

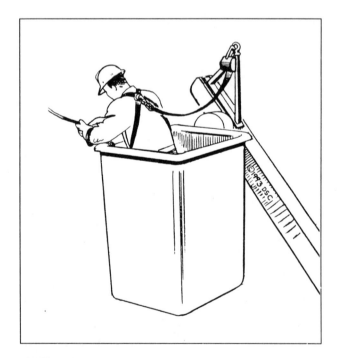

FIGURE 9.5
Utility bucket truck fall protection. Anchorage points should be located at the same height as the harness D-ring; the lanyard should be as short as possible to reduce slack.

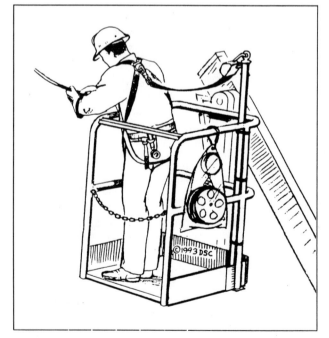

FIGURE 9.6
Construction Aerial Lift. Proper anchorage points, capable of withstanding the OSHA 2:1 factor, should be used. The platform must not be able to tip under any reasonable scenario.

outrigger into a concrete crack that may cause tipping and eject the worker without warning.

There are many ways to fall from the bucket – besides tipping the platform system over completely – which equates to anchorage failure (and which must be avoided at all costs by proper use of outriggers and proper leveling before use). Hence the need for fall arrest equipment.

In many ways, the applications are similar to suspended scaffolds used on the side of buildings for maintenance. Both are required to have lifelines for each worker. (See Figures 9.5 and 9.6.)

Where should the personal fall arrest equipment be attached, to the basket or the boom? Some companies with scissor–type lifts have used a central eyebolt mount where the lanyard is attached at foot level. The purpose of this arrangement is to restrain the worker from being able to use the midrail as a stepping point to reach up between a truss member, for example, and thus leave the basket or render the sides or railings ineffective. Other single or two-person platforms have an anchorage point on the railing (basket) or boom. This alternative complies with OSHA 1910.67(c)(2)(v). Relevant ANSI A92 standards have similar wording.

There are arguments for both positions, depending on the age of the lift and provision by the lift manufacturer, or additional features welded to the basket or boom or strapped to the boom. Fiberglass buckets point to the boom as anchorage, but many employers have drilled holes and threaded lanyards in a makeshift way, which, in the author's opinion, is not proper.

However the anchorage point may be arranged, the point must be used under strict rules. For example, never loop the lanyard around the railing so that the lanyard or device may be cut during a worst–case fall. A direct attachment is preferred. Strap attachments around booms are useful for maintaining dielectric properties, but suffer from loosening, sliding and weathering over time. Another problem is that whenever the midrail (if present) is used as a step, the free fall distance increases by 1-1/2 ft., enough to exceed the 6–ft. rule in most cases . . . and more so, of course, if the worker steps out!

It's important to note that the use of external anchorage points by aerial lift users is prohibited by OSHA 1910.67(c)(2)(iii) and 1926.556(b)(2)(iii) for extensible and articulating boom platforms.

What effect does moving workers from belts to lanyards have on the available anchorage points at waist height? A big difference in fall distance, if the worker uses a 6–ft. lanyard. The free fall distance will potentially reach 7 1/2 ft. This would be illegal in Michigan, and in the USA at large. Reduction to 4-ft. lanyards or use of properly–mounted retractable lanyards will help solve this problem.

What will happen in the event of a fall, and is it possible for the aerial platform to tip over? A critical question is, What happens at the worst case position of maximum reach at the lowest angle of reach permitted by the aerial device manufacturer (if it's telescopic and articulating)? Test for the value of the anchorage point stability (not strength) by statically pulling from the proposed anchorage point toward the ground in a simulated direction of a fall.

☞ The only way, it seems, to deal with this question is to provide an engineered fall protection system for each type of aerial device, where the maximum arrest force (dynamic rating) of a fall arrester deceleration device is less than one half of the anchorage tip strength on the boom.

Look to OSHA 1910.66 Appendix C for guidance in these general industry standards.

Another hazard is the distance of fall from the platform (worst case). The potential impact zone, with a 6–ft. shock absorbing lanyard, is 11 ft. below the bottom of the platform.

Recommendations

☞ The bottom line is that sturdy, shoulder–height anchor points should be considered if practical, along with (retractable) lanyards with a specific maximum arrest force suitable for the application. The anchor point must be labeled with a warning sign as to its purpose and as a reference to specific engineering drawing data depicting permitted fall arrest equipment and limitations on use.

Ladders

There are several types of recognized ladders for industrial and construction use:

- Stepladders
- Wood and aluminum portable ladders, including extension ladders
- Fixed ladders, which are an integral part of a structure
- Job–made ladders
- Fiberglass ladders
- Alternating tread type ladders

These and other ladders are described, by type of ladder, in the ANSI A14 standards. The author recommends a close reading of the Selection, Care and Use sections in these standards. OSHA requirements for ladders are found in 1926.1050–1053 and 1910.27.

Normally, it is recommended that ladders be placed at an angle of about 75 degrees (or a ratio of 4:1 for the working length compared with distance from the ladder support base). This angle minimizes tipping (when the ladder is too steep) and slipping (when the ladder is too flat). In addition, the climber, when facing the ladder, has a support to fall onto, which may allow enough reaction time to grab a rung.

Nevertheless, falls from ladders are a major source of injury in industry and construction. A search for positive fall protection is necessary in the future. The key ingredients of fall protection are the securing of the ladder from appreciable movement and an anchorage point for a fall arrest system.

Stepladders, by their nature, have a stable angle and are self-supporting when properly used, but have very little opportunity to be secured from tipping. Therefore, the height limitation for such usage should be minimized, possibly to a maximum of 6 ft. working height (or an 8-ft. stepladder). Within reason, railed stepladders with depressible casters offer more opportunity for access to height.

Stepladders are intended to be used as work platforms more than other types of ladders, because they present a more secure footing. Portable ladders have rungs with very little structure to stand on, and so require a worker to use at least one hand at all times for securely maintaining balance. This means that ladders can be dangerous when used for work involving the hands, either for lifting, carrying, holding, manipulating, or other purposes, particularly while moving.

Stepladders can have alternating treads for secure

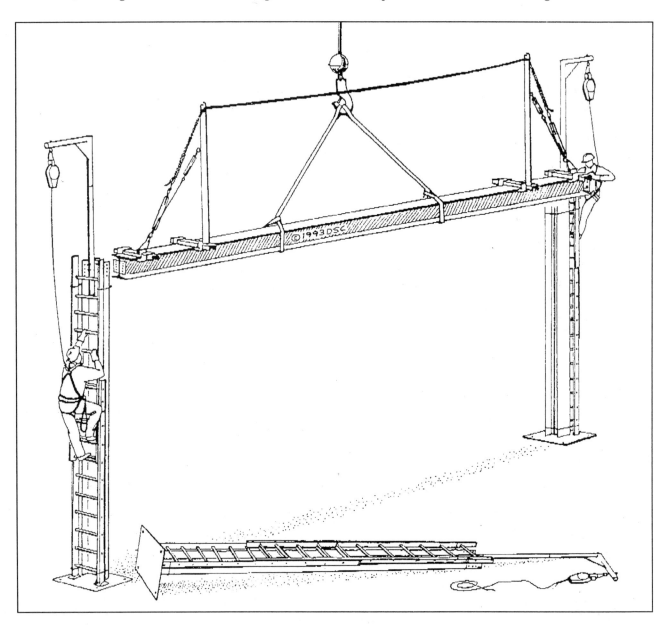

FIGURE 9.7
Practical access up the column in steel erection connection work.

APPLICATIONS

foot placement between 50 and 70 degrees from the horizontal. When railed and permanently secured, these present a better option for safer climbing in confined areas, than do standard ladders with horizontal rungs. These are classified as alternating tread stairs by OSHA, in the proposed 1910 Walking and Working Surfaces (10 April 1990).

In the construction industry, ladders often are required with longer lengths and are put to severe tests in handling, placement and usage. Therefore, the use of rugged job–made ladders customized for the location has become the choice of safety professionals over commercially available wood and aluminum ladders.

☞ When fall protection is used, in addition to good ladder practice, ladders should be positioned and secured vertically. At the very least, ladders used at an angle should be railed to minimize the possibility of swing falls, where impacts or long suspension can reasonable be predicted.

Job–Made Ladders

Job–made ladders often are used as a means of access to the next floor of a construction site, and are designed to be much sturdier than a portable ladder or extension ladder. Rules for construction and the use of job–made ladders are provided in OSHA 1926.1053 and ANSI A14.4.

Job–made ladders are through ladders, meaning the side rail extension above the landing permits stepping directly onto the landing from the top rung. The hands are used to pull the body forward, provided the side rails are no bigger than "2-by-4" at that part of the ladder. It is important that the top step is flush with the landing to avoid tripping when descending, and to avoid the enticing sidestep around the side rail. The size of side rails on job–made ladders is too large, including "2-by-4" lumber, to hold with any degree of graspability for swinging the body to the side. For this reason, guardrails must be positioned close to the job–made ladder, but without touching it, with a gap too small for a worker to pass through.

Fall protection while accessing up or down job–made ladders and portable ladders is provided in part by securing the ladder at the top and bottom, while the worker leans with his or her body against the 4:1 slope required by OSHA. The ANSI A14.4 standard permits the slope to be varied from that point to where the ladder is vertical. The author suggests that when the ladder is sloped more steeply than 4:1, fall protection with an independent fall arrest system is necessary, and proposes that a properly anchored retracting lifeline be used in conjunction with a full body harness. Figure 9.7 illustrates how fall protection can be achieved in steel erection connection work.

Summary

According to OSHA 1926.1053(a)(6)(i), all fixed and portable metal ladder steps or rungs manufactured after March 15, 1991 are required to be corrugated, knurled, dimpled, coated with skid–resistant material or otherwise treated to minimize slipping.

☞ Climbing ladders should be done with the free use of both hands and feet, to allow three–point control at all times, including access and exit.

OSHA permits the use of the ANSI A14 ladders' standards to meet the requirements of OSHA 1926.1053(a)(1).

Through portable and job–made ladders must have an extension to the side rails of 36 in. above the landing. Side–stepping should only be permitted if the side rails can be grasped effectively. The ideal diameter is 1 1/2 in. for graspability.

Confined–Space Fall Protection

Millions of workers in the USA are exposed to hazards in confined spaces each year, according to the National Institute for Occupational Safety and Health. And each year, approximately 50,000 emergency responses occur for occupational confined space incidents.[10]

Approximately 300 occupational fatalities per year result from such incidents.[11] And about half of these fatality victims are would–be rescuers.[12]

Definition

According to the OSHA standard for permit–required confined spaces, 29 CFR 1910.146, a confined space is defined as "an enclosed space which:

1. is large enough and so configured that an employee can bodily enter and perform assigned work;
2. has limited or restricted means for entry or exit;
3. is not designed for continuous human occupancy; and
4. has one or more of the following characteristics:

   • contains or has known potential to contain a hazardous atmosphere;
   • contains material with the potential for engulfment of an entrant;
   • has an internal configuration such that an entrant could be trapped or asphyxiated by inwardly converging walls, or a floor which slopes downward and tapers to a smaller cross–section; and
   • contains any other recognized serious safety or health hazards."

According to OSHA 1910.146, "a rescue team shall be available to respond to emergencies in the confined space."

Rescue personnel are highly dedicated, continuously trained and very willing. They also are becoming more apprehensive about confined–space entry in industrial plants. "DMD" is one term which reflects what one fire–rescue veteran describes as any liquid in the plant – dimethyl death.

The key issue, however, is timeliness. Other types of rescue personnel are skilled in mountaineering, climbing and rescue techniques. They too have a time problem. Plant and safety managers usually rely on rescue personnel for handling confined–space emergencies. They may neglect training the work crew in proper planning techniques for effective self-rescue and for the reduction or control of fall hazards prior to entry.

Retrieval or Rescue

Many workers who enter confined spaces confuse fall protection and related retrieval systems with equipment for rescue. For example:

- a harness becomes a wristlet;
- a lifeline becomes a rope;
- an anchorage point becomes a tie–off;
- connectors becomes knots;
- a rescue winch becomes a pulley;
- a system becomes a tool.

It is evident that connection is made for rescue purposes only and not for fall protection.

Many people feel that rescue planning has to occur after the incident. Thus little or no preparation is made by the work crew until the emergency is in progress. Fall protection is forgotten or deemed unimportant or inconvenient. Rescue and medical aid may wishfully be delegated to others with the skills and training. The problem is that there are too many rescue scenarios for the rescue squad, let alone an outside fire company, to face efficiently and to ensure the health and welfare of all concerned.

An outside fire company crew may be unfairly put at risk because, despite training frequency, few if any plant scenarios will have been "dry–run". In an emergency, if outside rescuers are unfamiliar with the plant's fall–protection procedures and equipment, their own separate equipment for rescue must usually be brought in to the scene.

Plant scenarios include potential exposure to toxic and/or inflammable chemicals, and thus the rescuers would have to address protective clothing and respiratory needs specific to an individual confined space.

The OSHA confined–space standard 1910.146 and the ANSI Z117.1 confined–space standard highlight the process for entry of confined spaces with proper procedures. However, little has been said about claustrophobia, heart attack or stroke as additional hazards to be dealt with in confined–space fall prevention and post–fall rescue.

The issue becomes one of time. Can the respiratory–relief assistance be in place within the critical four minutes? Can the capabilities of a hospital emergency room be made available within one hour? If the on–site personnel can arrange for retrieval themselves, it can reduce the time in which a rescue squad can respond with respiratory and other appropriate assistance.

Fall Arrest

We can take guidance from the OSHA 1910.66 Appendix C fall arrest system requirements, which are presently applicable only to powered–platform scaffolds used in the maintenance of building exteriors. The 1910 standard requires consideration of post–fall rescue methods: "The employer shall provide for prompt rescue of employees in the event of a fall or shall assure the self–rescue capability of employees." (Section 1, paragraph (e)(8)).

Fall arrest equipment with retrieval capability will only be helpful where there are vertical entries. Even then, the entrant should be immediately below the access point to allow winching to occur without emergency rescue entry.

For horizontal confined–space entrances, or those with both vertical and horizontal components, rescuers need a way to transport a victim to either a vertical lift position or alternatively to a horizontal exit. Some methods of projecting lifeline with retrieval features are available for horizontal entries at elevation.

Adding lower manway entrances with 24 in. to 30 in. openings is a trend for tank owners, which make foreseeable rescues much easier, if only because more exit options are available.

Some Crucial Considerations

Should fall–protection planning be required before entry to any confined space with a fall hazard?

If so, does that apply to the rescue squad, fire department or other outside rescue team?

What problems does proper fall protection for potential victims eliminate, and what scenarios will it not solve? For example: two people are in the confined space, with one standing by; or, alternatively, 10 people are in the confined space with one person standing by; etc.

If everything is done correctly, according to the current standards and proposals, what still can occur related to fall hazards?

APPLICATIONS

What percentage of rescues would be eliminated if work–crew preparation was reasonably done to provide for self–rescue or work–crew rescue?

How do the fire–trained rescue squad and the mountaineering–trained rescue squad differ in their approaches to confined space rescue?

Summary

Fall arrest equipment should be used at all times when a fall hazard of more than 6 ft. cannot be eliminated. The maximum free–fall distance should be 2 ft. for most confined spaces with limited size but which otherwise meet the criteria of OSHA 1910.66 Appendix C. Fall equipment with an integral retrieval feature should be considered.

Two of the hardest rescue problems to solve in confined spaces are the distillation columns and vessels with catalyst trays. Models should be created out of scaffolding or column section, with the rough dimensions of the column or vessel, and training should be regularly applied towards achieving even the most difficult rescue in the shortest time.

The most important confined–space recommendations are:

1. Entry is permitted only when the minimum size opening or dimension is 24 in.
2. Respiratory aid is available within four minutes.
3. Retrieval–device mechanical advantage is 4:1 or higher.
4. Free–fall distance potential is 2 ft. maximum.

Winches for Access and Retrieval in Confined Spaces

Many important additions to work safety were achieved with the OSHA 1910.146 permit-required confined space regulation issued in January 1993. None is more important than the consideration for extrication in the last few paragraphs of the standard, 1910.146(k). It is here that OSHA calls for the following requirements, applicable to employers who have employees enter permit spaces to perform rescue services:

1910.146(k)(3) To facilitate non-entry rescue, retrieval systems or methods shall be used whenever an authorized entrant enters a permit space, unless the retrieval equipment would increase the overall risk of entry or would not contribute to the rescue of the entrant. Retrieval systems shall meet the following requirements:
(i) Each authorized entrant shall use a chest or full body harness, with a retrieval line attached at the center of the entrant's back near shoulder level or above the entrant's head. [Second sentence omitted.]
(ii) The other end of the retrieval line shall be attached to a mechanical device or fixed point outside the permit space in such a manner that that rescue can begin as soon as the rescuer becomes aware that rescue is necessary. A

mechanical device shall be available to retrieve personnel from vertical-type permit spaces more than 5 feet deep.

OSHA intends to make other standards for fall protection applicable to confined spaces and is generally applying to this end its 1910.66 Appendix C, which thus becomes the key standard until other industry standards are adopted, especially in confined spaces because harnesses have always been the body support of choice.

In the year since this standard's promulgation, many organizations have invested in tripods, lifelines and winches for vertical entry. Many questions remain to be answered by OSHA relating to various confined space scenarios.

Although some confined spaces are not appropriate for tripod use due to the size of their opening or to workplace geometry, lifelines and winches can be used, along with a variety of davits and brackets suited to the application and appropriately designed into the workplace.

A mixture of rope rescue equipment coming from mountaineering, fire rescue and safety equipment manufacturers needs clarification as to purpose in general industry and construction.

This section is designed to address the fundamental need to extricate a worker from a confined space due to heart attack, stroke or heat stress whether permit-required or not under OSHA regulations or the ANSI Z117.1 standard.

If a four-minute limit is seen as the benchmark for stabilizing or retrieving a worker from any foreseeable hazard or personal emergency, then it becomes obvious that most rescues within that time limit will have to become the domain of trained work crews, not trained rescue workers. And as extrication becomes more difficult in existing baffled towers or in columns with catalyst trays, so the need to keep extremely well-trained general purpose rescue personnel on hand increases dramatically. Nothing is more welcome to a rescue team than the realization that they do not have to enter the confined space to bring out a victim. Therefore, the definition of fall arrest and retrieval equipment features for use in confined spaces and usable by trainable work crews becomes a critical necessity.

One of the most important tools necessary to a successful confined space program is the winch. And the best way to begin discussion on this crucial role that the winch plays is to address 11 critical fall arrest and retrieval considerations.

Questions...

1. Can retracting lifelines with integral two-way winches be used for access to and from confined space with or without lifelines?
2. Must access hoists for confined space use be UL listed/classified to meet OSHA standards?

3. When do OSHA's Boatswain's Chair regulations apply to confined space?
4. What minimum size opening is permitted for entry using a harness to support a worker?
5. What is the depth limit for manual winching under emergency conditions?
6. Can a single tripod be used for access and lifeline support?
7. What is the proper strength of tripods and lines for this application?
8. What anchorage point should be used when a tripod is not applicable?
9. How should confined space attendants be protected from falls?
10. Should entrants always be attached to a lifeline?
11. Should access hoists/winches be used for suspending loads?

Hoist/winch systems used for lifting workers from confined spaces have been evaluated to meet industry safety requirements. This evaluation is in lieu of any future OSHA Instruction Standards on such systems, or any OSHA regulation, or any ANSI Z359 Standard on Personnel Riding Systems or Work Positioning for confined space application.

It's important to note that the terms "hoist" and "winch" are often used interchangeably. In this particular text, however, "winch" is reserved for emergency retrieval purpose and "hoist" is used for suspension access purpose, also known as work positioning. The term "lifeline" is intended to mean a fall arresting system as defined by OSHA 1910.66 Appendix C or ANSI Z359.1, and in most cases a self-retracting lifeline device to avoid foreseeable fall collisions. Other terms are defined in OSHA 1910.66 Appendix C and OSHA 1910.146 regulations.

...and Answers
Here is a point-by-point response by the author to the 11 critical questions asked in the section just above.

1. (a) ☞ Emergency retrieval winches that are integral or non-integral in self-retracting lifelines must be for emergency and training use only; they are not to be used for ordinary/regular access suspension.

   (b) A fall-arrest lifeline is not necessary for emergency retrieval operations. However, for retrieval demonstration and training sessions, winches must be backed up with an additional fall arrest lifeline.

2. & 3. A fall-arrest lifeline is not necessary for emergency retrieval operations; however, for retrieval demonstration and training sessions, winches must be backed up with an additional fall arrest lifeline.

(a) OSHA's Boatswain's Chair regulations are applicable to confined space access systems when the access is "top-to-bottom" without planned "stop-start" work suspension.

(b) Confined space "top-to-bottom" access hoists are not required to be UL listed/classified as a single-point adjustable suspension scaffold. A back-up fall arrest lifeline must be used with a confined space access hoist.

(c) OSHA's single-point adjustable suspension scaffold standards may apply to hoists for "stop-start" activities such as brick-pointing and painting.

(d) Access hoists may be used for retrieval if they are practical for the situation.

4. (a) A full-body harness may be used for narrow vertical openings 18 in. or less in dimension. In such cases, suspension means and fall-arrest lifeline can be attached to the same harness but at different locations on the harness. Thorough inspection routines must be followed for the harness stitching and wear points.

   (b) Boatswain's chairs should be used for suspension instead of harnesses when openings equal or exceed 18 in. A harness should additionally be used for fall arrest attachment to a lifeline.

   (c) Boatswain's chairs may be unsuitable for emergency retrieval use when confined space dimensions are less than 18 in. width. Proper training procedures are critical; the four-minute limit for retrieval/stabilization should be applied.

5. Winching over 50 ft. manually is reasonable for non-IDLH atmospheres based on a lifting rate averaging 12 ft. per minute. For the possibility of heart attack or stroke, the time to reasonably lift a victim to the opening should be less than four minutes. When power features such as pneumatic or electric power are used in a confined space with a boatswain's chair or a harness, then a manual backup mode is required. A torque-limiter is needed on the power system for lifting to avoid placing high forces on a victim snagged on an obstruction.

6. ☞ A single tripod may be used for both a vertical entry access support and a fall arrest lifeline anchorage. Tripod attachments must be reasonably independent of each other or without a recognized failure mode based on the opinion of a qualified person. Note that "reasonably independent" means that no recognized hazard exists for that situation where both load line and lifeline could fail simultaneously.

APPLICATIONS

7. (a) A tripod must have a minimum ultimate strength of 3,600 lbs. for fall arrest and access use. Under fall arrest conditions, the tripod must have a safety factor of at least 2 documented by the manufacturer or a qualified person.

(b) All tripods used for confined space access and retrieval must be the "locking-leg" type to reduce the opportunity for collapse by lateral movement at the surface, such as during victim movement away from the opening.

(c) Chains at the base of the legs are only required when the manufacturer's conditions for meeting OSHA anchorage strength requirements cannot be achieved without such support. Chains may provide a tripping hazard unless they are slack. Tripods can sometimes be bolted to large-diameter flange vertical sloped openings.

(d) A davit system should be used for vertical openings that exceed a tripod manufacturer's limit for use. Wall mount, floor mount, drum mount and truck trailer hitch mount are available options. At least 3 ft. of headroom is required in order for a rescuer to access a victim under the armpits from a reasonably stable and secure position.

(e) Lines used for fall arrest should be 3,600 lbs. minimum strength. Lines used for work positioning under the UL requirements for scaffold hoists should support 6,000 lbs. minimum.

8. A 7-ft.-high tripod or quadpod may be useful for vertical openings up to 36 in. diameter of approximately 36 in. maximum height, if feasible with the tripod design. Larger vertical openings such as vaults with rectangular doors require davit systems. Horizontal openings require system or rescuer evaluation of the hazards to avoid abrasion injuries as a result of sliding when pulling to retrieve.

9. Attendants should be protected from falls into vertical access manholes within 6 ft. of an opening greater than 12 in. diameter. If the chosen anchorage is a tripod, then the tripod must be secured against moving if it's accidentally pulled laterally.

10. Entrants should be attached to a lifeline when the lifeline can arrest a fall safely. However, when the lifeline is angled such that a potentially injurious swing fall can be produced, then the usage is incorrect. Any lateral movement more than 5 ft. from the vertical edge of the entranceway or such that the lifeline touches any obstruction should not be permitted under most work scenarios, unless a second attendant who is a concurrent entrant is present and within easy reach of the entrant(s) who have a work purpose. Entrants making lateral

movement can be detached from a fall arrest lifeline or rescue lines. However, a means of moving the victim under a vertical opening should be devised before a rescuer re-attaches a retrieval line for emergency lifting. The capacity to retrieve more than one worker within a reasonable time is predicated upon pre-planning the use of equipment to suit the number of entrants and upon the particular features of the specific confined space. It is important to note that a synthetic line attached to a worker is very useful when rescuers are trying to locate an entrant, such as in smoke-filled electrical vaults involving lateral movement, or with cable lines in underwater diving situations where normal gravitational forces do not apply. A fall arrest lifeline should not be used for any other purpose, such as those just mentioned, in order to eliminate any confusion regarding the capability of the fall arrester device, which later might be called into question following an incident investigation.

11. A manual hoist designed for lifting or lowering a worker may be used to lift or lower a load, such as a pump, up to the rated safe working load limit. An emergency backup winch also serving as a lifeline can be used for lifting a nominal load, such as tools, in an emergency, up to 310 lbs. total weight. It is vital that all loads be known. Any load over 310 lbs., or any type of load repeatedly lifted, should meet OSHA material handling requirements. A load should not be permitted to be lifted above a worker if there is any reasonable possibility that it could fall for any reason and foreseeably strike the worker. For difficult situations involving stable loads, load fall arresters are available for a backup.

Fall Arrest and Emergency Retrieval
The OSHA 1910.146 Standard published January 14, 1993, is entitled "Permit-Required Confined Spaces for General Industry."[14] This standard requires that employers subject to general industry standards designate whether a confined space is permit-required or not permit-required. Permit-required confined spaces over 5 ft. in depth are required to have harness systems available, with a mechanical device, for the purpose of emergency retrieval should the occasion require it and if it is practical to do so. Training is required at least annually.

Fall arrest systems are expected to be cross-referenced in a future OSHA General Industry Standard.

There is no requirement specified in OSHA 1910.146 for the emergency winch (mechanical device) except that 1:1 manual pulling power is inadequate for retrieval. Some mechanical advantage is implied, and although the OSHA minimum limit of 4:1 mechanical advantage was withdrawn from the draft standard, this or a higher mechanical advantage is appropriate. Presumably, because of OSHA's duty to provide minimum standards for employers to achieve a safe workplace, OSHA would have the winch be reliable in its use and not be subject to breakdown in time of need, and also have workers trained on the winch system to sufficient confidence for emergency preparedness. Such periodic training in the field is usually sufficient to validate the winch for the prospective emergency use if it's in a ready-to-use condition and close at hand when the emergency arises.

The ANSI Z117.1-1989 Standard on Confined Spaces contains 12.3.1, which states that "Fall Arrest Systems shall be worn by personnel entering confined spaces as determined by a qualified person (sic)." In combination with the OSHA 1910.146 requirement and ANSI Z359.1, this standard indicates that harnesses should be full-body type, and not chest harnesses, for a dual fall arrest and retrieval use.

Emergency retrieval from vertical-entry confined spaces becomes much more difficult when the size or shape of the opening decreases below 18 in., which is the width of a typical shoulder or pelvis. Although aperture widths as small as 13 in. are known in industry, the range of possible rescuers for such an opening decreases dramatically and the time for rescue increases dramatically. The four-minute rule for extrication appears to be a reasonable guideline for training purposes to determine whether the method of entry is valid and whether a non-human method of accomplishing the task is feasible.

Some self-retracting lifeline fall arrest devices have integral winches designed for activation for emergency retrieval. The question arises whether winches can be used to raise or lower workers as a means of access when their primary purpose is emergency retrieval. If so, can they be used without a lifeline? The answer to both questions is no. These integral winches cannot be used for regular access because of design limitations. The use of a single line support on such devices is only permitted for emergency retrieval purpose, and thus a backup lifeline should be used whenever training is planned and conducted. If an employer wishes to use a two-way (up/down) retracting lifeline integral winch for ordinary (regular) use, vertical access (with an additional lifeline), then he or she should consider whether the manufacturer endorses that type of regular use.

Access Into Confined Spaces

Should access hoists be UL classified (or equivalent) for confined space personnel use?

At this time, OSHA has no requirements for access hoists or winches for personnel use into or out of confined spaces. But searching for relevance into current

OSHA regulations finds that OSHA 1926.451 and the nearly analogous 1910.28 scaffolding regulations are the closest applicable standards one might possibly apply. OSHA's proposed 1910.30(c)(2) also can be considered.

The following current standards should be considered, if relevant:

OSHA 1926.451(k) and 1910.28(i) Single-point Adjustable Suspension Scaffolds — The wording of the standard indicates an assumption that a cage or basket is integral with the hoist and that railings are to be provided. The equipment is to be used in accordance with the manufacturer's instructions, thus presumably requiring the users to each have a lifeline. The OSHA Construction Standard particularly requires a type tested and listed by Underwriters' Labs or Factory Mutual Engineering Corp. The General Industry Standard calls for testing and listing by a nationally recognized testing laboratory consistent with 1910.7 (and 1910.399 Subpart S Electrical).

OSHA 1926.451(j) and 1910.28(l) Boatswain's Chairs — The wording in these standards addresses a seat supported by slings attached to a suspended rope designed to accommodate one worker in a sitting position. No requirements are made for the hoist system employing such a seat. A lifeline is required.

Both sets of OSHA standards reference the ANSI A10.8-1969 construction industry standard. The particular ANSI standard currently applicable for hoists and boatswain's chairs is A10.8-1988.

In addition, Underwriters' Labs has prepared test method standard UL 1323 for scaffold hoists used for personnel lifting based on the OSHA and ANSI A10.8 standards. UL-classified manually-operated winch systems are labeled as to load capacity only, and not with regard to application, such as for confined spaces. UL is silent on the suitability for a particular application.

OSHA's proposed standard 1910.30(c)(2) calls for 1/4-in. diameter cable for suspension ropes for scaffolds.

Confined Space Worker Suspension Issues

Getting into and out of confined spaces with vertical openings entails some special considerations.

a. *Access with or without ladder/stairs/steps.* A fixed or portable ladder or steps are often provided in vertical openings for manholes requiring access for maintenance, and for larger manhole openings, stairs are sometimes practical. In such cases, an access hoist is not necessary for personnel use. However, a retrieval line is required by OSHA. A fall arrest lifeline, preferably with retrieval, is a candidate for use in vertical entries even though ANSI A14.3-1992 on Fixed Ladders does not require a ladder safety device for ladders up to 24 ft. depth,

APPLICATIONS

because ANSI Z117.1 Confined Spaces requires the wearing of a fall arrest system by an entrant as determined by a competent person.

Where no ladder or stairs or steps or a reliable feature in the confined space is provided for stepping and holding, then a boatswain's chair or harness and hoist is reasonable. A separate lifeline and retrieval capability is still required.

b. *Confined space opening size 24 in. or more.* An ideal opening should be 3 ft. minimum dimension at any point in the confined space where a worker may travel. The opening, during maintenance operations, should lead to a vertical space in distillation columns and vessels with catalyst trays, so that workers will not be trapped behind a circuitous route for retrieval, which could compromise the life safety of a first responder. New designs should not be less than 30 in. minimum clear dimension. Boatswain's chairs appear practical for most openings greater than 24 in. minimum dimension. A separate discussion is required for manways and horizontal openings.

Note: OSHA's proposed 1910.22(a)(4) standard requires a minimum opening of 24 in. for non-pressurized manholes and manways in new construction.

c. ☞ *Openings 18 in. to 24 in. minimum dimension.* For openings larger than 18 in. minimum dimension, for the temporary support of one person up or down a manway, shaft or column, a boatswain's chair or seat should be practical. Harnesses should not be used for vertical suspension when the confined space minimum dimension exceeds 18 in. The nature of both harness support and seat support is very confining, inflexible and unsuitable for a long, confined space, suspended workstation except under unusual work conditions. Note: Boatswain's chairs require a seat of 17 in. minimum width to support the seat area of the average American worker.

OSHA's proposed Appendix A to section 1910.30 recommends 9 in. x 17 in. minimum.

d. *Openings less than 18 in. least dimension.* Vertical openings less than 18 in. may be accessible only by harness suspension requiring dual use for both suspension and lifeline support, which OSHA has indicated [personal communication] it would accept. Harnesses used for both suspension and fall arrest use must be inspected by a competent person after each session of use for unusual wear and tear and to reorganize the straps if necessary.

Confined space openings and passageways narrower than 18 in. dimension should only be used for entry when crew or on-hand emergency response personnel can reasonably be sure that workers can be extricated or stabilized within a four-minute time period of incident occurrence. This must be determined through discussion and training. If this test cannot be passed, automatic or mechanical means for accomplishing the work must be sought without an entry being made.

e. *Unorthodox entry methods.* Head-down suspension by the feet, or suspension by the arms using wristlets and other such methods, are unreasonable for entering confined spaces because of improper support for the worker's body. This principle applies no matter how short the entry period or what its purpose. The only exception might apply in special situations for which a worker has been specifically trained and where the procedure is properly documented.

The question is, what rule, if any, is governing regarding suspension?

Since the use of a hoist/winch for personal lifting/lowering in a harness or seat constitutes boatswain's chair operations, the latter regulations should rule. However, there is no guidance for the winch or hoist in that section of either 1910 or 1926 OSHA standards. Thus we are forced to make a prudent selection.

That selection is based upon whether the winch/hoist should comply with OSHA single-point suspension scaffold requirements for testing by a nationally-recognized test laboratory when used for access only, "top-to-bottom".

There is a distinct difference between two situations that demands a distinctly different approach to current standards.

Because most seat or harness confined space operations usually are for only brief worker suspension, and because most confined space access (for example, in sewers) is from "top-to-bottom" or vice-versa, fitting that brief specific time usage, then such operations are for access only and thus do not require that the winch/hoist meet the requirements of OSHA 1910.28(i) or 1926.451(k).

However, if the winch/hoist is used on a repeated basis to provide work positioning, stopping regularly at points along the way, and this is the regular (not occasional) use of the winch/hoist, then this use constitutes "stop-start" operations. Thus there is more of a need to comply with the OSHA scaffold standards for a single-point adjustable suspension scaffold in this case. Examples are sewer brick pointing or repair, and tank cleaning.

UL Standard 1323 defines "hoist, manually powered," as a hoist in which the hoisting power is derived directly from the operator. This is very rarely the case in permit-required confined space operations where the required attendant would be the primary operator of the winch/hoist in most tripod or davit systems in use today and certainly if the emergency retrieval feature is integral.

Specifications for Confined Space Access
Following are ten specifications for manual winch/hoist access and retrieval devices for use in confined space access.

1. Minimum cable breaking strength 3,600 lbs. "top-to-bottom" access use; 6,000 lbs. for "stop-start" work operations.
2. Operation up only, or up and down; designed to lift one person up to 310 lbs. in weight, including tools (consistent with OSHA's fall arrest system weight limit in 1910.66 Appendix C).
3. Maximum load 600 lbs. that can be raised by reasonable manual effort.
4. Operation for 500 cycles without loss in winch efficiency at maximum load (1,000 cycles for work hoist).
5. Capacity to hold six times the maximum load through accessories such as tripods or davits. Note: Tripods should be tested on a flat concrete floor; a chain or cable between legs may be required on slippery floors during use.
6. Equipped with a feature to prevent rapid handle movement, fast unspooling, or uncontrolled descent. Any neutral mode must have an overspeed lock that has been performance tested.
7. Capable of lifting 310 lbs. weight, 50 ft., within four minutes, with a mechanical advantage of 4:1 or greater (the range 6:1 to 8:1 is preferred).
8. Salt spray pre-conditioning in areas subject to salt corrosion.
9. Not be used when depths exceed 50 ft. in IDLH atmospheres without a controlled power attachment. Note: Additional respiratory protection and emergency rescue/medical services may be required in some situations.
10. A personal fall arrest system is required for all hoist/winch use except emergency use. All parts must be reasonably independent. The tripod should be capable of supporting 3,600 lbs. minimum on the surface where it is required to be used. A single tripod may be used for both suspension and lifeline when the connections to the tripod are free from a recognized failure mode based on an evaluation by a competent person familiar with the worksite. A harness may be used for suspension and fall arrest in narrow holes marginally less than 18 in. dimension space.

☞ A fall arrest system in manholes must control falls within 2 ft. of activation and decelerate to a stop within 42 in. under test conditions described for self-retracting lanyards and lifelines in OSHA 1910.66 Appendix C and ANSI Z359.1 Fall Arrest Systems.

The exception is boilers and other large spaces with clear space greater than 20 ft. This type of project may use rope grab systems unless a Competent Person (OSHA 1910.66 Appendix C) says otherwise.

It should be noted that a manual mechanical device can be utilized at 10 to 20 ft./minute lift rate optimally under demonstration conditions. Remember that the object of the retrieval process is to extricate the worker within four minutes, the time limit rule-of-thumb for onset of brain damage from oxygen deprivation. Therefore, when manually powered hoists are used to provide access from more than 50 ft. depth, a pneumatic operation should be the primary lifting force.

Another factor for the 50 ft. limit is the static muscle work duration for upper-body cranking at approximately 30 lb. nonstop for several minutes (5:1 ratio with 12-in. lever arm). Rohmert in 1973, and Scherrer & Monod in 1960, showed that 75% of muscle power is lost in 2 1/2 to 3 minutes without a recovery rest period during intensive activity. Muscle strength rapidly deteriorates to approximately 20% of its original power. (See Figure 9.8.) This leads to the conclusion that use of a winch with a ratchet feature may be more efficient than use of one with only a rotary crank feature.

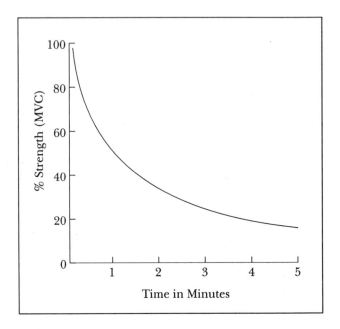

FIGURE 9.8
This graph illustrates the intensity/duration relationship for static muscle work (after Rohmert, 1973; Scherrer & Monod, 1960).[13]

APPLICATIONS

A manual operation should back up the pneumatic or electric function. A torque limiter (max. 450 lb. slip force) should be applied to all electrical or pneumatic personal lifting operations to avoid the full force of the power source plus mechanical advantage, causing damage to the worker or property.

Summary

Confined space fall arrest systems should meet the requirements of OSHA 1910.66 Appendix C and ANSI Z359.1-1992 until OSHA standards are fully in place by specific industry.

Fall arrest systems combining with or integrating emergency retrieval devices must be chosen carefully to meet the needs of a specific confined space category, seclected work method, the number of entrants, the degree of work crew and attendant training, and the proximity and readiness of on-site or off-site rescue teams. Regular training cannot be overemphasized.

OSHA Permit-required Confined Space programs call for identification and evaluation of permit spaces before entry. Collapse from heart attack, stroke or heat stress inside any type of confined space also should be addressed by employers.

It should be noted that the ANSI Z359 committee has begun work on the Z359.2 Positioning and Restraint Systems standard and on the Z359.3 Personnel Riding standard. But until a standard is developed for confined space access hoists, all hoists should be suited for their intended purpose of human lifting/lowering and backed up by a lifeline independent of the hoist mechanism, cable and seat. Access hoists for work positioning should be designated as top-to-bottom type or as stop-start type to determine proper specifications.

Notes

1. OSHA STD Instruction 3-11.1 March 3, 1982.

2. OSHA 49CFR 214.103(a), October 1, 1992.

3. Division of Motor Vehicles, State of Delaware. Driver's Manual. (1989 revision).

4. "Safety Guidelines for Window Cleaning." IWCA, Chicago, IL. 1992.

5. Ontario Ministry of Labour. "Guidelines for Roof Anchorage for Fall Arrest Systems." Regulations for Window Cleaning, Ontario Regulation 527/88.

6. Rodney Square Engineering Co., Wilmington, DE. Gabriel Fieni.

7. Ellis, J. Nigel. "Suspended Scaffolding: Proper Protection Reduces Fall Injuries." Occupational Health & Safety (January 1988).

8. Al Monaco, personal communication, 1987. American Manufacturing Co., Lafayette LA.

9. "Scaffold Fall Protection". Video by Dynamic Scientific Controls, 3101 N. Market St., Wilming-ton, DE. 1992.

10. NIOSH Criteria Document on Working in Confined Spaces 80-106, based on 2448 shipyard confined space accidents per year (p.19). Also, Moran/Ellis estimates based on conservative ratios of death to injury in U.S. industry (p.22).

11. NIOSH testimony of John Moran at OSHA Confined Space hearing, Docket S-019, November 1, 1989; supplementary submission February 23, 1990.

12. NIOSH Alert: Request for Assistance in Preventing Occupational Fatalities in Confined Spaces, January 1986, NIOSH. 86-110.

13. National Information Group. Contract Report #91-227-330, "Physiological Bases for Manual Lifting Guide". Springfield, VA. January 15, 1990.

Additional References

OSHA 1910.66 Appendix C.

OSHA 29 CFR 1910.146 Permit Required Confined Spaces October 10, 1989.

Stephens, Hugh. "Safer Tank Entry." *Professional Safety* (May 1979); 32-35.

Review Questions

1. An extension ladder is laid against an outside wall on a residence for painting by a handyman who is a part–time employee. The working length is 25 ft. and the distance from the base of the ladder to the wall is 7 ft. As you drive past, you observe the work in progress, and it disturbs you that the worker uses one hand while he climbs the ladder, holding the paint sprayer nozzle and line with his other hand. How should you, the safety supervisor, approach this person in order to teach him more safety?
   a. Suggest that he pull up the paint line on a string after maintaining a firm hold on the ladder while climbing.
   b. Provide rear braces to the top of the ladder to spread the load and inhibit tipping.
   c. Stop the work until his supervisor has thoroughly trained him in safe ladder techniques.
   d. Allow ladders for access only and prohibit actual work on a ladder unless that ladder is secured at the top.

2. For many years, a carpentry company has provided services for applying installation of trusses and sheeting (decking) for $150,000 to $300,000

homes under construction at residential developments. The industry has been unanimous in voicing strong opposition to fall protection on the grounds of unfeasibility due to lack of structural stability. You are determined to make headway in this seeming impasse to progress and to start a trial program as follows:

a. Truss separation and securing is your first fall protection goal and everything follows from this.

b. Attack the roofing phase because workers have something to stand on.

c. Require decking of the top floor to provide a working surface.

d. Sheeting operations are your first goal.

3. A worker offshore is being lifted in order to detach a faulty environmental sampling system using the blocks of the rig (a jack–up type engaged in drilling 12 miles off the Texas coastline). He is being lifted in a harness designed for climbing assist which is made from sturdy cotton purchased approximately 12 years earlier. Suddenly, one witness hears a ripping sound and the worker (225 lbs.) falls from the harness to his death on the drill floor. Subsequent analysis shows corroded wire supports and rotted canvas. You are the manufacturer of this harness. What defense do you have in the light of future litigation?

a. The worker's brother said that during the previous week the victim was worried about somebody doing him in because of his race.

b. Because the device was worn well beyond its intended lifetime, the employer is responsible for failure to inspect/maintain it.

c. The device is being incorrectly used.

d. No lifeline was used.

4. Your field people are calling to have you approve a residential roofing lifeline device which one OSHA compliance officer called inadequate for fall arrest. The manufacturer of the device states that the device can be either work positioning or fall arrest as a "universal" fall protection device. You:

a. Recommend that leaning on the line is permitted provided balance is maintained.

b. Check whether the anchorage can take 5,000 lbs.

c. Advise that if leaning off–balance occurs, a separate fall arrest lifeline is required.

d. Insist that a two–rope system be used.

5. Your new annual report shows several striking photographs of the public works construction projects you have completed in the past year. The Board is immensely proud to include this, but points out that almost every photo showing work being done has workers exposed to long falls over 6 ft., with workers wearing belts and lanyards attached to rebar. What do you do?

a. Call stockholder relations and warn them that some calls may be received and that they should forward these calls to you.

b. Tell your colleagues that these photographs were published without your review.

c. Review your construction fall protection rules with the Superintendent of Construction.

d. Request to review all photographs of operations before they are used in any future reports.

6. A warehouse works 18 hours per day and 364 days per year. You are the loss control engineer assigned to inspect several warehouses in your region. You are surprised to find that the snaphook gates of nearly all short lanyard devices in each warehouse are taped open, bent open, and have springs removed, and that the anchorage point bolts are hardware store purchased, with wingnuts in some cases. You approach management, who convince you that workers will be fired if they do not use their lanyard devices, and advise you that workers are complying with the posted signs. Your response is to do the following:

a. Write up management as having a poor safety program.

b. Point out that fall protection is being misused.

c. Advise the underwriter about the severe risk at the insured's warehouse location.

d. Return with your manager for a second inspection.

SAFETY RULES AND MAINTENANCE

No fall protection system can make up for a poor work method. Good fall arrest equipment that is incorrectly used is sometimes worse than no equipment at all.

❖ Aerial lifts

❖ Fall arrest equipment

❖ Guardrails

❖ Safety nets

❖ Scaffolds

❖ Steel erection

❖ Stockpickers

❖ Design and construction fall protection planning

❖ General industry fall protection planning

Administrative Rules and Fall Arrest Maintenance

OSHA's definition of a Competent Person (1910.66 Appendix C) is as follows:

A person who is capable of identifying hazardous or dangerous conditions in the personal fall arrest system or any component thereof as well as in their application and use with related equipment.

☞ When fall protection of any kind is provided, the project's competent person must teach workers the limitations to that system's effectiveness.

Safety Rules for Aerial Lifts

- Operators must have an effective procedure for leaving the platform when elevated.
- The anchor point should be at the same height as the operator's harness D-ring. The lanyard in most designs should be no more than 4 ft. long.
- Anchor points should be capable of withstanding twice the maximum arrest force of the fall arrest device to avoid the possibility of tip-over. Unauthorized anchor points must not be used.
- Never use the midrail as a step.

Safety Rules for Using Fall Arrest Equipment

- Never attach two pieces of fall arrest equipment together by any means unless the manufacturer has authorized such an attachment in writing.
- Never attach fall arrest equipment snaphooks together unless authorized in writing by the manufacturer.
- Never detach yourself from your fall arrest equipment at height, where a fall exposure may exist because of unstable flooring.
- Never use fall arrest equipment as a work tool unless your equipment is specifically designed for work positioning. If it is, you must have a fall arrest system in addition to the work positioning equipment.

Safety Rules for Guardrails

Guardrails are the primary means of fall protection in industry and construction.

- Do not step on, climb, straddle, use as a ladder, lean over or lean through a guardrail. Guardrails are used only as a same-level barrier to protect a worker from an exposed edge fall hazard. The guardrail's top rail is at a height of 42 in. Any opening under the top rail of up to 19 in. is permitted for industrial or construction use, but as little as 5 in. is permitted in some commercial building codes.
- Do not use guardrails as anchor points for fall arrest equipment, unless they are approved by a structural engineer for that specific purpose. There must be an engineering drawing showing what specific locations are suitable as anchor points, and what equipment, by rating, may be used and how it is to be attached. In addition, the worker must be trained in recognition of approved anchor points.

Safety Rules for Safety Nets

- Never use a debris net for personnel use unless a personnel net is incorporated. Clean out debris frequently.
- Never use a personnel net more than 25 ft. below the work surface
- Use nets with an 8 ft. minimum extension width for nets positioned at the same level as the work, up to 5 ft. below the work surface.
- Use nets with 10 ft. minimum extension width for nets positioned at 5 to 10 ft. below the work surface.
- Use nets with 13 ft. minimum extension width for nets positioned at 10 to 25 ft. below the work surface.
- Clearly identify by signs or labels whether the net is for personnel protection, or debris, or both. Otherwise, a worker is entitled to assume it is for both. Workers will assume it is if no sign states otherwise.

Note: Refer to proposed OSHA 1910.28(h)(3) on safety net criteria.

Safety Rules for Scaffolds

- The scaffold should be tied in at the first level, to avoid the possibility of tip-over, before fall arrest equipment is used. It should be tied in every 26 ft. thereafter, as per OSHA requirements.
- Frame scaffolds must be pinned before fall arrest equipment is used.
- Scaffold designs should be modeled if anchorage strength is less than 5,000 lbs. and if shock absorbing equipment is used.

SAFETY RULES AND MAINTENANCE

- Use picks or planks as a barrier to protect the worker from falling off and outside the scaffold enclosure.
- Secure all legs with pins before fall arrest equipment is attached to the frame or used.
- Do not permit angled falls beyond 45 degrees. Swinging impacts can be injurious. Keep anchorage points higher by proper sequence of erection to method to match the work methods.

Safety Rules for Steel Erection

- Waist height to overhead height cables erected at the ground or shake-out level can provide protection for predictable routes.
- Plan the routes of travel up and around the structure and stick to them.
- Check to see whether harnesses have abraded or cut webbing under the buttocks from cooning (straddling) work methods.
- Do not work connecting steel in unusually windy or wet weather conditions.
- Approve workboots for use on specific walking surfaces.
- Do not permit free climbing of columns. Instead, use ladders equipped with fall arrest gear.
- Do not walk on beams that are less than 6 in. flange in width.
- If possible, plan erection at ground level by discussing it with the fabricator, and then lifting it into position. This all but eliminates fall hazards.
- For decking work (the most dangerous phase of steel erection based on fatality records), plan the location of bundles of decking so that a platform can be erected immediately next to the first bundle and widened without the necessity of carrying or dragging deck panels along steel beams or further than 20 to 30 ft. A fall protection plan can be established to complement the selected work method.

Safety Rules for Stockpickers

- A boom is required for positioning the anchorage overhead to minimize swing falls while standing on the platform.
- Never stand or put your weight on a rack. Your fall arrest system cannot protect you if the surface collapses. Note: Pallets, particle board, plywood and metal surfaces are inherently unstable if unsecured, and racks frequently take punishing collisions with material handling equipment. These both con-

tribute towards destabilizing the rack system.
- Never step across an opening of more than 12 in. Your fall arrest device may not be able to prevent you from receiving severe injuries from a fall.
- Retractable lines are preferable to straight lanyards, which may get trapped under packages more easily. This causes the user to unhook at heights in order to disentangle him/herself, thereby permitting fall exposure.
- Prohibit moving across to the other side of the rack for any reason, a practice which encourages the worker to disconnect the lanyard and stretch while unprotected at heights.
- Inspect and maintain — with logs — all fall arrest equipment and anchorages on a monthly basis, based on heady use. Withdraw any equipment from use immediately if it is in less than an "as-new" or "as-designed" condition. Compare the equipment with the owner's engineering drawings, showing installation and details.

Safety Rules for Design and Construction Fall Protection Planning

- Each workers which anchorages are allowed, and then prohibit the use of all others without written approval.
- Demonstrate the approved methods of fall protection.
- Warn workers against swing fall hazards.
- Do not permit jury-rigged fall systems or unauthorized equipment on site.
- Do not allow knotted systems for fall arrest or fall anchorage attachments.
- Require 42 in. minimum height parapets on all commercial buildings when planning life-cycle – from construction to demolition – fall protection.
- Install perimeter cables designed for fall arrest use before decking is installed, if feasible.
- Use the quick-release method for column slings after initial connection.

Safety Rules for General Industry Fall Protection Planning

- Do not use guardrails as anchorages unless approved by engineering.
- Never use pipevents as anchorages.
- Do not allow knotted systems for fall arrest or fall anchorage attachments.

- Teach tie-backs for both scaffold suspension and lifelines
- Require building managers to install permanent roof anchors.
- Require footpaths and catwalks for main allowed routes of travel on roofs, especially those with no or low parapets.
- Require permanent warning lines at 6 to 10 ft. from the edge of a roof with no or low parapets.

- Instruct when harnesses are to be attached to fall arrest devices and when they are unnecessary.

It is very important to note that this list of safety rules is not complete.It is merely an indication of the need for very clear rules for the use and inspection of fall arrest equipment, in order for that equipment to be effective.

TRAINING

Individual test records are the
starting point of a claim that a
worker has been trained.

❖ Training to meet OSHA safety regulations
❖ Supervisor training
❖ Employee training

Training to Meet OSHA Safety Regulations

Training is a very subjective matter, and its adequacy for a given project can always be criticized. Yet, it is vital that employees and subcontractor representatives are able to accurately relate the degree of safety and health training they have received.

Employees should be instructed to be responsive and to tell the truth when questioned about their training by compliance officers during a site visit. If they do not tell about the training they have received, it is possible that their employer will be cited by OSHA for failure to train under 1926.21(b)(2) for construction projects.

On a wider front, OSHA compliance officers look to see if employers are following OSHA Instruction Standard 3-1.1, applicable presently to the construction industry, in their safety and health program, as follows.

Answer yes or no for each of the following checkpoints to gauge your compliance.

Management Commitment and Leadership

1. Policy statement is formed: goals are established, issued and communicated to employees.
2. Program is revised annually.
3. Management participates in safety meetings and inspections; agenda items in meetings showing safety issues have been raised for discussion.
4. Commitment of resources is adequate.
5. Safety rules and procedures are incorporated into site operations.
6. Management observes safety rules.

Assignment of Responsibility

1. Knowledgeable and accountable safety designer is on site.
2. Supervisors' (including foremen) safety and health responsibilities are understood.
3. Employees adhere to safety rules.

Identification and Control of Hazards

1. Periodic site safety inspections include supervisors.
2. Preventative controls are in place (PPE, maintenance, engineering controls).
3. Action is taken to address hazards.
4. Safety committee is established where appropriate.
5. Technical references are available.
6. Procedures are enforced by management.

Training and Education

1. Supervisors receive basic training.
2. Specialized training is given when needed.
3. Employee training program exists, is ongoing, and is effective.

Recordkeeping and Hazard Analysis

1. Records of employee illnesses and injuries are maintained and posted.
2. Supervisors perform accident investigation and propose corrective action.

GUIDANCE FOR AN EFFECTIVE FALL PROTECTION PROGRAM INCLUDES BOTH SUPERVISOR AND EMPLOYEE FALL PROTECTION TRAINING

Supervisor Fall Protection Training

- Read policy statement.
- Read rules line by line; explain to employees.
- When is fall protection required?
- When is fall protection not required?
- Examples; application slides.
- Project planning; site visit/engineering.
- Company video (10 minutes).
- Hands-on session with fall arrest/work positioning equipment; testing know-how.
- Responsibility: crew selection/instruction.
- Responsibility: safety review/methods.
- Responsibility: enforce citation policy.
- Frequent observation of crew.
- Safety is the supervisor's responsibility!

Employee Fall Protection Training

- Read policy statement.
- Read fall protection rules line by line.
- When is fall protection required?
- When is fall protection not required?
- Examples; application slides.
- Project planning: Who? When?
- Company site video (10 minutes).
- Hands-on session with fall arrest/work positioning equipment.
- Citation policy reviewed and discussed.
- Must pass performance evaluation (written test or personal review).
- Observation and enforcement procedures.
- Refresher training policy.
- Owner/general contractor's main business message: Make profits from fall protection.

FIGURE 11.1

An effective fall protection program depends upon training for both supervisor and worker.

TRAINING

3. Injuries, near misses, and illnesses are evaluated for trends and similar causes, and corrective action initiated.

First Aid and Medical Assistance

1. Supplies and medical services are available.
2. Employees are informed of medical results.
3. Emergency procedures and training are available where needed.

Review Questions

1. Your contractor training program consists of a plant video and a questionnaire reflecting your knowledge of evacuation procedures, emergency phone numbers and numerous do's and don'ts relating to work on site. The fall protection section in the video consists of a few seconds emphasizing the requirement to wear belts when exposed to fall hazards. However, your new plant policy requires the use of harnesses throughout the plant for fall hazard exposures. What should your additional fall protection training for contractors include at this time?
   a. Orally correct the video message by emphasizing harnesses.
   b. Require that contractors meet OSHA proposed construction regulations 29 CFR 1926 Subpart M (published November 25, 1986) on fall protection.
   c. Bring in a vendor to demonstrate his fall protection products.
   d. Demonstrate the proper wearing of a harness; list available anchor points on site and note those which are not for use; make available an engineering contact for structural strength information.

2. Your normal procedure has been to use knuckle boom aerial platforms to get to piperack locations in difficult locations. However, one particular location cannot be reached with the lift, and that's where your workers have to be for a pipe leak on that same day you find out the location is inaccessible. What one thing do you hope your maintenance crews remember from your last fall protection training session?
   a. Tie off portable ladders.
   b. Use lifelines when exposed to a fall hazard.
   c. Build scaffolding for safe access.
   d. Install a safety net first.

3. For 40 years, your plant practice has been to exempt scaffold erection from fall protection unless railings cannot be used uniformly, or the erection starts above ground. How do you change this practice to provide more safety for erectors/users of ground-built scaffolds?
   a. Circulate a date by which time fall protection is expected and required.
   b. Model, with engineering assistance, scaffold fall protection.
   c. Train scaffold builders with a hands-on fall protection equipment demonstration.
   d. ☞ Show a video of several different types of scaffold structure being built with fall protection.

4. OSHA in your region has started to enforce OSHA 1926.1053 ladder or ramp requirements on forms where the step up or down is greater than 19 in. How can you comply?
   a. Require the use of a ladder on all form work.
   b. Require that forms be redesigned to have step distances less than 19 in.
   c. Require that only one main access to form scaffolds be used.
   d. Require that lifelines be used on all forms at height.

5. Your company has evolved model training programs for workers at risk, supervisors, engineers and trainers. After training is well underway at numerous plants, an employee who has been trained suffers a fatal fall through a roof opening. Your legal department decides to pay OSHA willful citation fines totaling $20,000, and now, in the "intentional tort" lawsuit that follows, your training programs are used as evidence that you did not train the victim. What defenses do you have?
   a. The employee saw a video six times showing how and why to wear a harness.
   b. The company is protected under state workers' compensation laws; the employee assumed the risk; contributory negligence.
   c. The employee put the harness on and experienced hanging in it as part of aerial lift training.
   d. The employee saw a video, experienced suspension, was tested, and was shown how to install equipment for the roof application.

POSTSCRIPT

"We measure safety by the number of exposures, not the number of accidents."

T. ALLEN McARTOR, ADMINISTRATOR, FEDERAL AVIATION ADMINISTRATION, SPEAKING ON NBC'S "MEET THE PRESS" AUGUST 22, 1987

Today, leading companies strive to provide a workplace safe from recognized hazards for their employees, using personal protective gear – such as clothing protection, eye protection, head protection and foot protection – in addition to machine guards, and recently adding Material Safety Data Sheets (MSDS) to facilitate chemical label warnings awareness.

Fall hazards are the last major safety hazard to be addressed, and we need to think beyond the limited belt/lanyard concept for protection.

I hope that this second edition of *Introduction to Fall Protection* will be of assistance to those who are dedicated to this end. In fact, many helpful ideas from first edition readers already have been added into this edition.

To quote the business policy of one major US corporation, "We'll do it safely or we won't do it."

That's the spirit!

GLOSSARY OF TERMS

The definitions in this glossary are, for the most part, the author's presentation of the current standards, rewritten for clearer understanding. When a standard is quoted, its title is given.

A

Absail: The mountaineering term for descent control.

Access: Means of reaching a workstation, physically or mechanically.

Acrometry: The study of the geometry of elevated workstations, used for planning fall protection security.

Activation Distance: The distance traveled by a fall arrester (FA) or the amount of line played out by a self-retracting lanyard/lifeline device (SRL) from the point of onset of a fall to the activation point where the fall arrester begins to apply a braking or stopping force. This activation point may occur where the fall arrester engages the lifeline or, in the case of an SRL, where an internal brake engages (ANSI Z359.1-1992).

Aerial Lifts: Mechanical devices such as manlifts, man baskets, scissor lifts and bucket trucks used for access to heights. (The term "skip" is reserved for materials use on construction sites.)

Anchorage: A secure point of attachment for lifelines, lanyards or deceleration devices, and which is independent of the means of supporting or suspending the employee (OSHA 1910.66 Appendix C). Also, a secure means of attachment to which the Personal Fall Arrest System (PFAS) is connected (ANSI Z359.1-1992).

Angled Descent: An emergency descent at an angle away from a structure to avoid additional hazards, such as fire or explosion.

Arresting Force: The amount of force exerted on a worker or test weight when a fall protection system stops a fall. The amount usually expresses the peak force experienced during the fall. (See *Maximum Arrest Force*.)

Attendant: A standby person for confined space entry. An additional attendant might also be an entrant for monitoring purposes.

B

Block: See *Retracting Lifeline*.

Body Belt: A strap with means both for securing it around the waist and for attaching it to a lanyard, lifeline, or deceleration device (OSHA 1910.66 Appendix C). Also, a strap that a worker can secure around the waist and to which the worker can attach a lanyard or device for work positioning. Note: ANSI Z359.1 has not recognized the body belt for use in a fall arrest system.

Body Harness: A design of straps that may be secured about the employee in a manner to distribute the fall arrest forces over at least the thighs, pelvis, waist, chest and shoulders, with means for attaching it to other components of a personal fall arrest system (OSHA 1910.66 Appendix C).

Body Restraint System: A single or multiple strap device, such as a body belt, chest harness or full body harness, that can be secured around a worker and attached to a load-bearing anchorage in order to restrict travel and limit the fall hazard.

Body Support: A component comprised of a strap or straps suitably arranged and assembled to support the human body during and after fall arrest. It generally includes adjustable means for fastening it about the body and means for attaching it to other components or subsystems of the PFAS (ANSI Z359.1-1992). Note: This standard addresses only personal fall arrest systems incorporating a full body harness.

Boatswain's Chair/Seat: A workseat equipped with a seat strap and body belt, used for positioning. Also known as a *bosun chair*.

Buckle: Any device for hooking the body belt or body harness closed around the employee's body (OSHA 1910.66 Appendix C).

Bungee Cord: An clasticized rubber cord.

C

Cable: Wire rope. In this text, wire rope is used for lifelines. When fixed vertically (secured at top and bottom), cable serves as part of a vertical climbing protection system. When fixed horizontally, a cable may be part of a hazardous lifeline system.

Cable Grab: A fall arrest device that locks by either inertia or a cam lock (locking arm) when a free fall is sensed. It is attached to a worker directly or by a lanyard that slides up or down a fixed cable or vertical cable lifeline.

Car Restraint Belt: A lap belt, shoulder strap, or combination of the two (seat harness) that is designed to restrain a victim during a collision and distribute arresting forces over the victim's body.

Carabiner: An oblong ring snaphook (Europe:

karabinier), often erroneously called a D-ring. Also, a connector component generally comprised of a trapezoidal or oval-shaped body with a normally closed gate or similar arrangement, which may be opened to permit the body to receive an object and, when released, automatically closes to retain the object (ANSI Z359.1-1992).

Carrier: A track of flexible cable or rigid rail secured to a fixed ladder or structure on which a ladder safety device (climbing sleeve) moves up and down with the climber. Should a fall occur, the device is designed to lock onto the carrier to arrest the fall.

Catenary Line: A flexible line hanging freely between two fixed points under its own weight. See *Horizontal Lifeline.*

Chest Harness: An arrangement of straps that secures around the chest and shoulders, and to which a lanyard is attached. It is usually used for restraint or possibly emergency retrieval, but never for fall arrest.

Chest-Waist Harness: An arrangement of straps that secures around the chest, shoulders, and waist, with a D-ring in the center of the back. It is used for limited free-fall arrest or restraint.

Climbing Assist: A counterbalance weight system that minimizes fatigue by reducing the weight of a belted worker on long ladder or structure climbs.

Competent Person: A person who is capable of identifying hazardous or dangerous conditions in the personal fall arrest system or any component thereof, as well as in their application and use with related equipment (OSHA 1910.66 Appendix C). Note: The OSHA Competent Person definition (1926.650 and 1926.32(f)) also requires that a competent person have the authority to take prompt corrective measures to eliminate hazards.

Confined Space: A space in which hazardous gases, vapor mists, dusts, or aerosols can accumulate, or an oxygen-deficient atmosphere can occur. This can happen because of its location, construction, contents, or the activity that goes on within.

Connecting Means: A device or lanyard used to connect a body support to an anchorage, so that it provides protected mobility for an elevated work task.

Connector: A device that is used to couple (connect) parts of the system together. It may be an independent component of the system (such as a carabiner) or an integral component of part of the system (such as a buckle or D-ring) sewn into a body belt or body harness, or a snaphook spliced or sewn to a lanyard or self-retracting lanyard (OSHA 1910.66 Appendix C). Also, an ironworker who attaches major structural elements during steel erection.

Continuous Fall Protection: The design and use of a fall protection system so that no exposure to an elevated fall hazard occurs. This may require more than one fall protection system or a combination of prevention or protection measures.

Controlled Descent: A descent automatically controlled at a constant rate of speed by a device that requires no manual operation.

D

D-ring: A connector used integrally in a harness as an attachment element or fall arrest attachment and in lanyards, energy absorbers, lifelines and anchorage connectors as an integral connector (ANSI Z359.1-1992). Note: A D-ring is sometimes referred to as a carabiner snaphook in the mountaineering equipment industry.

Danger: Combination of hazard and risk that yields a qualitative measure of exposure of a person or a system to harm, injury, damage or loss.

Deceleration Device: A mechanism such as a rope grab, retracting lifeline or shock absorbing lanyard that absorbs or dissipates energy during a fall arrest.

Deceleration Distance: The vertical distance between the user's fall arrest attachment at the onset of fall arrest forces during a fall, and after the fall arrest attachment comes to a complete stop (ANSI Z359.1-1992).

Descent Control: A device used to control descent that requires manual operation. The user must constantly maintain control of the device for it to perform properly. Different body weights require different settings.

Dog Line: A horizontal lifeline attached (usually) to the back of a swinging scaffold. A lanyard is usually attached to the dog line.

Double-Locking Snaphook: (An old term.) See *Locking Snaphook.*

Double-Pass Friction Buckle: A device that retains its position on webbing by friction and requires two passes over the center bar to have a reliable hold.

Drop Line: A vertical lifeline secured to an upper anchorage for the purpose of attaching a lanyard or device. (Used in A10.14-1975).

Dynamic Rating: The arresting force a manufacturer reports after conducting an OSHA force test. (See *Maximum Arrest Force.*)

E

Egress: A means of escape from a workstation; for

GLOSSARY

177

example, stairs, a door or an escape device. Note: Not to be confused with the National Fire Protection Association's (NFPA 101) definition of egress.

Elevated Fall: An uncontrolled drop from one level to another.

Ellis' Rule: The vertical component of a swing fall should not exceed 6 ft. or the maximum free fall distance permitted by the authority having jurisdiction.

EMR: Experience Modification Rate. The EMR reflects employer performance in accident prevention under state Workers' Compensation laws.

F

Fall Distance: The distance from the location of a worker's support prior to a fall and the place where the worker finally comes to a complete stop.

Fall Equipment: Any equipment designed for fall arrest or escape, as cited in this book.

Fall Arrest System: A tested device and components that function together as a system to arrest a free fall and minimize the potential for compounding injury. See *Personal Fall Arrest System.*

Fall Hazard: Any position from which an accidental fall may reasonably produce injury.

Fall Prevention: Any same-level means used to reasonably prevent exposure to an elevated fall hazard. Floors, walls, guardrails and area isolation are means of fall prevention.

Fall Protection: What is done to effectively address fall hazards.

Fall Protection Equipment: See *Fall Arrest System.*

Fall-Restraint System: A lanyard or device that is designed to restrain a worker in order to prevent a fall from occurring.

Fixed Anchorage: A stationary point of attachment for lanyards, lifelines or devices that is capable of supporting at least twice the maximum potential force in each fall protection system that may be used. See *Anchorage.*

Force Factor: The ratio of the arresting force on a rigid metal test weight to the arresting force on a human body having the same weight, both falling under identical conditions.

Force Test: An OSHA test designed to measure the maximum arrest force in a fall protection equipment system.

Free Fall: The act of falling before the personal fall arrest system begins to apply force to arrest the fall (OSHA 1910.66 Appendix C).

Free Fall Distance: The vertical displacement of the fall arrest attachment point on the employee's body belt or body harness between onset of the fall and just before the system begins to apply force to arrest the fall. This distance excludes deceleration distance, and lifeline and lanyard elongation, but includes any deceleration device slide distance or self-retracting lifeline/lanyard extension before their operation and before full arrest forces occur (OSHA 1910.66 Appendix C).

Friction Buckle: A device that retains its position on webbing by friction.

Full Body Harness: An arrangement of straps that can be secured around the body, and to which a lanyard or device can be attached. A full body harness is designed to distribute arresting and suspension forces over the buttocks, pelvis, thighs, chest and shoulders, and is used for personal fall arrest.

G

Gate: A snaphook closure that swings closed to secure.

Guardrail: See *Railing, Standard.*

H

Hand Line: Used to raise tools to an elevated work position. Also, a horizontal line used to help maintain balance. Never to be used for fall protection.

Handrail: A narrow rail for grasping with the hand for support (Webster's New Collegiate Dictionary, 9th ed.). Also, a bar or pipe supported on brackets from a wall or partition, as on a stairway or ramp, to furnish persons with a handhold in case of tripping (OSHA 1926.502(c)).

Hardware: Snaphooks, D-rings, buckles, carabiners, adjusters, and O-rings that are used to attach the components of a fall protection system to each other.

Harness: Also known as chest harness, chest-waist harness, and mountaineering harness. See *Full Body Harness.*

Hazard: Condition with the potential to incur harm; an agent, energy or characteristic that can cause physical damage to personnel or property. Attributes of a physical object that statistically or dynamically presents a continuing threat of harm, injury, or loss to a person or system.

Horizontal Lifeline: A rail, rope, wire or synthetic cable installed horizontally and used for attachment of a worker's lanyard or lifeline device while moving horizontally. It is used to control dangerous pendulum-like swing falls.

Horizontal Lifeline Accessway: A combination of a slip-resistant walkway and an elevated fall hazard control system.

I

Independent Anchorage: A point of attachment that is not part of the working/walking surface or equipment rigging points.

K

Keeper (Lock): Latch hold to manually control a snaphook gate action in a locking snaphook. It is also used to refer to any snaphook moving part.

Kernmantle: A core-sheathed rope sometimes used as a lifeline in industry (mountaineering term).

L

Ladder Climbing (Safety) Device: A device or climbing sleeve connected to the front D-ring on the climber's body belt or full body harness that slides up and down a rigid rail or cable. Should a fall occur, the device is designed to lock by inertia or cam action to arrest the fall.

Ladder, Fixed: A ladder that cannot be readily moved or carried because it is an integral part of the building or structure. There are side-step fixed ladders and through-fixed ladders.

Ladder, Job-Made: A ladder that is fabricated by employees, typically at a construction site, and is not commercially manufactured. Job-made ladders can be single or double cleat design, with the latter offering a center rail to allow simultaneous two-way traffic ascending and descending to a specific access point.

Ladder, Portable or Portable Extension: A ladder that can be readily moved or carried. Self-supporting ladders are stepladders. Non-self supporting ladders are lean-to design.

Lanyard: A flexible line of rope, wire rope, or strap used to secure the body belt or body harness to a deceleration device, lifeline, or anchorage.

Lifeline: A component consisting of a flexible line for connection to an anchorage at one end to hang vertically (vertical lifeline), or for connection to anchorages at both ends to stretch horizontally (horizontal lifeline), and which serves as a means for connecting other components of a personal fall arrest system to the anchorage (OSHA 1910.66 Appendix C). A vertical lifeline usually extends an anchorage point onto which a rope grab is attached.

Lineman's Belt and Strap: A waist belt worn close to the hips in conjunction with a strap, used for leaning and work positioning. A lanyard may also be a work-positioning device.

Loadline: The line which supports the weight of a person on a scaffold or boatswain's chair or for work positioning.

Locking Snaphook: A connecting snaphook that requires two separate forces to open the gate — one to deactivate the gate lock or keeper, and a second to depress and open the gate, which automatically closes when released. It is used to minimize roll-out or accidental disengagement when attached to other components of a fall arrest system.

Low-Pitched Roof: A roof having a slope less than or equal to 4 in 12 (OSHA 1926.502(p)(3)).

M

Man Baskets: Crane- or derrick-suspended personnel platform used for the hoisting of personnel when the platform is hoisted on the loadlines of cranes or derricks.

Maximum Arrest Device (MAD): A deceleration device or fall arrest system meeting OSHA regulations.

Maximum Arrest Force (MAF): The peak force measured by the test instrumentation during arrest of the test weight in the dynamic tests set forth in this standard (ANSI Z359.1-1992). (See *Dynamic Rating.*)

Monkey Line: See *Horizontal Lifeline.*

N

Non-locking Snaphook: A connector that requires only one force to open the gate, and that is sometimes subject to roll-out.

P

Parachute Harness: See *Full Body Harness.* (The original parachute design was used to hold a victim vertical in a manhole.)

Personal Fall Protection System: A system used to arrest an employee in a fall from a working level. It consists of an anchorage, connectors, a body belt or body harness, and may include a lanyard, deceleration device, lifeline, or suitable combinations of these (OSHA 1910.66 Appendix C).

GLOSSARY

Positioning Belt: A single or multiple strap that can be secured around the worker's body to hold the user in a work position. Examples are a lineman's belt, a rebar belt, a window cleaner belt and a saddle belt.

Positioning System: A system employing a boatswain's chair or saddle belt and used in conjunction with a loadline to descend to or reach a workstation; i.e., a lineman's belt and strap.

Q

Qualified Engineer: An individual with a degree from an accredited institution or a professional certificate who is capable of design, analysis, evaluation, specification and system safety planning in the areas needed for fall hazard control.

Qualified Person: A person with a recognized degree or professional certificate and with extensive knowledge and experience in the subject field, who is capable of design, analysis, evaluation and specifications in the subject work, project, or product (OSHA 1910.66 Appendix C). Note: The OSHA Qualified Person definition (1926.32[1]) has similar wording.

Quick Release Buckle: A multiple component device that can be disengaged with one positive action and whose releasing mechanism is positively locked in normal use.

R

Railing, Standard: A vertical barrier erected along exposed edges of a floor opening, wall opening, ramp, platform, or runway to prevent the fall of persons (OSHA 1926.502(k)).

Rebar Belt: A work-positioning support for use on steel bar reinforcing rods while adding and tying new rods (ANSI A10.14 Type II).

Reconditioning of Fall Arrest Devices: A manufacturer's maintenance program to inspect and repair fall equipment.

Restraint Line: A line from a fixed anchorage or from between two anchorages to which a worker is secured in order to prevent the worker from walking or falling off a low-pitched roof or surface to a lower level. Not a fall arrest system.

Retracting Lifeline: A fall arrester whose integral line extends as a worker moves downward and automatically retracts as the worker moves up toward the unit, eliminating slack. Retracting lifelines can have a centrifugal locking mechanism, or alternatively, a centrifugal braking mechanism (also known in Europe as "block") for controlled descent.

Retrieval Winch: A hoisting device designed for personal raising and/or lowering in emergency situations.

Risk: The probability of a loss occurring expressed as a percentage or as a fraction. Also, the non-sequentialized chance that a person or system is exposed to harm, injury or loss.

Roll-out: The unintentional disengagement of a snaphook caused by the gate being depressed under torque or contact while twisting or turning. A particular concern with single-action (non-locking) snaphooks that do not have a lock.

Rope: This term may refer to wire rope or synthetic rope (usually the latter in this text when discussing lifelines).

Roof Tie-Backs: Fixed anchorage points suitable for the attachment of lifelines or rigging equipment for use with suspended scaffolds, as a backup to primary anchorage points.

Rope Grab: A fall arrester that is designed to move up and down a lifeline suspended from a fixed overhead anchorage point to which a worker's belt or harness is attached. In the event of a fall, the rope grab locks onto the compatible rope through compression to arrest the fall.

S

Saddle Belt: A single or multiple strap that can be secured around the body, usually having a sub-pelvic strap for support under the buttocks while climbing or descending in a sitting position.

Safety Belt: A generic term originally used for means of body support.

Safety Factor: The ratio of the calculated strength or deceleration of a load-bearing member or material to the maximum load or deceleration the component is expected to sustain in actual use.

Safety Line: See *Lifeline*.

Safety Sleeve: See *Ladder Climbing Device*.

Self-Retracting Lanyard (SRL): This term has been adopted by the ANSI Z359 committee to include the following: retracting lifelines, retractable lifelines, self-locking anchorages (UK), and self-retracting lifelines/lanyards (OSHA 1910.66 Appendix C). The rationale has gone beyond the fact that lanyards are typically short lines and lifelines are longer lines. The retractable lanyard term was selected because the device connects directly from the anchorage to the body support.

Self-Retracting Lifeline/Lanyard Device: A deceleration device which contains a drum-wound line that may be slowly extracted from, or retracted onto, the drum under slight tension during normal worker movement, and which, after onset of a fall, automatically locks the drum and arrests the fall (OSHA 1910.66 Appendix C).

Shock Absorber: A component of a fall protection system that dissipates energy by creating or extending the deceleration distance.

Shock-absorbing Lanyard: A flexible line of webbing, cable or rope that has an integral shock absorber and is used to secure a body belt or harness to a lifeline or anchorage point.

Single-Action Snaphook: A connecting snaphook that requires a single force to open the gate, which automatically closes when released.

Single-Pass, Fixed-Bar Friction Buckle: A device that retains its position on webbing by means of a single threading of the webbing over the fixed center bar.

Skip: A mechanical box for elevating materials used on construction sites and mining facilities.

Sleeve: A fall arrester used for rail or cable ladder safety devices/climbing protection equipment.

Sliding Back D-ring: A D-ring that is attached to a body support by threading the webbing through an integral slot. The sliding action is used for adjustment or on a harness to absorb energy during a fall arrest, as well as to position the body upright for suspension and retrieval.

Slip: A sliding motion that occurs when the friction between the supporting surface and the opposing surface of the foot or foot gear is inadequate.

Snaphook (Snap-hook, OSHA): A connector comprised of a hook-shaped member with a normally closed keeper, or similar arrangement, which may be opened to permit the hook to receive an object and, when released, automatically closes to retain the object. Snaphooks are generally one of two types: (1) the locking type, with a self-closing self-locking keeper, which remains closed and locked until unlocked and pressed open for connection or disconnection, or (2) the nonlocking type, with a self-closing keeper, which remains closed until pressed open for connection or disconnection (OSHA 1910.66 Appendix C). A carabiner is a special type of snaphook.

Stair Railing: A vertical barrier erected along exposed sides of a stairway to prevent falls of persons (OSHA 1926.502(i)).

Static Line: Also known as a messenger line. See *Horizontal Lifeline*.

Strength Member: Any component of a fall protection system that could be subject to loading in the event of a fall.

Strength Test: An OSHA test designed to measure approximately twice the force expected in the normal use of fall equipment.

Suspended Scaffold: A single point or multiple point work platform used for powered or unpowered access up and down the side of a structure.

Suspension Belt: A single or multiple strap that can be secured around the worker's body as an independent work support for escape, rescue or retrieval.

Swing Fall: A pendulum-like motion that can result from moving horizontally away from a fixed anchorage and falling. Swing falls generate the same amount of energy as a fall through the same distance vertically but with the additional hazard of colliding with an obstruction or the ground.

Synthetic Fibers: A manufactured fiber such as nylon, polyester or polypropylene.

T

Tail Line: See *Lanyard*.

Tie Off: To secure the end of a lanyard to an anchorage point. Note: An anchorage point is sometimes referred to as a *tie-off point*.

Tongue-Buckle: A connector that requires an integral tongue to be pushed through a grommeted hole in the webbing or strength member of a belt or harness to retain its position on the webbing.

Total Fall Distance: The sum of free fall distance and deceleration distance plus any elongation of the system or anchor. This should also include reversible rope lifeline stretch if appreciable.

Trolley Line: See *Horizontal Lifeline*.

W

Waist Belt: See *Body Belt*. Not to be confused with a tool belt, which is not for fall arrest.

ANSWERS TO REVIEW QUESTIONS

Chapter 1
1. d
2. b
3. c
4. b
5. a

Chapter 2
1. c
2. a
3. d
4. d
5. c

Chapter 3
1. b
2. a
3. d
4. b
5. d

Chapter 4
1. d
2. a
3. d
4. c
5. d

Chapter 5
1. c
2. c
3. c
4. b
5. d

Chapter 6
1. c
2. d
3. d
4. d
5. a

Chapter 7
1. c
2. a
3. a
4. d
5. b

Chapter 8
1. c
2. c
3. c
4. c
5. d
6. a
7. a

Chapter 9
1. c
2. d
3. d
4. c
5. d
6. d

Chapter 10
1. c
2. b
3. a
4. b
5. c

Chapter 11
1. d
2. b
3. d
4. d
5. c

APPENDICES

APPENDIX A-1:
Fall Protection, Escape and Rescue Standards

OSHA 1910.5 General Industry Provisions apply where specific rules do not address a hazard. Also, some states with local OSHA rules may have stricter requirements than federal rules. ANSI Standards and equipment manufacturers' instructions are advisory, but may be used to support a 5(a)(1) OSHA citation.

General Description	OSHA Construction Industry	OSHA Other & Maritime	References
Anchorage Strength	1910.66 Appendix C	1926.104(b)	ANSI A10.14-1991 ANSI Z359.1-1992 ANSI A120.1-1992
Building Exterior Maintenance - see Powered Platforms, Scaffolds			
Catch Platforms - also see Roof Lifelines	1910.28(s)(3)	1926.45(u)(3)	- -
Confined Space	1910.146	1926.21(b)(6) 1926.352(g) 1926.353(b)	ANSI Z117.1-1989 NIOSH 86-110 NIOSH 80-106
Crane Safety Standards - Cab Egress	- -	1926.550(a)(13)	
a. Overhead and Gantry Cranes			ANSI B30.2-1990
b. Hammerhead Tower Cranes		1926.550(c)(2)	ANSI B30.3-1990
c. Portal, Tower and Pillar Cranes			ANSI B30.4-1990
d. Monorails and Underhung Cranes			ANSI B30.11-1988
e. Controlled Mechanical Storage Cranes			ANSI B30.13-1991
f. Manbasket		1926.550(g)	ANSI A10.28-1990
Egress Standards	1910.35-38		
a. Emergency Action Plan	1910.38a	1926.35	
b. Emergency Egress From Elevated Work Stations			NIOSH 76-128(1975)
(i) Workover Rigs			OSHA Instruction STD. 1-2.1
(ii) Off-Road Machines			SAE J185-1981
(iii) Chimney Cage Hoists			OSHA Variances, "Rust Engineering Co." (1973 et.al.)
(iv) Tramways, Lifts & Toys			ANSI B77.1-1982
(v) Mobile Offshore Drilling Units			USCG 108.527
(vi) Grain Elevators	1910.272 Appendix A-11 1910.272(d)		
c. Fixed Ladders	Standard 1- 1.12		NSC Data Sheet #606
Electrical Maintenance	- -	1910.269(g) The Electric Power Generation Transmission and Distribution: Electrical Protective Equipment: Final Rule.	
Fall Protection-Current (status 2/93)	Standard 1-1.13 1910.129-131 (proposed 4/10/90)	1926 Subpart M (proposed 11/25/86)	ANSI A10.14-1991 ANSI Z359.1-1992
Fall Protection (offshore)	- -	- -	USCG 142.42

APPENDIX A-1 | **185**

General Description	OSHA Construction Industry	OSHA Other & Maritime	References
Floor & Wall Openings	1910.23	1926.500	ANSI A12.1-1973 A1204-1989
Grain Handling & Storage	1910.272	- -	- -
Ladder Safety Devices a. Storage Cranes	1910.27(d)(5) 1910.131 (proposed 4/10/90)	1926.450(a)(5) 1926.1053	ANSI A14.3-1992 FAA Interim Federal Spec. RR-S-001301 (1967) Mil-S-87966 (USAF) (1980) OSHA (Instruction STD 1-1.3 ANSI B30.13-1977
Lineman Body Belts (Telecommunication, Power Transmission) Oil & Gas Drilling & Servicing	1910.130 (proposed 4/10/90) 1910.270 (proposed 12/28/83)	1926.959	- -
Personal Protective Equipment	1910.132(a)	1926.28(a) 1926.95(a)	49 CFR 214.103(a)
Platforms	1910.23 1910.132	1926.500	- -
Powered Platforms	1910.66 Appendix C	- -	- -
Process Safety Management	1910.119	1926.64	- -
Railroad Bridge Fall Protection	- -	- -	49 CFR 214.1-5 49 CFR 214.101-107 Federal Railroad Administration/DOT 49 Transportation, Subpart B, Bridge Worker Safety standards, Fall Protection General
Rescue Standards a. Confined Spaces b. Excavations c. Grain - see also Grain Handling & Storage d. Power Transmission and Distribution	1910.146	1926.651(g)(2)(ii) 1926.651(h)(1) 1926.651(l)(1)	ANSI Z117.1-1989 NIOSH #80-106 (1979) ASTM C478.85 Pre-cast reinforced concrete manhole spec. Construction training manual NIOSH 9/85

INTRODUCTION TO FALL PROTECTION, SECOND EDITION

General Description	OSHA Construction Industry	OSHA Other & Maritime	References
Rescue Standards (cont.)			
e. Pulp and Paper	1910.261(b)(5) 1910.261(g)(2)(iii) 1910.261(g)(15)(iii)		
f. Respiratory Protection	1910.134(e)(3)(iii)		NIOSH #78-193A (1978)
g. Sand Foundry			ANSI Z241.1-1981
h. Trenching		1926.652(f)	
i. Ventilation in Tanks	1910.94(d)(11)(v)		
j. Welding in Confined Spaces	1910.252(e)(4)(iv)		
k. Working Over Water		1926.106(c)	
Roof Lifelines	1910.28(s)(3) 1926.500(g)	1926.451(u)(3)	- -
Safety Belts/Lanyards/Lifelines **Fall Protection Requirements**	1910.66 Appendix C	1926.104 1926.107(b)1(c)	California Construction Safety Orders,Title 8, Article 24 MIL-STD-1212 (1967) FAA TSO-C22f Construction Safety Code ASP, Anjou, Quebec
a. Aerial Lifts	1910.67(c)(2)(v)	1926.556(b)(2)(v)	ANSI A92.2-1979
b. Bell Bottom Pier		1926.652(f)	
c. Boatswains Chairs	1910.28(j)(4)	1926.451(1)(4)	ANSI A39.1-1987 California's General Industry Safety Orders Title 8, Article 24 (1976)
d. Crawling Boards or Chicken ladders	1910.28(t)(3)	1926.451(v)(2)	
e. Concrete and Masonry Construction		1926.701(e)(2)	
f. Cranes		1926.550(c)(2)	
g. Harnesses(Military)			MIL-H-24460SH(1981)
h. Longshoring	1910.16(a)	1918.32:96	
i. Low Lift and High Lift Trucks			ANSI B56.1-1988
j. Power Transmission and Distribution	1910.268	1926.951(b) 1926.959	
k. Pulp Paper and Paperboard Mills	1910.261(b)(5) 1910.261(f)(4) 1910.261(g)(2)(iii) 1910.261(g)(4)(i) 1910.261(q)(15)(iii) 1910.261(e)(18)		ANSI A14.1-1981
l. Sawmills	1910.265(d)(4)(ii) 1910.265(c)(21)(i) 1910.265(c)(21)(ii)(c)		
m. Scaffolds			
(i) Float or Ship	1910.28(u)(6)	1926.451(w)(6)	
(ii) Needle Beam	1910.28(n)(8)	1926.451(p)(9)	ANSI A10.8-24.6-1988
(iii) Window Jack	1910.28(r)(3)	1926.451(t)(3)	
(iv) Pump Jack		1926.451(y)(11)	
(v) Roofing Brackets		1926.451(u)(3)	
(vi) Suspended		1926 Subpart L	California General Industry Safety Orders, Title 8, Article 24(1976)

APPENDIX A-1   **187**

General Description	OSHA Construction Industry	OSHA Other & Maritime	References
Safety Nets (cont.)			
(vii) Swinging	1910.28(g)(9)	1926.451(i)(8)	ANSI A10.8-1989
(viii) Single Point	1910.28(i)(9)	1926.451(k)	ANSI A39.1-1987
n. Shipyard Employment		1915 Subpart E	
o. Silos, Hoppers, Tanks, Bins		1926.250(b0(2)	ANSI Z241.1-1981
p. Telecommunications	1910.268(g)(1)		
q. Tunnels and Shafts		1926.800(h)(3)(v)	
r. Type T Powered Platforms	1910.66(d)(8)		ANSI A120.1-1992
s. Welding, Cutting, Brazing	1910.252(e)(1)(i) 1910.252(e)(4)(iv)		
Safety Nets	1910.23(e)(3)(ii) (proposal 4/10/90)	1926.105 1926.750(b)(1)(ii)	New York City Construction Code, Article 19, Section 61-1983 NSC Data Sheet #608 ANSI A10.11-1989 49 CFR 214.103(a) 49 CFR 214.105(c)
Safety Training & Education	1910.66 App.C, Sec. III	1926.21(b)(2)	--
Stairs and Ladders	1910.24-.27	1926.501 1926.1050-1053	ANSI A1264.1-1989 ANSI A14.1-5
Steel Erection-Multi-tiered Buildings		1926.750(b)(1)(ii) 1918.32(c)	ANSI A10.13-1989 NBSIR 85-3271 Corps of Engineers EM385-1.1 OSHA Bulletin 2254
a. Steel Erection (Interior Falls)		1926.750(b)(1)(ii)	
b. Steel Erection (Exterior Falls)		1926.105 1926.750(b)(2)(ii) &(iii)	
Tree Trimming	--	--	ANSI Z133.1-1982
Foreign Standards	--	--	
a. Australian Lifelines			AS 1891 (1976)
b. Australian Safety Belts			AS 1891 (1976)
c. Canadian Safety Belts and Lanyards for Construction and Mining			CSA Z259.1-M1976
d. Canadian Full Body Harness			CSA Z259.10-M1990
e. Canadian Fall Arresting Devices & Lifeline			CSA Z259.2-M1979
f. Canadian Shock Absorbing Lanyard			CSA Z259.11-M1992
g. Canadian Lineman's Body Belt & Strap for Linemen			CSA Z259.3-1978
h. European Fall Protection Standards			EN341-365(1992)
i. Japanese Safety Belts for Linemen			JIS T 8165 (1979)
j. Japanese Safety Belts for Miners			JIS M 7624 (1974)
k. New Zealand			NZS 5811 (1981) Part 1 & 2

NOTE: Some ANSI and State Standards refer to portions of ANSI A10.14-1975 for fall equipment specifications, which have been updated in the 1991 Standard. Users can alternatively refer to equipment specifications and testing in OSHA 1910.66 Appendix C and ANSI Z359.1-1992. OSHA is applying the 1910.66 Appendix C fall arrest standard across all industry and construction in lieu of less advanced "safety belt" requirements. Also see Fall Protection - Current Status, above.

Standards in this Appendix provided courtesy of A.M. Best Co., Oldwick, N.J.

APPENDIX A-2:
Calculation of Vertical Fall Arrest Forces

The need to know whether present fall protection systems meet OSHA or other regulatory requirements can set the initial stage for overhaul of a company's fall protection program and work methods review.

Design, installation and application of fall arrest equipment are discussed by Chen Wang, a former OSHA official, in "Free Fall Restraint Systems", published in 1977 by the American Society of Safety Engineers – as well as by Harold Steinberg in "A Study of Fall Safety Equipment", published by the National Bureau of Standards (NBS) that same year.

A paper by Andrew Sulowski, covering forces encountered in fall arrest systems, based on guidance provided to Ontario Hydro and published in *National Safety News*, was used as the basis for the force calculations that are illustrated in this Appendix.[1,2]

Calculation of Maximum Arresting Force

Equations 2-1 and 2-2 below can be used to estimate the Maximum Arresting Force (MAF), denoted as F_N or F_P respectively. Anchorage points are deemed reasonably inextensible (refer to OSHA 1910.66 Appendix C; CSA Z259; ANSI Z359.1, and European (EN) standards).

Equation 2-1 can only be applied using metric units. The falling mass, M, must be shown in kilograms; the rope modulus, K_N, must be in newtons/square millimeters; and the lanyard/lifeline length and the free fall distance in meters. The result provides an estimated MAF in newtons.

Please refer to Figures A2.4 and A2.5 for additional rope modulus factors and considerations.

Equation 2-1:
MAF in newtons = F_N (metric)

$$F_N = (W_{kg} \cdot g + 4.5 \sqrt{W_{kg} \cdot f \cdot K_N}) \cdot \frac{a \cdot b \cdot s}{c}$$

Where:
a = fall arrest device reduction factor, (Table 1 in Figure A2.1)
b = body support reduction factor, (Table 2 in Figure A2.2)
c = rigid weight/manikin factor, (Figure A2.5)
f = fall factor (h/L), ratio
g = gravitational acceleration, 9.8 m/s²
F_N = maximum arresting force, N (newtons)
h = free fall distance, m

K_N = lanyard tension modulus, N/mm² (Figure A2.4)
L = lanyard/lifeline length, m
s = shock absorber reduction factor, (Table 3 in Figure A2.3)
W^{kg} = mass, kg

Note: Modulus E (N/mm²) = K_N

k, the spring constant, = A•E (area x modulus)

and

$$c = \frac{A \cdot E}{L} = \frac{k}{L}$$

Equation 2-2, below, allows the user to apply English units, which are converted from the metric by factors already included in the equation. The fall factor f is a ratio (L/h) and no correction factor is needed.

Equation 2-2:
MAF in pounds = F_P (English)

$$F_P = (0.031 W_P \cdot g + 1.012 \sqrt{0.003125 \ W_P \cdot f \cdot K_P}) \cdot \frac{a \cdot b \cdot s}{c}$$

Where:
a = fall arrest device reduction factor, (Table 1 in Figure A2.1)
b = body support reduction factor, (Table 2 in Figure A2.2)
c = rigid weight/manikin factor, (Figure A2.5)
f = fall factor (h/L), ft
g = gravitational acceleration, 32.2 ft/sec²
F_N = maximum arresting force, lbf
h = free fall distance, ft
K_P = lanyard/rope tension modulus, psi (Figure A2.4)
L = lanyard/lifeline length, ft
s = shock absorber reduction factor, (Table 3 in Figure A2.3)
W_P = weight of mass, lbs

Note: Modulus E (psi) = K_P

Table 1

Fall Arrester Device Reduction Factor: a

Wire and aramid line	0.7
Nylon and polyester	0.9
Friction	0.7
Mechanical lever	1.0
No fall arrester	1.0

FIGURE A2.1

APPENDIX A-2 **189**

Table 2

Body Support Reduction Factor: b	
Body belt (1.5" and 2")	0.9
Body harness	0.8

FIGURE A2.2

Table 3

Shock Absorber Reduction Factor: s	
Tear stitches	0.6
Tear fabric (synthetic)	0.6
Tear fabric (wire rope)	0.7
No shock absorber	1.0

FIGURE A2.3

Examples

The following sample fall arrest problems and their resulting calculations are the author's interpretation of Andrew Sulowski's work, with the addition of conversion factors in Equation 2-2, which allow the user to work in English units to obtain a solution in pounds force (lbf).

Example 1a

A 220-lb. welder was exposed to an elevated fall hazard. He had been issued a 6-ft., 5/16-in. diameter (6 x 21) wire rope lanyard with a fiber core, and a 1 3/4-in. body belt with a single back D-ring. When the welder slipped and free fell 6 ft., the wire rope lanyard arrested his fall. What was the maximum arrest force (MAF) experienced by the welder?

Applying Equation 2-2:

$$F_P = (0.031 W_P \cdot g + 1.012 \sqrt{0.003125\ W_P \cdot f \cdot K_P}) \cdot \frac{a \cdot b \cdot s}{c}$$

Where:

W_P = 220 lbs.
h = 6 ft.
L = 6 ft.
f = $\frac{h}{L} = \frac{6}{6} = 1$
K_P = 13,000,000 psi (USS Wire Rope Engineering Hand Book)
a = 1
b = 0.9
s = 1
c = 1.7
$\frac{a\ b\ s}{c}$ = $\frac{1 \cdot 0.9 \cdot 1}{1.7}$ = 0.5294

$F_P = (0.031 \cdot 220 \cdot 32.2 +$
$\quad 1.012 \sqrt{0.003125 \cdot 220 \cdot 1 \cdot 13,000,000}) \cdot 0.5294$
$\quad = 1718$ lbf

The value of 1,718 lbs. far exceeds the 900 lbs. limit required by OSHA (1910.66 Appendix C). Thus the welder should be minimally equipped with a shock absorber component to add to the wire rope lanyard. Values of a = 0.7 and s = 0.7 will bring the system into compliance technically. A harness also should be required.

Example 1b

Now that same welder is freshly provided with a 5/8-in. (16mm) diameter nylon rope lanyard (sheathed in leather for slag burn protection), as well as a shock absorber component. He is wearing a harness. He is subjected to a 6-ft. (1.8m) free fall on his 6-ft. (1.8m) lanyard. What is the maximum arrest force (MAF) seen by this system, in both pounds force and in newtons?

Applying Equation 2-1:

W_p = 100 kgs
h = 1.8 m
L = 1.8 m
f = 1
K_n = (32,000N/mm 2) (Figure 1)
a = 0.7
b = 0.8
s = 0.6
c = 1.3
$\frac{a\ b\ s}{c}$ = $\frac{0.7 \cdot 0.8 \cdot 0.9}{1.3}$ = 0.2585

$F_N = (9.8 \cdot 100 + 4.5 \sqrt{100 \cdot 1 \cdot 32,000}) \cdot 0.2585$
$\quad = 2334$ Newtons

The welder is far better protected from impact injury with this new equipment.

Applying Equation 2-2:

W_P = 220 lbs.
h = 6 ft.
L = 6 ft.
f = 1
K_P = 4,464,415 psi
a = 0.7
b = 0.8
s = 0.6
c = 1.3
$\frac{a\ b\ s}{c}$ = $\frac{1.7 \cdot 0.8 \cdot 0.6}{1.3}$ = 0.2585

$F_P = (0.031 \cdot 220 \cdot 32.2 +$
$\quad 1.012 \sqrt{0.003125 \cdot 220 \cdot 1 \cdot 4,464,415}) \cdot 0.2585$
$\quad = 515$ lbf

Example 2

A construction worker exposed to a 120-ft. elevated fall hazard is issued a body belt connected to an 11-ft.-long, 5/8-in. diamter, 3-strand nylon lanyard. (See Figure A2.4.) The worker is instructed to connect the snaphook of the lanyard to an eye bolt installed on the structural steel 9 ft. above the work surface. The extra-long lanyard is needed to provide mobility. The worker weighs 220 lbs., including his tools. His body belt D-ring is 4 1/2 ft. above the work surface. Calculate the MAF – F_P – in pounds force that this worker would experience if a fall occurs.

Example 3

A fall arrest system consisting of a 1/2-in.-diameter, 3-strand, nylon vertical lifeline is rigidly anchored 5 ft. above a fall arrester rope grab, which is closely connected to the lifeline (using the same type of rope as the lifeline) to the D-ring on a 2-in.-wide belt worn by a worker weighing 220 lbs., including his tools. Assuming the free fall distance will be approximately 3.5 ft., what is the MAF this worker will experience if a fall occurs?

But First, Some Additional Considerations, by Factor

Before solving Examples 2 and 3 above, refer to Figures A2.4 and A2.5, and for Example 2 in particular, refer to A2.6. Also note the following additional considerations.

h = free fall distance. This usually is twice the U-shaped slack of a lanyard. However, for clearance calculation, be sure to add approximately 3.5 ft. for a belt and 5 ft. for a harness in order to ensure clearance for the worker's limbs hanging below the D-ring.

L = active length of the lanyard or combined lifeline/lanyard length. The longer this line, the longer the stretch that has to be included when calculating clearances.

a = fall arrester device reduction factor. In general, the reduction of the maximum arresting force (MAF) by a fall arrest device (FAD) is the result of several phenomena, out of which dissipation of the fall energy due to friction between the FAD and the vertical lifeline is a primary contributor. The reduction factor, a, is defined as the ratio of the MAF in a fall arrest system (FAS) with the FAD, to the MAF in a FAS without a FAD, under the same fall conditions, with all other elements of the FAS being the same. An

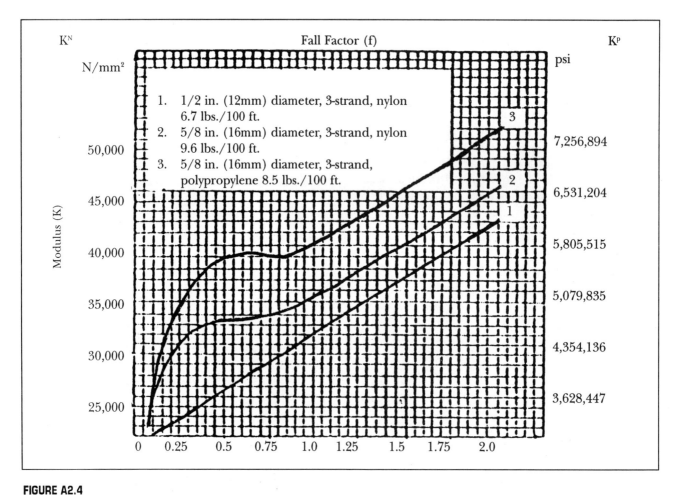

FIGURE A2.4
Rope Modulus, K, versus Fall Factor, f
Note: Modulus for 5/16-in.-diameter wire rope cable (6 x 21) is 13 million psi.

APPENDIX A-2

inertial wire rope grab can have a reduction factor of 0.7, and a synthetic rope grab can have a value as high as 0.9 if there is no slip. When no fall arrest device is included in the system, use a factor of 1. These factors have been experimentally determined for each device. When the exact value of a is not known, then the highest one for the particular type of FAS should be employed.

b = body support reduction factor. This is based on laboratory drop tests, and can have the following values: body belt 0.9, body harness 0.8.

c = rigid weight (solid test weight) to human weight reduction factor. This is based on experimental results and has a value of 1 when a harness is used. When body belts are used, the value approaches 1 when the fall distance is closet to, or

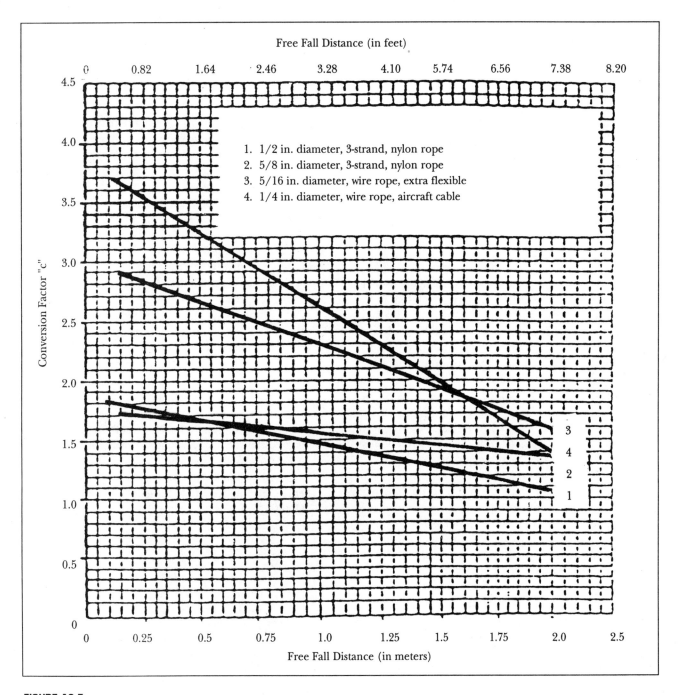

FIGURE A2.5
Rigid weight/manikin conversion factor 'c'. Illustration for use with Example 3.
Note: Most body belts are worn at a 38 to 42 in. height.

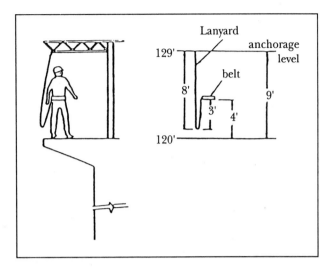

FIGURE A2.6
Illustration for Example 2.
Note: Most body belts are worn at a 38 to 42 in. height.

W_P = 220 lbs.
h = 3.5 ft.
L = 8.5 ft.
f = 0.41
K_P = 3,628,447 psi
a = 0.9
b = 0.9
s = 1
c = 1.5

$F_P = (0.031 \cdot 220 \cdot 32.2 + 1.012 \sqrt{0.003125 \cdot 0.41 \cdot 220 \cdot 3{,}628{,}447}) \cdot \frac{0.9 \cdot 0.9 \cdot 1}{1.5}$
= 671 lbf

exceeds, 6 ft. For shorter falls, the factor for body belts at 3 ft. is 1.5 when used with nylon lanyards. And when wire rope lanyards are employed, a factor of 3 is recommended. It should be noted that OSHA has adopted a 1.4 safety factor in its 1910.66 Appendix C.

s = shock absorber reduction factor. This is used to provide additional shock absorption to that in the lanyard. Most independent shock absorbers reduce the fall-arresting force on the body to a range of between 600 to 800 lbs. force. Within the overall strength of the shock absorber, the values generally range from 0.4 to 0.7. When very long falls are anticipated, the capacity of the absorber must be checked.

K = rope modulus (stretch). In this text, the term "modulus" is used to indicate the stretch measured when rope is subjected to various loads. There is little correlation between "modulus for stretch" and the term "tension modulus" normally used for engineering calculations, unless the area of the stress member, angle of twist of the rope, and length of the lanyard/vertical lifeline are included in the calculation, and yield strengths are not exceeded.

Apply Equation 2-2 to Examples 2 and 3 (top of second column). When used to estimate the arresting force for a specific application using this method for lanyard and robe grap systems attached to a firm anchor, Sulowski's work has indicated that these calculations should provide MAF estimates that are accurate to within +/- 5%.

Summary

In summary, the person doing the calculations and making the recommendations should keep the maximum arresting force as low as possible, and certainly below the limit of 8 kN (1,800 lbf) currently included in the OSHA regulations for full body harnesses, or 4 kN (900 lbf) when using body belts.

Most vertical arrest force problems can be minimized by the use of shock-absorbing mechanisms in the system and by using the manufacturer's MAF specifications while ensuring the capacity of the shock-absorbing lanyard is within limits by properly limiting the length of the free fall.

The author has proposed and designated the term "dynamic rating" to signify maximum arrest force meeting OSHA regulations for labeling purposes.

Notes

1. Sulowski, Andrew C. "In Fall Arresting Systems...Assessment of Maximum Arrest Force". *National Safety News* (April 1981): 50-53.
2. Sulowski, Andrew C. "Formula for Maximum Arrest Force in Fall Arresting Systems." Report 80-191 for Ontario Hydro.

References

1. David Ferguson, Ferguson Consulting Company, Wilmington DE, reviewed this Appendix in its 1988 draft, and corresponded in January 1993 with Andrew Sulowski concerning the metric and English presentations and interpretations from Sulowski's "Fall Protection Principles" publication.

APPENDIX A-3:
Calculation of Horizontal Lifelines Forces

Introduction

The proper engineering of horizontal lifelines is a critical necessity for protection against fall hazards while moving. Many perimeter cables can be used as horizontal lifelines if they meet certain fall arrest criteria. Appendix 2 can be used to estimate forces in vertical fall arrest systems unless a shock absorber force limit approach is employed in the system, in which case that force limit can be used. If no criteria are available, the force limit or maximum allowed dynamic force by jurisdiction having authority should be used (e.g. OSHA 1910.66 Appendix C, 1,800 lb. for harnesses). Also, for an engineered fall protection system, OSHA would allow the static strength of an anchorage point to exceed the peak anticipated dynamic load by a factor minimally of 2:1. This applies to vertical and horizontal systems.

Nomenclature

(See also Figure A3.1 and Figure A3.2)

A	=	Net cross sectional area of cable.
DLF	=	Dynamic Load Factor.
E	=	Modulus of elasticity in tension.
f_1	=	Vertical deflection (sag) of cable under own weight only.
f_2	=	Vertical deflection of cable under both own weight and concentrated center load.
f_3	=	Dynamic deflection (sag) of cable.
f_4	=	Final sag when all weights are at static equilibrium (1,2 and 3 weights 220 lb. each suspended).
F	=	Weight of individual concentrated load at center span.
L_1	=	Length of cable when supporting its own weight.
L_2	=	Length of cable when supporting its own weight and concentrated center load.
S	=	Horizontal distance between supports.
s	=	Chord length of sub-span between center load and support (Equation A3.7).
t_1	=	Horizontal component of cable tension and tension at mid-span when supporting own weight only.
t_2	=	Cable tension at mid-span after center load is applied.
T_1	=	Cable tension at either anchorage when supporting cable weight only.

T_2	=	Cable tension at either anchorage after center load is applied.
T_3	=	Dynamic tension at either anchorage (Maximum Arrest Force (MAF)).
T_4	=	Final end-force at either end when all weights have come to rest and static equilibrium is achieved (three weights of 220 lb. each).
w	=	Weight of cable per unit length.
β	=	Angle between the horizontal and the tangent to the cable curve at the terminus.
γ	=	Parameter defined by Equation A3.11.
θ	=	Angle between the horizontal and the chord at half-span with center loading.
σ	=	Tensile stress in cable at terminus.

Analysis

The problem addressed in the following analysis is that of determining the deflection of a horizontal lifeline while arresting the fall of a person connected to the cable by a lanyard. In many applications, the maximum arresting force will be well defined, since the lanyard itself will contain a "shock absorber" that limits the force applied to the lifeline cable to that required to activate the shock absorber. It will be assumed in this appendix that force, F, is prescribed in this way.

The analysis presented here is based on equations for sag and cable tension in horizontal cables with self-weight loading, and with both self-weight loading and concentrated loading, which are found in the *USS Wire Rope Engineering Handbook*[1], but may otherwise be derived on the basis of conventional cable theory, such as presented by Finner[2] and Hibbeler[3]. It differs substantially from that of the previous edition of this book in that it treats more fully the deflection caused by both the loading of cable weight and arrested load, combined with the effects of stretching of the cable itself under load. A method of including the effect of cable inertial forces and total deflection is also presented.

The analysis is carried out by first determining the initial cable length when the cable loading is only its own weight. For this calculation, one must know either the initial sag at the center, or the cable tension at the attachment point. The sag after the arrested load is applied is next determined by combining two equations: one relating the final length to the final tension, and the other relating the change in cable length to the change in tension as the concentrated load is applied.

The center deflection or sag (f_1), the center tension (t_1), the terminus tension (T_1), and the cable length (L_1) under the initial, self-weight, loading are related by :

A3.1
$$f_1 = \frac{wS^2}{8t_1} \ or \ t_1 = \frac{wS^2}{8f_1}$$

A3.2
$$t_1 = \left[T_1^2 - (\frac{wS}{2})2 \right]^{1/2}$$

A3.3
$$L_1 = S \left[1 + \frac{w^2S^2}{24t_1^2} \right] \ or \ L_1 = S \left[1 + \frac{8f_1^2}{3S^2} \right]$$

It is seen that if either the initial sag or the support tension is measured, then the initial length of the cable can be calculated using either version of Equation A3.3.

The equations which relate cable tension, sag, and length after the application of a center load, in addition to the cable self-weight are as follows:

A3.4
$$f_2 = \frac{S(2f+wS)}{8t_2}$$

A3.5
$$L_1 = 2 \left[s + \frac{w^2(s/2)^3}{24t_2^2} \cos^3\theta \right], \ where$$

A3.6
$$\tan\theta = \frac{f^2}{S/2}, \ and$$

A3.7
$$s^2 = S^2/_4 \left[1 + \frac{(2F+wS)^2}{16t_2^2} \right]$$

Each of the above sets of equations expresses the deflected shape which the cable must assume in order that the conditions of static equilibrium be satisfied. They do not contain conditions reflecting changes in cable length resulting from cable stretching due to extensional flexibility.

The link between the two sets of equations expressing equilibrium, prior to and after the addition of the arrested load, F, is provided by an equation that relates the lengths of cable before and after the center load is applied.

If the cable is very stiff extensionally, then stretching can be neglected and:

A3.8
$$L_2 = L_1$$

For cables that may stretch appreciably, the following load-extension relationship is employed:

A3.9
$$L_2 - L_1 = (t_2 - t_1) - L_1/_{EA}$$

The above equation (A3.9) assumes that the cable tension is constant along its length, an assumption which is satisfactory for cables with small sag.

Equations A3-5 and A3-6 may be combined to phrase L2 in terms of t2 in the following manner:

A3.10
$$L_2 = S\gamma \left[1 + \frac{w^2(s/2)^2}{3\gamma^4 t_2^2} \right], \ where$$

A3.11
$$\gamma = \left[1 + \frac{(2F+wS)^2}{24t_2^2} \right]^{1/2}$$

To find the sag after the center loading is applied, Equation A3.10 is combined with Equation A3.8 or A3.9. The value of t2 which satisfies the resulting equation is determined. L2 is then found from Equations A3.8 or A3.9, and f2 from Equation A3.4. It is recommended that the equation for t2 be solved using a programmable calculator or a computer, as it is highly transcendental.

Finally, the final cable tension and the cable stress at the support are given by:

A3.12
$$T_2^2 = t_2^2 + \left(\frac{F+wS}{2} \right)^2$$

A3.13
$$\sigma = T_2/_A$$

Cables with Shock Absorbers

When the horizontal cable contains a "shock absorber" device, which opens when the cable tension reaches a predetermined value, then the above procedure must be modified. In the method employed here, no attempt is made to model the complete dynamic interactions among the falling worker, the lanyard shock absorber, and the cable shock absorber. The initial cable length and tension are calculated as described above. The shock absorber extension during loading is then added to this result and this new length, used as L_1 in Equations A3.8 or A3.9 for the calculation of t2.

Dynamic Effects

All of the above analysis is "quasi-static", in that inertial forces arising from accelerations of the cable mass are neglected. These inertia loads, however, can have a substantial effect on the total cable deflection. The maximum displacement of a cable under a suddenly applied load can be up to twice what it would be if the load were applied very slowly.

This phenomenon can perhaps best be explained by considering a simple dynamic system consisting of a single mass supported by an elastic element, or spring, of stiffness k. If a load, F, is applied very slowly, the

APPENDIX A-3

spring stretches by an amount F/k. If the same load is applied suddenly, the mass is first accelerated and then carried beyond its static equilibrium displacement by virtue of its acquired inertia, before being brought to rest by the stretched spring. If the force remains applied for up to one-half of the period of free vibration of the spring-mass system, the maximum displacement of the mass is twice the static displacement.

The stretched wire has both stiffness and mass, and therefore behaves dynamically analogously to the simple spring-mass system discussed above. Although the cable has an infinity of natural frequencies, it can be shown that as the duration of loading approaches one-half the period of largest natural period of free vibration, dynamic cable displacement becomes twice that predicted for static loading. Periods of natural vibration of cable ranging in length from 20 to 150 ft. are of the order of the duration of the loading pulse exerted by the lanyard arresting the fall of a worker. For this reason, it is recommended that the cable sag calculated for static loading, which is the difference between f_2 and f_1, be multiplied by a factor, called the dynamic load factor (DLF), in order to account for the above described dynamic effects. The following table, Figure A3.12, gives the recommended DLF for both 1/2-in. steel cables of length ranging from 25 to 150 ft. The DLF increases with decreasing cable length because the longer cables have longer fundamental periods of free vibration, and therefore a smaller ration of pulse duration to natural period. Although the DLF is greater for shorter cables, these have the least static deflection.

Cable length (ft.)	Dynamic Load Factor (DLF)
50 and less	2.0
75	1.80
100	1.60
125	1.40
150	1.20

FIGURE A3.12

The DLF for both RTC 5/8-in. Permacable®[1] cable and 5/8-in. twisted strand polyester rope of any length up to 150 ft. is 2.0. These cables have smaller periods of free vibration because of their lower mass density.

Sample Problem

Consider a 1/2-in. steel cable which, as noted in the *USS Wire Rope Engineering Handbook*[2], has a cross sectional area of 0.101 in². The span is 150 ft. and the initial sag is 1.0 ft. The cable has the following properties and loading, shown in Figure A3.13:

$w = 0.42$ lb./ft., $E = 12\times10^6$ psi., $F = 650$ lb.

From Equation A3.1	$t_1 = 1181.25$ lb.
From Equation A3.2	$T_1 = 1181.67$
From Equation A3.3b	$L_1 = 150.0178$ ft.

Next solve for t_2.

From Equation A3.11 $\quad \gamma\left[1+\dfrac{77.407\times10^3}{t_2^2}\right]^{1/2}$

From Equation A3.10 $\quad L_2 = 150\gamma\left[1+\dfrac{330.75}{\gamma^4 t_2^2}\right]$

Equations A3.9 & A3.10 are solved simultaneously for L_2 and t_2 yielding: $\quad L_2 = 150.365$, and $t_2 = 4000$ lb.

From Equation A3.4	$f_2 = 6.39$ ft.
From Equation A3.12	$T_2 = 4016$ lb.

FIGURE A3.13

Since the DLF is 1.2 for a 150-ft. cable, the total dynamic sag is $(6.39 - 1.0) \times 1.2 + 1.0 = 7.46$ ft. The tensile strength of a 1/2-in. steel cable is 22,800 lbs., and the factor of safety is 5.7 based on T_2.

The anchorage cable tension, T_3, corresponding to the total dynamic sag, f_3, may be calculated by using Equations A3.4 and A3.12 by replacing f_2, t_2, and T_2 by f_3, t_3, and T_3 respectively. For the present example, this results in a dynamic anchorage tension of 3,444 lbs. force. Since this is substantially less than the final resting tension, T_2, it is recommended that T_2 be used for cable strength safety factor calculations. Of course, appropriate strength reduction factors should be applied to account for locally high attachment point stresses.

Sample Results

A computer program has been written to carry out the preceding calculations. Results obtained by using this program are presented graphically in a special section at the end of this Appendix. These graphs – Figures A3.1 - A3.11 – illustrate the relationships among the various parameters appearing in the analysis.

All of the results are for a 1/2-in. steel cable with a tensile modulus of 12×10^6 psi.

Figure A3.3 illustrates the relationship between initial tension and initial sag as given by Equations A3.1 and A3.2. Figures A3.4 and A3.5 show how the static sag, f_2 and the dynamic sag, f_3 vary with initial cable tension, T_1 for cables of various lengths with a center load of F equal to 650 lbs.

Figure A3.6 illustrates the dependence of the static anchorage cable tension on initial tension for the same center load. It is especially noted that, for smaller cable lengths, increasing the initial tension beyond 500 lbs. has only slight effect on the sag, while the final tension is increased significantly by further increase of T_1.

Figure A3.7, which shows how f_2 varies with T_2, results from combining Equations A3.4 and A3.12. The same graph may be used to represent the relationship between f_4 and T_4 for three 220-lb. weights at rest at the center of the cable.

Figures A3.8 through A3.11 show the effect of cable shock absorber opening length (δL) on the static and dynamic sag and cable tension. In each of these figures, the sag or tension is plotted against the opened length of the shock absorber. Figures A3.8 and A3.9 illustrate how the static and dynamic sag increase with shock absorber opening, while Figures A3.10 and A3.11 show the corresponding decreases in cable tension.

Summary

Wire cable diameters of 5/16 in. may be reasonable for some spans in general industry, but should be minimally 3/8 in. for construction because of the greater chance of damage from collisions and misuse. For example, 1/2-in. (diameter) perimeter cables may be used as horizontal lifelines after having been engineered and sketched on engineering drawing showing the usage in detail, along with written description of the installation, methods and limitations of use.

Supports for perimeter cables should not be washers because of the inability to control the flux temperature and because of production of a brittle joint subject to sudden failure when leaned against or stood on for access (a foreseeable misuse). In addition, threading wire cables through washers or other eyebolts will not allow continuous movement past such supports. Rope perimeter lines should not be permitted due to flexibility sufficient to permit a person to fall through or over such lines. However, when designed as a horizontal lifeline restraint, such lines may be entirely permissible within 6 to 10 ft. of an exposed edge.

Based on testing, engineered horizontal lifelines are capable of absorbing the force of several workers falling, and up to three workers have been tested with both weights and personnel with little effect on maximum arrest force at cable termination (T_3). A 20% increase in force per worker (up to three workers) is believed satisfactory. It should be noted that configurations of use of horizontal lifelines must be designed so that the fall of one worker does not reasonably cause another worker to fall from his or her work position. Horizontal lifelines must not be used by workers to support their balance or weight at any time. Horizontal lifelines are for emergency fall arrest use only. Also to be noted: Use a second suspension system for supporting the weight of the scaffold, tools, etc.

Notes

1. Permacable® is a registered trademark of Research & Trading Corp., Wilmington, DE.
2. *USS Tiger Brand Wire Rope Engineering Handbook.*
3. Finner, R.T. Mechanics of Solids. Blackwell Scientific Publications, Boston. 1989.
4. Hibbeler, R.C. Engineering Mechanics: Statics. Macmillian Co., New York. 1992.
5. This work has been contracted to Dr. Herbert Kingsberry, Professor of Mechanical Engineering, University of Delaware, Newark, DE.
6. Additional data are available upon request from the author, including metric equivalence not available at the time of printing, and other examples for different materials, different diameters and different constructions shown graphically.

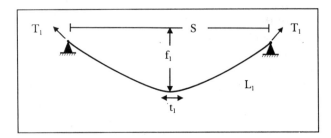

FIGURE A3.1
Self Weight Sag and Tension

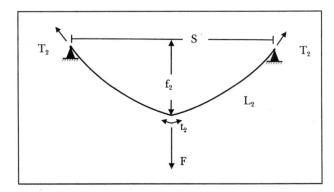

FIGURE A3.2
Center Load, Self Weight Sag and Tension

APPENDIX A-3 **197**

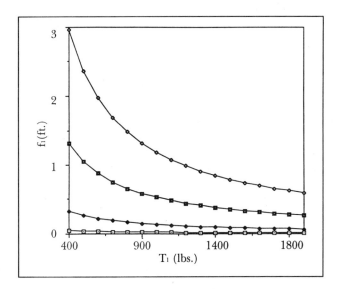

FIGURE A3.3A & B
Initial Sag vs Initial Tension
1/2-Inch Steel Cable, F = 650 Lbs.

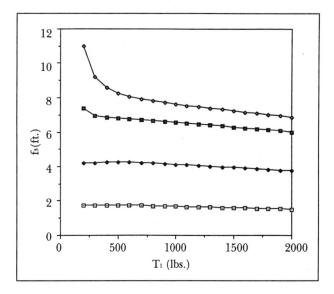

FIGURE A3.5
Final Dynamic Sag vs Initial Tension
1/2-Inch Steel Cable, F = 650 Lbs.

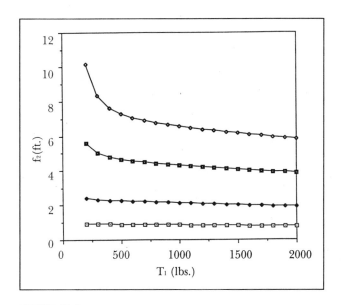

FIGURE A3.4
Final Sag vs Initial Tension
1/2-Inch Steel Cable, F = 650 Lbs.

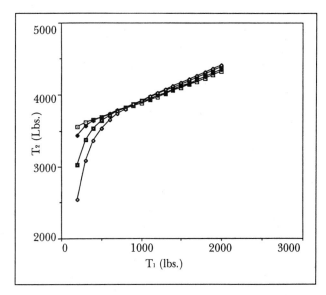

FIGURE A3.6
Final Tension vs Initial Tension
1/2-Inch Steel Cable, F = 650 Lbs.

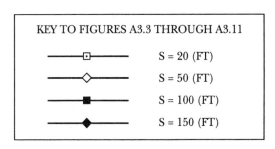

198   INTRODUCTION TO FALL PROTECTION, SECOND EDITION

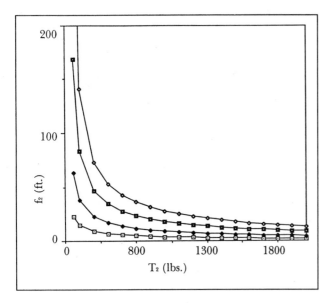

FIGURE A3.7
Final Sag vs Final Tension
1/2-Inch Steel Cable, F = 650 Lbs.

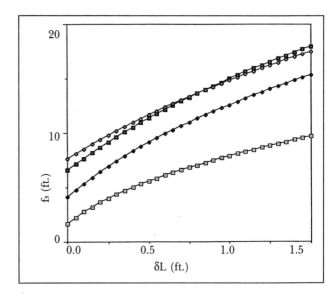

FIGURE A3.9
Final Dynamic Sag vs Length of Shock Absorber
1/2-Inch Steel Cable, T_1 = 1000 Lbs, F = 650 Lbs.

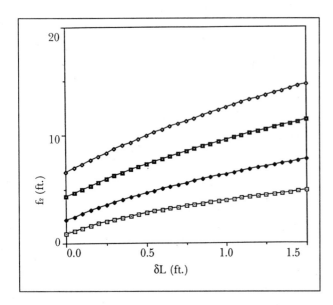

FIGURE A3.8
Final Sag vs Length of Shock Absorber
1/2-Inch Steel Cable, T_1 = 1000 Lbs, F = 650 Lbs.

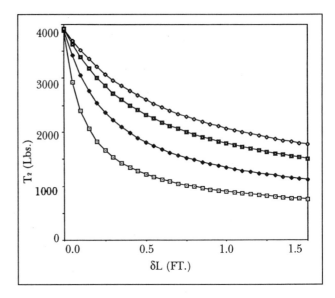

FIGURE A3.10
Final Tension vs Length of Shock Absorber
1/2-Inch Steel Cable, T_1 = 1000 Lbs, F = 650 Lbs.

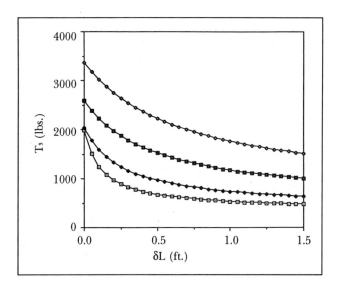

FIGURE A3.11
Final Dynamic Tension vs Length of Shock Absorber
1/2-Inch Steel Cable, T_1 = 1000 Lbs, F = 650 Lbs.

APPENDIX A-4:
Equipment Installation and Use Engineering Guide

The engineers who prepare the work site for use of fall arrest equipment have a responsibility to review their designs and work methods with the responsible safety manager. Approval for fall arrest equipment attachment means much more than being able to sustain a static leaning force of 200 lbs. specified for perimeter protection. It means the equipment must be capable of sustaining a free fall or maximum arresting force (MAF). This Appendix provides guidance needed to install and use these systems.

Section 1: Vertical Lifeline Criteria

(See Appendix A-2)
Note: All anchorage designs should be approved by a qualified engineer who is a specialist in this field (OSHA 1910.66 Appendix C).

a. Vertical anchorage points should have a 5,000-lb. minimum static strength per person, except for retracting lifelines, which should have a minimum static strength of 3,000 lbs. For engineered systems, the anchorage should support a minimum of twice the maximum arrest force anticipated by the fall arrest equipment (obtained from manufacturer's data or by testing). ANSI Z359.1 refers to 3,600 lbs. minimum for standard fall arrest systems.

b. Fall arrest maximum force measurements can be established using equipment manufacturer-supplied test data recorded with equipment that has an instrumentation sensitivity range of 0.1-125 Hz, and that is free from interfering anchorage test point resonance. Refer to ANSI Z359.1-1992.

c. Consider application of horizontal lifelines as discussed in Section 2 of this Appendix and in Appendix A-3. Perimeter catenary lines can only be used as horizontal lifelines when specifically designed for the purpose.

d. Anchorage point height should be shoulder height or higher when harnesses are used, but never less than waist height for all persons standing or working exposed to fall hazards within several feet because of wind gusts, slips, or collapse.

e. All buildings requiring window cleaning by scaffold or boatswain's chair equipment should have specific lifeline anchorage points that are engineered for each person and drop position. Consider roof pad-eyes welded into plates attached to the building structure and labeled as to purpose.

Similar planning is required for suspended scaffolding used for other applications, and during building construction.

f. Consider the length of the anticipated fall stopping distance produced by fall equipment. Also consider the consequence of swing falls from anchorage points not installed directly overhead.

g. Do not allow backup lifeline systems to substitute for adequate access to the workstation. If a lifeline system is used to support the worker's balance, it is no longer a backup system. Elevating platforms, scaffolds, or walkways must be considered.

Section 2: Horizontal Lifeline Criteria

(See Appendix A-3)
Note: All horizontal lifeline designs should be approved by a qualified engineer who is a specialist in this field (OSHA 1910.66 Appendix C).

Installation Height and Erection Tension Requirements

The following determines horizontal lifeline (HLL) installation height recommendations so that the line can be easily attached to the lanyard while not interfering with the movements of the user. It is recommended that the horizontal lifeline be installed at 7 ft. above the working surface, with erection sag limited to 1 ft. The erection tension on the HLL serves two purposes. First, it controls the sag when installed to erection tension. Secondly, as described in Appendix A-3, the erection tension is tied to the HLL tension and sag when a fall occurs; and the line is loaded with MAF. A method for setting HLL erection tension is provided in Section 4 of this appendix.

Note that when nylon fiber ropes are used for horizontal lifelines, they tend to stretch following installation and tensioning. Retensioning is recommended on these following every period of use. This problem is minimized when polyester and aramid fiber, wire or ropes are used. All HLL tensions should be checked every seven days.

The following formula, using the Friction Factors shown in Table 1 in Figure A4.1 can be used to establish torque values for tensioning a HLL:

$$T = \frac{t_e \bullet F \bullet d_e}{12}$$

Where:
T = Torque
t_e = Tension
F = Friction Factor; see Table 1, Figure A4.1
d_e = Nominal diameter of the eye bolt

Table 1 - Friction Factors

Plain Bolts (factory lube only)	0.20
Lightly Oiled	0.15
Plated Smooth Chrome	0.15
Galvanized (hot dip)	0.13
Graphite/mineral oil	0.10

FIGURE A4.1

The following example illustrates a typical application of this method:

A rigger is assigned to erect a HLL with an initial (erection) tension (t_e) of 2,000 lbs., using a 3/4-in. hot-dipped galvanized steel eye bolt.

Apply the equation

$$T = \frac{2000 \cdot 0.13 \cdot 0.75}{12}$$

to find that Torque = 16.25 foot lbs.

Following erection of the HLL, the worker would restrain the eye bolt from turning with a spud wrench. Using a common torque wrench, the worker would turn the nut to the calculated value (16.25 foot lbs.). This would set the 2,000-lb. initial tension on the HLL. In order to lock the nut in place, a second nut would be installed and jammed against the torqued nut to lock it in place.

System Forces With More Than One Worker

Assume, for the purpose of engineering calculation, that one or more workers are attached directly to a horizontal lifeline. There are two approaches to this situation.

a) *Static Treatment.* The HLL must support 5,000 lbs. per person applied perpendicularly to the line. This assumes that all persons dynamically compound the force in a few milliseconds' range of time, and that forces may approach 5,000 lbs. in a single-person fall. The standard addressed the problem in this manner. However, it may be impossible to use the criteria for some common or lightweight structures, such as wood frame building trusses, scaffolds, antennas and aircraft.

b) *Dynamic Treatment.* This approach considers the probability of more than one person falling and dynamically impacting a horizontal cable in the same few critical milliseconds range. See Figure A4.2. Since typical lanyard arrest forces peak in the five-millisecond duration range (for example, at 50% wave height), the chance that forces are going to be superimposed is extremely unlikely, so much so that for design purposes, it can be ignored for most applications up to four persons. But note that factors leading to the conclusion that the superimposition of dynamic forces is remote include these variances: location on the line, weight, center of gravity of the worker, harness or belt, and length of device or lanyard. Practical tests done with two or three workers falling "simultaneously" gave an accumulated maximum force at the terminations of 2,500 lbs., although the workers personally impacted vertically at approximately 600 lbs. each. For design purposes, because the accumulation of forces can give a slight increase, a factor of 0.2 per person, as a result of both theory and testing, should be added. There certainly is no basis for an accumulated factor of 1.0 per person. A conservative design approach need not exceed 0.5.

However, if, for example, 10 or 20 workers were to fall "simultaneously" in a span, then the probability of superimposition of forces increases, but still not to a factor of 1.0 per person. Even in these cases, use of lanyard shock absorbers makes the theoretical chance of superimposition such a small number that the danger of overloading safety cables is very low. The main concern is that the fall of one worker would cause the cascade-like fall of many others. The key, then, is to limit the force each worker can maximally exert on the system, and limit the number of workers between supports to two or three. Then, for several workers, a horizontal lifeline span originally designed for one worker can be considered.

Vertical fall test results of shock absorbing lanyards show that shock absorption typically occurs over 200 to 300 milliseconds. Yet the superimposition probability among the numerous peaks is still very low. For design

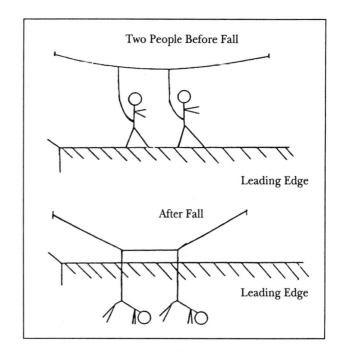

FIGURE A4.2
The dynamics of two falling workers.

purposes, the line usage should be limited to four workers within one span.

One caution here is that the termination of wire ropes by wire rope clips/clamps must be assembled correctly. Based on dynamic tests, this is known to be a critical necessity for successful use under dynamic stress to avoid failure. Ideally, longer mechanical grips and field swaging should be used for cable terminations when possible. Wire rope clip assemblies are not easily testable because of too many torque variables, which usually cannot be diagnosed.

Note that for terminating perimeter cables that only have to withstand a static load of 200 lbs. with minimal deflection, wire rope clips may be adequate. Therefore, when a perimeter cable is used as a horizontal lifeline, more reliable terminations should be used.

Another caution: the running of retracting lifelines on horizontal lifelines requires reasonably taut lines so that these devices can run freely overhead to maximize swing fall consequences, unlike for attachment of lanyards. A cable sag approximately 5 ft. from a termination of approximately 12 in. or less has been shown to give smooth running, which rules out catenary suspensions.

Yet another caution is that the material of the horizontal lifelines meet the circumstances of the work site. For steel erection, 1/2-in. steel is to be preferred over smaller cables or the more easily handled 5/8-in. synthetic ropes, in order to withstand foreseeable collisions without damage to suspended beams or other heavy objects. Yet, at other worksites without steel erection, synthetic lines are a major advantage regarding weight and speed.

Section 3: Lifeline Termination Requirements

Concerning terminations and anchorage points, it's important to look at the nominal break strength and other values for cable and ropes as follows.

Wire cable terminations can be made to equal or exceed the nominal cable break strengths, and synthetic ropes terminated by splices eyes can develop close to 100% the break strength of the rope.

However, just because a 1/2-in. steel cable may be used does not necessarily mean that the anchorage points should withstand 18,000 lbs. for a horizontal lifeline anchorage.

The British Standard for Lifeline Anchorages[1] requires approximately 5000 lbs. minimum axial strength for attachment of fall arrest devices. The installed eyebolt must be able to withstand a force of 2200 lbs. in the direction of fall, for vertical fall arresting systems meeting the BS5062 standard.

If we consider the maximum vertical maximum arrest (MAF) force of 900 lbs., it represents a retracting lifeline on a horizontal lifeline system. The test results indicate that properly terminated 5/16-in. cable can adequately handle these forces. Where horizontal systems are not subject to potentially damaging side impacts of loads, then smaller cables or ropes can be used. Either way, the calculated or tested dynamic loads, not casual impacts on the cable by suspended loads, should determine anchorage point strength.

Wire Cable and Synthetic Rope Lines in Shear

Values shown in Figure A4.3 represent recommended minimum strengths for system evaluation for cables 06 $T_{(Br)}$ and ropes (0.8_{Br}) estimated.

Line tensile strength (T_{Br}) is reduced by factors relating to line construction, size of cable, angle of line, tension T_1 in the line, and configuration of runner when maximum arrest force (MAF) is applied. Note that the runner can represent a connector, such as a pulley, hook or ring, used to attach a lanyard or fall arrest device. The key factor is the line construction: the more flexible the line, the more line shear strength (T_{shear}) approaches T_{Br}. Thus, 7 x 19 constructions are

Table 2 - Minimum Requirements for Anchorage Point Strength

Minimum requirements for anchorage point strength	Est. Dynamic Stretch	Description	Typical Break Strengths Wt./100 ft.	Tensile (T_{Br})	T_{shear}
	0.5%	5/8-in. steel cable (16mm)	715 lbs.	33,000 lbs.	19,800 lbs.
	0.5%	1/2-in. steel cable (12mm)	458 lbs.	18,000 lbs.	10,800 lbs.
5,000 lbs. min.;	1.0%	3/8-in. steel cable (10mm)	243 lbs.	10,300 lbs.	6,180 lbs.
refer to	1.0%	5/16-in. steel cable (8mm)	17 lbs.	7,500 lbs.	4,500 lbs.
Appendix A-3	5.0%	5/8-in. Permacable™ (16mm)[2]	22.5 lbs.	16,000 lbs.	12,800 lbs.
Minimum	10.0%	5/8-in. polyester rope (16mm)	12 lbs.	12,400 lbs.	9,920 lbs.

FIGURE A4.3

Note: In shear cables (T_{shear}) = $0.6T_{Br}$ est.; ropes $0.8\ T_r$ est.

APPENDIX A-4

preferable over 1 x 9 wire cable constructions, provided a pulley is used (pulley diameter = 24d for 7 x 19 and 40d for 1 x 9 where d = diameter of the wire cable). Individual systems should be tested in shear by the engineer designing the fall arrest system in order to determine the correct factor.

For more complete definitions of terms used in this Appendix, see Appendix A-3.

Notes

1. Permanent Anchors for Industrial Safety Belts and Harnesses, BS5845: 1980, British Standards Institute.

2. Permacable® is a registered trademark of Research & Trading Corp., Wilmington, DE.

References

1. Information appearing in this Appendix has been jointly developed by RTC (Research & Trading Corp.) and Invetek Inc.

APPENDIX A-5:
Outdated Fall Protection Methods

The natural fiber rope and leather belts once used for fall arrest strength members hopefully have seen their final days. They should all be gone from industry, all replaced with rot-resistant synthetics, for the benefit of workers.

Leather belts and straps are subject to drying out and cracking from lack of maintenance. They are simply too great a risk, unless composites or other materials can be used in combination with the leather to retain strength yet provide wearer comfort when requested.

The strength of manila was downgraded in the early 1970s by the Cordage Institute when 3/4-in. manila rope went from 5,400 lbs. break strength to approximately 4,800 lbs. because of the shorter-length fibers being used in the available ropes. Furthermore, manila will rot if left wet, and degradation due to light, oxygen and chemicals is much faster in manila than in most of the synthetic products currently on the market. However, please note: some polyethylenes and non-UV stabilized polypropylene ropes also may degrade rapidly in strong sunlight.

There is simply too much risk to both employer and employees to continue using leather and natural fiber rope strength members for fall arrest support.

Too much risk also is posed by using a rope cinched around a worker's waist in lieu of webbing strap belt and harness products. This is no way to address fall hazards on the job; the cinched rope may act as a noose. Ropes are too narrow for support, and may cut or restrict circulation following a fall. A 1 3/4-in. or 2-in. width of strap against the body for harnesses seems necessary to avoid rolling or twisting and yet help provide minimum support. For belts, a body pad of 3 in. to 6 in. helps spread the forces in a fall. By 1993, a reasonable proporation of American industry had changed to harnesses for fall arrest, again with approximately 1 3/4-in. webbing widths.

This Appendix on fall equipment materials should not be confused with applications of linemans' belts and straps used for positioning only, and where electric company training and maintenance programs are well developed and effective. Fall arrest systems are additional systems for backup safety.

Tie-Off Techniques — No Knots, Please!

Attaching two ropes to each other, or one rope back to itself around a post by the tying of knots, is a favorite past-time of boaters, mariners, and Boy Scouts down through the ages. Properly tied knots still may have a place in construction and industry when used for material handling or binding. But other more positive methods should be sought for almost all safety applications. There are two types of industrial-use knots, both of which present many potential knot problems.

Bend Knots

In industry, tree trimmers, fire fighters, and many construction trades have long tied knots in ropes in order to secure loads, to raise and lower tools, and for training. One type of knot used to secure is called a "bend", which is designed not to slip. Both ropes used in this knot bend to accomplish this frictional resistance; neither rope will slip.

A trend over recent years has been to replace lifeline rope termination knots with eye-splices, which can develop the full rated strength of a rope. Where the need for quickly-tied termination knots remains, the tracing figure 8 has been promoted by some fire training schools, such as Texas A&M, over the traditional bowline, because of greater residual strengths, and ease of tying and untying. Many bend knots designed around one diameter of rope can reduce rope strength by as much as 50%. However, the tracing or follow through figure 8 knot termination can maintain a much higher strength.

For these reasons, lifelines and lanyards for backup safety use never should be lengthened by tying knots to join two or more lengths together. The consequences will be unpredictable in a fall situation and the hazards increase, such as necessary temporary removal of the grab to by-pass the connection point. To the author's knowledge, this fact alone has caused at least one worker's death.

Wrapping lifelines around a roof-top structure – such as a pipe or air conditioner compressor and using it as a form of rigid block or bollard – continues to be a common anchorage practice. There is a need to move to a more advanced system of permanent well-identified roof eyebolts or eyepads, locking snaphooks, and eye-splice rope lifelines for minimum adequacy and reliability. Horizontal lifelines with shock absorbers are increasing in popularity for roof uses.

For example, tie-off by wrapping a lanyard or lifeline around an angle iron or girder is not a good practice, because unlike a smooth dockside bollard, structural steel has edges that may be sharp, and according to a Canadian Standards Association Hazard Alert, are getting sharp enough to cut a lanyard for an unwitting user in the event of a fall.

Hitch Knots

Another type of knot is called a "hitch", which is used primarily for two functions:

APPENDIX A-5 205

1. Hitching around an object. Fixing a rope around a sturdy object and back to itself by two half hitches (or other hitch) can be quick to tie, reliable to hold fast, and easy to untie. For a safety line, a knotting method of anchorage may be the only available method for a worker, unless slings or tiebacks are provided by the employer and building manager. But hitches, such as two or three half-hitches, can slide and tighten against the anchorage, which may thus expose the line to more sharp edges during dynamic stress, as compared to bend knots, which tighten and lock in place.

Tying both lifelines and lanyards to objects is not recommended for safety because the anchorage typically will be an untested ladder rung, railing or sharp angled steel. Tying lifelines and lanyards to objects may also denote non-continuity of protection, and lack of forethought, and may provide a false sense of security, whether they're intended for positioning, restraint or fall protection.

2. Hitching one rope to another. Here only one of the two ropes bends; one rope allows slippage. Hitches have been used for centuries for securing loads from slipping during hoisting. They can slide along another line easily by hand, but they lock tightly when the hitched line becomes loaded. Hitches have been used for safety by attaching slack rope lanyards to lifelines for fall protection when workers are moving vertically, such as on scaffolds. The merit is that no mechanical rope grab device is required, provided the user is skilled in tying the correct knot. Skilled users of the hitch, as expected, swear by the efficiency of the technique, but individual users can only speak for themselves and their own beliefs.

Arnör Larson, Rigging for Rescue, in British Columbia, Canada, has championed the triple hitch knot for mountaineering rescue work, and rightly so. When used with skill, using proper materials and techniques, this knot is very reliable. But the demerits of using hitches to provide reliable, personal fall protection are numerous in industry today. Factors include:

a. No reproducibility. A particular knot tied in the field and unsupervised cannot be certified "tested" to meet industry standards in a given jurisdiction.

b. Too many ways to tie the hitch knot! Combinations range from one turn over one turn (unreliable) to the minimum advised three over three (often referred to as the triple hitch), but the variables of using dog or bottom (hitch) line for loading, the reversal of the dog line, or the many degrees of knot tightness, produce dozens of methods for tying a similar locking knot, with no clear understanding by a supervisor or inspector of what is potentially safe and what is not adequately safe for fall protection.

c. Different diameters of lifeline with different widths or diameters of lanyard.

d. Different constructions of rope lifelines and lanyards (twists, braids, tubes, webs and wire cables).

e. Different hardnesses of lanyard rope lays.

f. Different directions of hitch with the lanyard rope twists parallel or perpendicular.

g. The effect of ice-stiffening of wet nylon lanyards, overnight for example.

h. The effect of weather degradation on each individual rope.

i. The effect of paint, oil or other worksite contaminants on frictional stiffness and other properties of lanyard.

j. Different materials for lanyard and lifeline.

Understandably, many older workers still prefer the concept of the hitch knot over the rope grab, but at best knot-tying is a personal skill that now has little or no proper place in today's company-wide fall protection programs.

Testing of Lanyard Hitch Knots

The Construction Safety Association of Ontario (CSAO) has done extensive dynamic testing (220 lbs./6 ft.) on hitch attachments of a lanyard (5/8-in. nylon) to a lifeline (5/8-in. polypropylene). Test results have shown good functioning under a wide range of conditions, with slippage to stop within 6 in., providing the hitch knot is tight enough to stay on the line without falling down, and that icy nylon lanyards are thawed before use. The triple hitch is the only sliding hitch recommended by CSAO when no mechanical rope grab is available.

The author's testing in this field has been on the static holding power of various hitch knots under increasing tension. A 5/8-in. polypropylene lifeline was used with a 9/16-in. spun nylon lanyard. Results showed that all knots need to be sufficiently tightened before gripping to the lifeline could occur. All knots with a single hitch slipped at 100 lbs. or less, regardless of how many dog loops and regardless of whether the hitch was at the top or bottom of the knot. Double hitch knots performed as well as triple hitch knots – whether single, double or triple dog loops were used and whether at the top or bottom of the knot–reaching 350 lbs. before slipping occurred. One conclusion that can be drawn is that the flexibility of the lanyard rope and the tightness of the knot are crucial to efficiency of either the double or triple hitch. Also, since most industrial lanyards are several feet long, not even the promise of subsequent descent after a fall by manipulating a reachable knot has much merit. While manually moving and holding the knot, a worker in

Ontario experienced a more-than-100 ft. fall because the lanyard could not become taut.

One of the strongest reasons not to rely on sliding hitch knots for personal back-up safety may be that the knot must be moved along the lifeline by hand and by design. If a fall occurs, the knot cannot tighten if it is gripped, and an uncontrolled fall will occur. This can be deadly because the first human reaction to falling is to grasp tightly onto the nearest object. This is a strong inherent reaction that is already exhibited in infancy and continues throughout life. Several times the author has heard of instances of this "death-grip" in workers' falls, occuring in much the same way that a drowning victim may inadvertently try to strangle his or her rescuer. Note that some mechanical rope grabs of the cam-friction kind have this same requirement to move the attachment manually, which can be dangerous because the exposure builds.

Put in the employer-employee context, the employer needs to be sure that the method of fall protection he or she provides is reliable for each and every worker. In the case of lanyard hitch knots, the employer can never truly know the degree of their reliability. One solution for the employer is to mandate the use of a practical commercial rope grab to meet the need for vertical movement, or for more advanced fall protection, mandate the use of retracting lifeline systems. The correct rope grab will either statically slip on the correct lifeline above 1,000 lbs. of tension, or otherwise hold the strength over 5,000 lbs., and will test similarly in a laboratory reproduction. Retractable lifelines have their own criteria, which can be tested reproducibly.

The question remains whether the correct triple hitch knot is better than nothing. The answer from this author is a conditional yes, provided the worker bears the total responsibility. If the worker cannot do so under the law, or is unwilling to do so, then a tested rope grab or other device must be used in a rope grab type system.

In summary, successful static or gradual loading of ropes by individual body weight should not be confused with the sudden stresses of a dynamic load while falling, especially when a human life is at stake and where sliding hitch knots could be a serious liability. Safety equipment should not rely on a worker's skill!

A falling worker, like the drowning victim, may clutch at straws.

There is just too little time to react in a fall.

Other Potential Knot Problems

Vertical lifelines, of 5/8 in. to 3/4 in. diameter, equipped with knots at periodic intervals, have been used as attachment points for lanyard snaphooks at different levels, particularly in elevator shaft work. The problem here is that for the worker to move, his or her lanyard must be unsnapped, exposing the worker to fall hazards for a brief time, which is continually repeated as part of the work method. This method also is an invitation for more than one worker to use the same lifeline without a clear idea of its capacity.

Lanyards have been shortened (deliberately or inadvertently) by means of knots to take up slack, perhaps to meet a maximum fall distance requirement. Overhand knots are not helpful in providing whatever shock absorption function a lanyard might have by design; this can lead to debate instead of problem solving when an accident occurs.

Sometimes workers may decide to knot, tape, or attach a clip to a retracting lifeline to provide a stop point for line retraction. A stop point may be reasonable in some applications.

But the use of knots anywhere in a fall protection system is a sign that the system's strength may have been severely compromised. These methods also can give rise, inadvertently, to very long falls, which may be catastrophic.

In other cases, workers decoratively pigtail their 6-ft. lanyards attached to safety belts to avoid a tripping hazard while the lanyard is not in active use. This practice probably inhibits such lanyards from being used in a fall hazard situation.

Short lifelines terminated with an overhead knot at the lower end (to hold a rope weight or to signal if a rope grab may run off) are problematic, because the overhand knot may capsize under stress. A figure 8 knot is better, but a lifeline which reaches the ground is the best policy. To adjust a lifeline's usage length, use a lifeline anchorage adapter.

Confined Space Rescue

The concept of one attendant standing by in case of emergency, ready to lift a victim out of a manhole or manway solely by using a rope, hopefully is retired! This is a dangerous practice: unless a specific technique has been practiced and a fall arrest device is used, it is entirely unfeasible and is probably impossible for training. Even using two or three persons to pull the rope is unfeasible, because the hand action reciprocation is so awkward as to be impractical. Furthermore, while heroic lifting of massive weights by an individual, often based on the rescuer's adrenalin level, is recorded from time to time in the press, such notions should be laid to rest with pre-planned training sessions that espouse the proper practical methods, which must be used under all foreseeable circumstances.

Winches with 4:1 minimum mechanical advantage are needed for retrieval, even from vertical openings as shallow as 3 ft. or 4 ft. A plan for completing the rescue within four minutes is crucial.

APPENDIX A-5 **207**

Air- or electric-powered winches with a slip clutch are needed for depths beyond 50 ft.

Anchorage Structures

Discussion of outdated fall protection methods using knots and ropes should address anchorage safety, as well.

Wooden members, including wood guardrails, may be sufficient on a temporary basis, but only if they have been certified by a registered professional engineer or tested in the field. Use of tree limbs — necessary for tree trimming — should follow the guidelines of ANSI Z133. Bamboo poles lashed together with narrow synthetic ties in 2 1/2-ft. to 3-ft. squares are still being used for scaffolding structures in some Far East countries, but these are used for perimeter access and for some perimeter protection. These should not be used as anchor material for reliable fall protection systems because of weather degradation and because they may be a non-standard structure at any given time in the future.

Ladder rungs or steps, guardrails or railings of any kind should not be used for fall arrest anchorages unless they are designed specifically for that purpose. Steel members should be used for anchorage point structures whenever possible. Masonry fittings can be suitable when used with through bolts and plate washers. Expanded anchor bolts should be specified by a register professional engineer. The British Standard BS5845: 1980, can assist engineers with specific guidelines.

The key point for anchorage safety is that anchorage members should not degrade over the lifetime of the overall structure to below the minimum strength required ($T_A \leq T_{AB}$) (See Appendix A-3).

No worker should be allowed to use any anchorage point that does not meet OSHA's safety requirements or has not been approved or modeled for anchorage use.

References

1. "Properties of Ropes of Dacron and DuPont Nylon," DuPont Technical Information Bulletin X-226. (February 1969): 4.

2. Ashley, Clifford W. The Ashley Book of Knots. Garden City NY: Doubleday & Co., Inc., 1944.

3. Hubacek, John (Texas A&M). "Figure 8 Knot Holds Up in Rescue." *Fire Engineering*, March 1983.

4. New England Ropes Splicing Guide. Form-SPG 686. New England Ropes, New Bedford, MA 02740.

5. Construction Safety Association of Ontario. "Special Investigation of the Triple Sliding Hitch." Test Report of April 27, 1983.

APPENDIX A-6:
OSHA Guidance on Fall Planning

The following text is a reproduction of OSHA 1910.66 Appendix C, from the Federal Register, Vol. 54, No. 144, Friday, July 28, 1989, Rules and Regulations.

III: Additional non-mandatory guidelines for personal fall arrest systems. The following information constitutes additional guidelines for use in complying with requirements for a personal fall arrest system.

(a) Selection and use considerations. The kind of personal fall arrest system selected should match the particular work situation, and any possible free fall distance should be kept to a minimum. Consideration should be given to the particular work environment. For example, the presence of acids, dirt, moisture, oil, grease, etc. and their effect on the system, should be evaluated. Hot or cold environments may also have an adverse affect on the system. Wire rope should not be used where an electrical hazard is anticipated. As required by the standard, the employer must plan to have means available to promptly rescue an employee should a fall occur, since the suspended employee may not be able to reach a work level independently.

Where lanyards, connectors, and lifelines are subject to damage by work operations such as welding, chemical cleaning, and sandblasting, the component should be protected, or other securing systems should be used. The employer should fully evaluate the work conditions and environment (including seasonal weather changes) before selecting the appropriate personal fall protection system. Once in use, the system's effectiveness should be monitored. In some cases, a program for cleaning and maintenance of the system may be necessary.

(b) Testing considerations. Before purchasing or putting into use a personal fall arrest system, an employer should obtain from the supplier information about the system based on its performance during testing so that the employer can know if the system meets this standard. Testing should be done using recognized test methods. Section II of this Appendix C contains test methods recognized for evaluating the performance of fall arrest systems. Not all systems may need to be individually tested; the performance of some systems may be based on data and calculations derived from testing of similar systems, provided that enough information is available to demonstrate similarity of function and design.

(c) Component compatibility considerations. Ideally, a personal fall arrest system is designed, tested, and supplied as a complete system. However, it is common practice for lanyards, connectors, lifelines, deceleration devices, body belts and body harnesses to be interchanged since some components wear out before others. The employer and employee should realize that not all components are interchangeable. For instance, a lanyard should not be connected between a body belt (or harness) and a deceleration device of the self-retracting type since this can result in additional free fall for which the system was not designed. Any substitution or change to a personal fall arrest system should be fully evaluated or tested by a competent person to determine that it meets the standard, before the modified system is put in use.

(d) Employee training considerations. Thorough employee training in the selection and use of personal fall arrest systems is imperative. As stated in the standard, before the equipment is used, employees must be trained in the safe use of the system. This should include the following: Application limits; proper anchoring and tie-off techniques; estimation of free fall distance, including determination of deceleration distance, and total fall distance to prevent striking a lower level; methods of use; and inspection and storage of the system. Careless or improper use of the equipment can result in serious injury or death. Employers and employees should become familiar with the material in this Appendix, as well as manufacturer's recommendations, before a system is used. Of uppermost importance is the reduction in strength caused by certain tie-offs (such as using knots, tying around sharp edges, etc.) and maximum permitted free fall distance. Also to be stressed are the importance of inspections prior to use, the limitations of the equipment, and unique conditions at the worksite which may be important in determining the type of system to use.

(e) Instruction considerations. Employers should obtain comprehensive instructions from the supplier as to the system's proper use and application, including, where applicable:

(1) The force measured during the sample force test;

(2) The maximum elongation measured for lanyards during the force test;

(3) The deceleration distance measured for deceleration devices during the force test;

(4) Caution statements on critical use limitations;

(5) Application limits;

(6) Proper hook-up, anchoring and tie-off techniques, including the proper dee-ring or other attachment point to use on the body belt and harness for fall arrest;

(7) Proper climbing techniques;

(8) Methods of inspection, use, cleaning, and storage, and

(9) Specific lifelines which may be used.

This information should be provided to employees during training.

(f) Inspection considerations. As stated in the standard (Section I, Paragraph (f)), personal fall arrest sys-

APPENDIX A-6

tems must be regularly inspected. Any component with any significant defect, such as cuts, tears, abrasions, mold, or undue stretching; alterations or additions which might affect its efficiency; damage due to deterioration; contact with fire, acids, or other corrosives; distorted hooks or faulty hook springs; tongues unfitted to the shoulder of buckles; loose or damaged mountings; non-functioning parts; or wearing or internal deterioration in the ropes must be withdrawn from service immediately, and should be tagged or marked as unusable, or destroyed.

(g) Rescue considerations. As required by the standard (Section I, Paragraph (e)(8)), when personal fall arrest systems are used, the employer must assure that employees can be promptly rescued or can rescue themselves should a fall occur. The availability of rescue personnel, ladders or other rescue equipment should be evaluated. In some situations, equipment which allows employees to rescue themselves after the fall has been arrested may be desirable, such as devices which have descent capability.

(h) Tie-off considerations. (1) One of the most important aspects of personal fall protection systems is fully planning the system before it is put into use. Probably the most overlooked component is planning for suitable anchorage points. Such planning should ideally be done before the structure or building is constructed so that anchorage points can be incorporated during construction for use later for window cleaning or other building maintenance. If properly planned, these anchorage points may be used during construction, as well as afterwards.

(2) Employers and employees should at all times be aware that the strength of a personal fall arrest system is based on its being attached to an anchoring system which does not significantly reduce the strength of the system (such as a properly dimensioned eye-bolt/snap-hook anchorage). Therefore, if a means of attachment is used that will reduce the strength of the system, that component should be replaced by a stronger one, but one that will also maintain the appropriate maximum arrest force characteristics.

(3) Tie-off using a knot in a rope lanyard or lifeline (at any location) can reduce the lifeline or lanyard strength by 50 percent or more. Therefore, a stronger lanyard or lifeline should be used to compensate for the weakening effect of the knot, or the lanyard should be reduced (or the tie-off location raised) to minimize free fall distance, or the lanyard or lifeline should be replaced by one which has an appropriately incorporated connector to eliminate the need for a knot.

(4) Tie-off of a rope lanyard or lifeline around an "H" or "I" beam or similar support can reduce its strength as much as 70 percent due to the cutting action of the beam edges. Therefore, use should be

made of webbing lanyard or wire core lifeline around the beam or the lanyard or lifeline should be protected from the edge; or free fall distance should be greatly minimized.

(5) Tie-off where the line passes over or around rough or sharp surfaces reduces strength drastically. Such a tie-off should be avoided or an alternative tie-off rigging should be used. Such alternatives may include use of a snap-hook/dee ring connection, wire rope tie-off, an effective padding of the surfaces, or an abrasion-resistance strap around or over the problem surface.

(6) Horizontal lifelines may, depending on their geometry and angle of sag, be subjected to greater loads than the impact load imposed by an attached component. When the angle of horizontal lifeline sag is less than 30 degrees, the impact force imparted to the lifeline by an attached lanyard is greatly amplified. For example, with a sag angle of 15 degrees, the force amplification is about 2:1 and at 5 degrees sag, it is about 6:1. Depending on the angle of sag, and the line's elasticity the strength of the horizontal lifeline and the anchorages to which it is attached should be increased a number of times over that of the lanyard. Extreme care should be taken in considering a horizontal lifeline for multiple tie-offs. The reason for this is that in multiple tie-offs to a horizontal lifeline, if one employee falls, the movement of the falling employee and the horizontal lifeline during arrest on the fall may cause other employees to also fall. Horizontal lifeline and anchorage strength should be increased for each additional employee to be tied-off. For these and other reasons, the design of systems using horizontal lifelines must only be done by qualified persons. Testing of installed lifelines and anchors prior to use is recommended.

(7) The strength of an eye-bolt is rated along the axis of the bolt and its strength is greatly reduced if the force is applied at an angle to this axis (in the direction of shear). Also, care should be exercised in selecting the proper diameter of the eye to avoid accidental disengagement of snap-hooks not designed to be compatible for the connection.

(8) Due to the significant reduction in the strength of the lifeline/lanyard (in some cases, as much as a 70 percent reduction), the sliding-hitch knot should not be used for lifeline/lanyard connections except in emergency situations where no other available system is practical. The "one-and-one" sliding hitch knot should never be used because it is unreliable in stopping a fall. The "two-and-two", or "three-and-three" knot (preferable), may be used in emergency situations; however, care should be taken to limit free fall distance to a minimum because of reduced lifeline/lanyard strength.

(i) Vertical lifeline considerations. As required by the standard, each employee must have separate lifeline when the lifeline is vertical. The reason for this is that in multiple tie-offs to a single lifeline, if one employee falls, the movement of the lifeline during the arrest of the fall may pull other employees' lanyards, causing them to fall as well.

(j) Snap-hook considerations. Although not required by this standard for all connections, locking snap-hooks designed for connection to suitable objects (of sufficient strength) are highly recommended in lieu of the non-locking type. Locking snap-hooks incorporate a positive locking mechanism in addition to the spring loaded keeper, which will not allow the keeper to open under moderate pressure without someone first releasing the mechanism. Such a feature, properly designed, effectively prevents roll-out from occurring.

As required by the standard (Section 1, paragraph (e)(1)) the following connections must be avoided (unless properly designed locking snap-hooks are used) because they are conditions which can result in roll-out when a nonlocking snap-hook is used:

- Direct connection of a snap-hook to a horizontal lifeline.
- Two (or more) snap-hooks connected to one dee-ring.
- Two snap-hooks connected to each other.
- A snap-hook connected back on its integral lanyard.
- A snap-hook connected to a webbing loop or webbing lanyard.
- Improper dimensions of the dee-ring, rebar, or other connection point in relation to the snap-hook dimensions which would allow the snap-hook keeper to be depressed by a turning motion of the snap-hook.

(k) Free fall considerations. The employer and employee should at all times be aware that a system's maximum arresting force is evaluated under normal use conditions established by the manufacturer, and in no case using a free fall distance in excess of six feet (1.8m). A few extra feet of free fall can significantly increase the arresting force on the employee, possibly to the point of causing injury. Because of this, the free fall distance should be kept at a minimum, and, as required by the standard, in no case greater than six feet (1.8m). To help assure this, the tie-off attachment point to the lifeline or anchor should be located at or above the connection point of the fall arrest equipment to belt or harness. Since otherwise additional free fall distance is added to the length of the connecting means (i.e. lanyard) attaching to the working surface will often result in a free fall greater than six feet (1.8m). For instance, if a six foot (1.8m) lanyard is used, the total free fall distance will be the distance

from the working level to the body belt (or harness) attachment point plus the six feet (1.8m) of lanyard length. Another important consideration is that the arresting force which the fall system must withstand also goes up with greater distances of free fall, possibly exceeding the strength of the system.

(l) Elongation and deceleration distance considerations. Other factors involved in a proper tie-off are elongation and deceleration distance. During the arresting of a fall a lanyard will experience a length of stretching or elongation, whereas activation of a deceleration device will result in a certain stopping distance. These distances should be available with the lanyard or device's instructions and must be added to the free fall distance to arrive at the total fall distance before an employee is fully stopped. The additional stopping distance may be very significant if the lanyard or deceleration device is attached near or at the end of a long lifeline, which may itself add considerable distance due to its own elongation. As required by the standard, sufficient distance to allow for all of these factors must also be maintained between the employee and obstructions below, to prevent an injury due to impact before the system fully arrests the fall. In addition, a minimum of 12 feet (3.7m) of lifeline should be allowed below the securing point of a rope grab type deceleration device, and the end terminated to prevent the device from sliding off the lifeline. Alternatively, the lifeline should extend to the ground or the next working level below. These measures are suggested to prevent the worker from inadvertently moving past the end of the lifeline and having the rope grab become disengaged from the lifeline.

(m) Obstruction considerations. The location of the tie-off should also consider the hazard of obstructions in the potential fall path of the employee. Tie-offs which minimize the possibilities of exaggerated swinging should be considered. In addition, when a body belt is used, the employee's body will go through a horizontal position to a jack-knifed position during the arrest of all falls. Thus, obstructions, which might interfere with this motion should be avoided or a severe injury could occur.

(n) Other considerations. Because of the design of some personal fall arrest systems, additional considerations may be required for proper tie-off. For example, heavy deceleration devices of the self-retracting type should be secured overhead in order to avoid the weight of the device having to be supported by the employee. Also, if self-retracting equipment is connected to a horizontal lifeline, the sag in the lifeline should be minimized to prevent the device from sliding down the lifeline to a position which creates a swing hazard during fall arrest. In all cases, manufacturer's instruction should be followed.

BIBLIOGRAPHY

Confined Space

Allison, W.W. "Confined Space Fatalities: Are Priorities for Preventive Actions Based on Facts or Emotions." *Professional Safety* (March 1986): 23-27.

_____. "Work in Confined Areas—Part 1: The Problem." *National Safety News* (February 1976): 45-50.

_____. "Work in Confined Areas—Part 2: Solutions to the Problems." *National Safety News* (April 1976): 61-67.

American National Standard Institute. *ANSI Z117-1-1989.* Published by American Society of Safety Engineers, Des Plaines, IL.

American Petroleum Institute. *Guide for Inspection of Refinery Equipment.* Washington, DC: API, 1978.

"Atmospheres in Sub-Surface Structures and Sewers." *National Safety News* (April 1979).

BioMarine Industries, Inc. *A Primer on Confined Area Entry.* Malvern, PA; BMI, 1975.

Campbell, Chris W. "All About Confined Spaces." *Professional Safety* (February 1990): 33-35.

Christy, Elizabeth. "Outfitted to Filter Out Respiratory Risk." *Occupational Health & Safety* (September 1993): 62-66.

Colanna, Guy R. "Confined Space Hazards Dictate Employee Training Improvements." *Occupational Health & Safety* (July 1987): 21-28.

Ellis, J. Nigel. "Plan Confined-Space Fall Protection Before and Beyond Required Rescue." *Occupational Health & Safety* (February 1992): 17-19.

Hans, Michael. "OSHA Closes In on New Confined Space Standard." *Safety & Health* (June 1991): 58-60.

Jorgensen, Ernest B. Jr. "Confined Space Entry." *Professional Safety* (February 1992): 22-26.

Krivan, S.P. "Confined Space Entry." *Professional Safety* (September 1981): 15-19.

_____. "Confined Space Entry—Can the Deaths and Injuries be Eliminated?" *Professional Safety* (September 1982): 15-19.

Loud, James J. "Hazards of Confined Spaces Required Clearly Defined Policies." *Occupational Health & Safety* (April 1985): 34-39.

Minter, Stephen. "Confined Spaces: Killers Without Clues." *Occupational Hazards Magazine* (February 1992): 57-59.

National Institute of Occupational Safety and Health. *Criteria for a Recommended Standard—Working in Confined Spaces.* 80-106. Washington, DC: NIOSH, 1979.

Occupational Safety and Health Administration. *Reports of OSHA Fatality/Catastrophe Investigations.* Washington, DC: OSHA, April 1982, August 1982, July 1985.

Pettit, Ted A., Lee M. Sanderson and Herbert I. Linn. "Workers/Rescuers Continue to Die in Confined Spaces." *Professional Safety* (February 1987): 15-22.

Preventing Accidents in Confined Spaces. Kemper Insurance Company, 1981.

Rekus, John F. *Complete Confined Spaces Handbook.* Boca Raton, FL: Lewis Publishers, January 1994.

Roychowdhury, Mahendra. "Entry Program for Any Industry." *Professional Safety* (February 1992): 16-21.

Smith, E.B. "Working in Confined Spaces." *Job Safety and Health* (November 1978).

Stephens, Hugh M. and Richard Tooth. "A New Tank Rescue Procedure." *Professional Safety* (May 1984): 15-18.

Wilson, Alan H. "Safe Work Rules for Manholes." *Transmission Distribution* (August 1977): 30-31.

Fall Statistics, Test Reports and Articles

Accident Prevention Manual for Industrial Operations, 8th ed. Chicago: National Safety Council, 1981.

American Petroleum Institute. *Oil and Gas Well Drilling and Servicing Operations.* API RP 54. Washington, DC: API, 1981.

Andres, Robert O., Keith Kreutzbert, and Eric M. Trier. *An Ergonomic Analysis of Dynamic Coefficient of Friction Measurement Techniques.* Ann Arbor: University of Michigan, College of Engineering, 1984.

Ardouin, G. *Experimental Studies on Safety Belts, Part I.* CIS 75-195. Paris: Centre Experimentaux de Recherches Des Batiments et Travaux Publics, August 1975.

Ardouin, G. *Experimental Studies on Safety Belts, Part II.* CIS 684-1973. Paris: Centre Experimentaux de Recherches Des Batiments et Travaux Publics, August 1975.

Associated General Contractors. "Prevention of Falls on Construction Projects." *The Constructor*. Washington, DC: AGC, 1963.

Ayoub, M.M. and Gary M. Bakkien. *An Ergonomic Analysis of Selected Sections in Subpart D, Walking and Working Surfaces*. #B-9-F-8-1320. Lubbock: Texas Tech University, Institute for Biotechnology, 1978.

The Boeing Company, Aero-Space Division. "Evaluation of Safety Belts, Lanyards and Shock Absorbers." *Safety Engineering* 2 (1967): 1886-09.

Brinkley, James W., et al. *Evaluation of Fall Protection by Prolonged Motionless Suspension of Volunteers*. Harry G. Armstrong Aerospace Medical Research Laboratory, Wright-Patterson Air Force Base, 1986.

British Standard Institution. *Specification for Industrial Belts, Harnesses, and Safety Lanyards*. BS 1397:1979. London: BSI, 1979.

Canadian Standards Association. *Fall Arresting Safety Belts and Lanyards for the Construction and Mining Industries*. Z359.1-1976. Toronto: CSA.

Chaffin, Don B., et al. *An Ergonomic Basis for Recommendations Pertaining to Specific Sections of OSHA Standard, 29 CFR, Part 1910, Subpart D, Walking and Working Surfaces*. Washington, DC: Department of Labor, Bureau of Labor Statistics, 1978.

Chaffin, Don B. and Terence J. Stobbe. *Ergonomic Considerations Related to Selected Fall Prevention Aspects of Scaffolds and Ladders as Presented in OSHA Standard 29 CFR 1910 Subpart D*. Washington, DC: Department of Labor, Bureau of Labor Statistics, 1979.

Chapanis, Alphonse. "To Err is Human, To Forgive - Design." Speech given at the American Society of Safety Engineers, Professional Development Conference, New Orleans, LA, June 1986.

Cloe, William. *Selected Occupational Fatalities Related to Powered, Two-Point Suspension Scaffolds/Powered Platforms as found in Reports of OSHA Fatality/Catastrophe Investigations*. Report #PB83194050, Springfield, VA: U.S. Department of Commerce, 1983.

Cohen, H.H. and D.M.J. Compton. "Fall Accident Patterns." *Professional Safety* (June 1982): 16-22.

Construction Safety Association of Ontario. *Current Research on Safety Belts, Lanyards, and Lifelines*. Research Publication No. 30, Toronto: CSAO, 1975.

_____. *Rope Grabbing Device*. Research Publication No. 13. Toronto: _____, 1973.

Cragle, A. "Plan for Access to Structures." *Transmission and Distribution* (February 1983): 38, 48.

Culver, Charles, Michael Marshall and Constance Connolly. "Analysis of Construction Accidents: The Workers' Compensation Database." *Professional Safety* (March 1993): 22-27.

Delaware Division of Motor Vehicles. *Driver's Manual*. State of Delaware: Rev. 1989.

"Don't You Fall." *Lifeline Magazine* (September/October 1975): 26-27.

Edison Electric Institute. "Lineman's Climbing Equipment." *Standard AP-2*. Washington, DC: Edison Electric Institute, 1972.

Ellis, J. Nigel. "Accidental Falls Cause Consternation; Protection Programs are Needed." *Northeast Oil Reporter* (April 1983).

_____. "Fall Protection: Equipment Selection and Program Development." *Best's Safety Directory, 14th-31st eds*. Oldwick, NJ: A.M. Best Company, 1973-1991.

_____. "Fall Protection: A Sound Investment." *Well Servicing Magazine* (July 1984): 14-16.

_____. "Fall Protection System Can Reduce Injuries from Falls." *National Safety News* (February 1985): 47-51.

_____. "Fall Protection for Tower and Antenna Climbers." *Communication News* 13, No. 6: 54H.

_____. "Fall Safety Equipment Up to Standards." *The American Oil & Gas Reporter* (June 1984): 18-20.

Ellis, J. Nigel and Howard B. Lewis. "Fall Protection—A Systems Approach Reviewing Types of Equipment." *Industrial Safety & Hygiene News Magazine* (December 1984): 57.

_____. "Fall Protection: Meeting the New Standard." *Western Oil Reporter* (April 1985): 51-58.

_____. "PW Technical File: 100% Fall Protection." *Purchasing World* (January 1985): 22-26.

"Emergency Action Planning." *Grain Storage and Handling* (June 1983): 15-24.

English, William. "Don't Fall Down on the Job." *National Safety* (February 1976): 82.

Gallagher, B.G. *Aerial Bucket Accident*. Toronto: Ontario Hydro.

Gallagher, Vincent A. "Unsafe Design: Fall and Machine

BIBLIOGRAPHY

Hazards." *Professional Safety* (December 1991): 22-26.

Hardesty, Charles, Charles Culver, and Fred Anderson. "Ironworkers Fatalities in Construction." *Occupational Hazards Magazine* (June 1993): 47-48.

Hearon, Bernard F. and James W. Brinkley. *Fall Arrest and Post-Fall Suspension: Literature Review and Direction for Further Research.* AFAMRL-TR-84-021. Armstrong Aerospace Medical Research Laboratory, Wright-Patterson Air Force Base, 1984.

Hewitt, J. "Roof Anchorage for Maintenance Workers." *The Safety Practitioner* (November 1984): 19-20.

Himmelrich, L.H. "Specialized Personal Protection...Advances in High Places Safety." *National Safety News* (October 1980): 52-53.

Himmelrich, L.H. and A.C. Sulowski. "Two Views of Fall Protection." *National Safety News* (June 1980): 8-10.

Hirsh, Tom. "Rescue Devices and Fall Protection." *National Safety News* (September 1956): 28-30.

International Labour Organisation. *Encyclopedia of Occupational Health and Safety, 3rd ed.* Edited by Luigi Parmeggiani, 829-836, 1960-1962, 2210-2212. Geneva, Switzerland: ILO, 1983.

Kelly, Susan-Marie. "Fall Protection Is Worth the Investment." *National Safety and Health News* (January 1986): 41-44.

Kingsley, Norman. "The Swami Belt: A Deadly Tie-In?" *Summit* 21 No. 6 (August 1975): 12-13.

Kravitz, Michael. "Should the Handicapped Standard for Change in Level Be Applied to Sidewalks and Crosswalks?" Abstract 451M, NAFE Seminar, Tucson, AZ, January 12, 1994.

L'Association Francaise de Normalisation (AFNOR). *Equipments Individuals de Protection contre Chutes.* NFS 710020. Paris: AFNOR, July 1978.

_____. "Fighting Falls with a Standard and Procedure." *National Safety News* (August 1983): 39-43.

Lahey, James W. "Nets: Watch That First Step." *National Safety News* (November 1983): 7-72.

Mosacchio, Carl. "The Construction Industry's Struggle for Safety." *Occupational Hazards* (October 1975): 33-35.

National Institute of Occupational Safety and Health. *Criteria for a Recommended Standard...Egress from Elevated Workstations.* NIOSH 76-128. Washington, DC: GPO, 1975.

National Institute for Occupational Safety & Health. *Preventing Workers Deaths And Injuries from Falls Through Skylights and Roof Openings.* Publication No. 90-100. Cincinnati, OH: Department of Health and Human Services, National Institute for Occupational Safety & Health, December 1989.

National Safety Council. *Harnesses and Accessories.* Chicago: NSC, 1952.

_____. "Falling Accidents." *National Safety News* (October 1977): 55.

_____. *Accident Facts.* Chicago: NSC, 1981-1993.

_____. *Falls on Floors.* Education Data Sheet No. 495 revised. Chicago: NSC, 1991.

Noel, Georges. *Study to Standardize Safety Equipment Used in Building and Public Works, Part II.* CIS-598, Paris: Centre Experimentaux de Recherches Des Batiments et Travaux Publics, 1975.

Occupational Safety and Health Administration. *Reports of OSHA Fatality/Catastrophe Investigations.* Washington, DC: GPO, May 1979, November 1979, April 1982.

Paler, Robert. "Don't Fall For It." *Nation's Business* (December 1985).

Philo, H. and R.L. Steinberg. "A Partial Revocation of the Legal License to Kill Construction Workers." *Trial Magazine* 15, No. 6 (June 1979): 24-28.

Research & Trading Corporation. *Fall Protection Tips, 2nd ed.* Wilmington, DE: RTC, 1992.

Roof Work: Prevention Falls. Guidance Note GS10. Her Majesty's Stationery Office, 1979.

Selected Occupational Fatalities Related to Miscellaneous Working Surfaces as found in Reports of OSHA Fatality/Catastrophe Investigations, April 1982.

Shand, T.G. "The Design of Modern Safety Belts and Their Users." *British Journal of Industrial Safety* 51 (1960).

"Safety Nets-Fall Protection for the Construction Industry." *National Safety News* (September 1982): 49-56.

"Shopping for Safety-Fall Protection." *National Safety News* (October 1982): 62-64.

Stanford University. *Tech Report 260.* Palo Alto, CA: Stanford University, 1981.

State of California, Department of Industrial Relations. "Personal Safety Devices and Safeguards." Article 10 of *Industrial Relations,* Sacramento: State of California, 1974.

_____. "Safety Belts and Nets." Article 24 in *Industrial Relations*, Sacramento; State of California, 1974.

Steinberg, H.L. *A Study of Personal Fall-Safety Equipment.* NBSIR 76-1146. Washington, DC: National Bureau of Standards, Institute for Applied Technology, Product Systems Analysis Division, 1977.

Sullivan, H.C. and C.P. Wickersham. "Fall Protection Device Prevents Serious Injury." *Chemical Processing* (October 1982): 140.

Sulowski, Andrew C. *Anthropomorphic Manikin Versus Rigid Weight Conversion Factor in Testing of Fall Arrestors.* Research Report No. 78-609-H. Toronto: Ontario Hydro, December 1978.

_____. "Assessment of Maximum Arrest Force in Fall Arresting Systems." *National Safety News* 123, No. 4 (1981): 50-53.

_____. *Evaluation of Fall Arresting Systems.* Research Report No. 78-98-H. Toronto: Ontario Hydro, March 1978.

_____. *Protection Individuelle Contre les Chutes de Hauteur).* France: Recontre d'Experts, Boulogne-Billancourt, OPPTBP, May 1982.

_____. "In Fall Arresting . . . Assessment of Maximum Arrest Force." *National Safety News* (April 1981): 50-53.

_____. The Safety Belt Question." *National Safety News* (February 1985): 44-46.

_____. "Selecting Fall Arresting Systems." *National Safety News* 20, No. 4 (1979): 55-60.

Texas Employers Insurance Association. *NSC Accident Facts 1985.* National Safety Council: Chicago.

Thus, R.F. "Engineering to Prevent Falling Accidents." *National Safety News* (November 1964): 26.

U.S. Department of Labor, Bureau of Labor Statistics. *Injuries to Construction Laborers.* Bulletin 2252. Washington, DC: GPO, 1986.

_____. *Injuries in Oil and Gas Drilling and Services.* Bulletin 2179, Washington, DC: _____, 1983.

_____. *Injuries Resulting from Falls from Elevations.* Bulletin 2195, Washington, DC: _____, 1984.

Ulysse, J.F. and Andrew C. Sulowski. "Fall Arresting Systems." *Professional Safety* (May 1982): 32-36.

Wang, Chen H. "Free Fall Restraint Systems." *Professional Safety* 22 (February 1977): 9-13.

Wexler, A. "The Theory of Belaying." *American Alpine Journal* 7 (1950): 379-405.

Yancey, C.W.C. *Perimeter Safety Net Projection Requirements.* NBSIR 85-3271. Washington, DC: GPO, November 1985.

Emergency Escape

"New Derrick-Escape Device Tested." *Well Servicing* (September/October 1983): 41-42.

Guardrails and Handrails

Fattal, S.G., L.E. Cattaneo, G.E. Turner and S.N. Robinson. *A Model Performance Standard for Guardrails.* NBSIR 76-1131, Washington, DC: GPO, 1976.

_____. *Personnel Guardrails for the Prevention of Occupational Accidents.* NBSIR 76-1132, Washington, DC: National Bureau of Standards, 1976.

National Fire Protection Association. *NFPA 101 Life Safety Code Handbook, 5th ed.* Edited by James K. Lathrop. Quincy, MA: NFPA, 1992.

Human Impact Tolerance

Aerospace Applications of Energy Absorption and Peak Force Reduction Devices. Technical Document No. 102-73. El Centro, CA: NPTR, 1973.

Armstrong, R.W. and H.P. Waters. "Testing Programs and Research on Restraint Systems." *SAE Transactions* (May 1972): 1023-1070.

Beeding, E.B. and J.D. Mosely. *Human Deceleration Tests.* AFMDC-TN-60-2. 1960.

Bierman, H.R. *Distribution of Impact Forces on the Human Through Restraint Devices. (U.S. Department of Commerce)* AD491-763. Springfield, VA: National Technical Information Service, 1971.

Bierman, H.R. and B.R. Larson. *Reaction of the Human to Impact Forces.* Navy Research Institute, 1946.

Brabin, E.J. "The Dynamic Properties of Seat Belt Webbing and End Fixings as Tested on the Pneumatic Accelerator." *MIRA Bulletin* 4 (July/August 1970): 4-11.

Dahnke, J.W., J.F. Palmer and C.L. Ewing. *Results of Parachute Opening Force Test Program.* TR 2-76. Washington, DC: Naval Air Systems Command, 1976.

Department of the Navy, Air Standardization Coordi-

BIBLIOGRAPHY

nating Committee. *Air Standardization Agreement on Ejection Acceleration Limits.* Air Standard 61/1. 1975.

"Human Tolerance to Extreme Impacts in Free Fall." *Aerospace Medicine* 34 No. 8 (August 1963).

King, W.R. and H.J. Mertz. *Human Impact Response: Measurement and Simulation.* 181-199. New York: Plenum Press, 1973.

Kourouklis, G., J. Gloney and S. DesJardins. *The Design Development and Testing of an Air Crew Restraint System for Army Aircraft.* 64-65. Technical Report 72-26. Ft. Eustis, VA: U.S. Armstrong Aerospace Medical Research Laboratory (USAAMRL), 1972.

Kroell, C.K., D.C. Schneider and A.M. Nakum. *Impact Tolerances and Responses of the Human Thorax.* T.E. Research Publication No. GMR-1167. Warren, MI: General Motors Corporation, 1971.

_____. *Impact Tolerances and Responses of the Human Thorax, Part II.* T.E. Research Publication No. GMR-1167. Warren, MI: General Motors Corporation, 1974.

Melvin, J.W., R.L. Stalnaker and V.L. Roberts. *Impact Injury Mechanism in Abdominal Organs.* New York: Society of Automotive Engineers, 1972.

Neathery, R.F. and T.E. Lobdell. *A Mechanical Simulation of the Human Thorax Under Impact.* T.E. Research Publication No. GMR-1420. Warren, MI: General Motors Corporation, 1973.

Neathery, R.F., C.K. Kroell and H.J. Mertz. *Prediction of Thoracic Injury from Dummy Responses.* Research Publication No. GMR-1918. Warren, MI: General Motors Corporation, 1975.

Noel, Georges, M. Amphoux, et al. *Safety Equipment in Construction and Public Works Transportation.* No. 362. Montreuil, France: Technical Institute for Construction and Public Works, 1978.

Reid, D.H. and J.E. Doerr, et al. "Acceleration and Opening Shock Forces During Free Fall Parachuting," *Aerospace Medical Bulletin* 42 (1971): 12-7-1210.

Roebuck, Kraemer and Thomson. *Engineering Anthropometry Methods.* New York: John Wiley and Sons, 1975.

Snyder, R.G. "Human Impact Tolerance." Paper #700398 presented at the International Automobile Safety Conference, 1970.

_____. *Occupational Falls.* UM-HSRI-77-51. Highway Safety Research Institute. Ann Arbor: University of Michigan, 1977.

Snyder, R.G., D.R. Foust and B.M. Bowman. *Study of Human Impact Tolerance Through Free Fall Investigation.* HSRI-77-8. Ann Arbor: University of Michigan, 1977.

Society of Automotive Engineers. *Mathematical Modeling Biodynamic Response to Impacts.* Sp-42. Warringdale, PA: SAE, 1976.

Stapp, J.P. "Human Tolerance to Severe, Abrupt Acceleration," *Gravitational Stress in Aerospace Medicine.* Boston: Little, Brown, 1961.

Van Cott, H.P. and R. G. Kinkade, eds. *Human Engineering Guide to Equipment Design.* 508-509. Washington, DC: American Institute for Research, 1972.

Viano, DC and C.W. Gadd. *Significance of Rate of Onset in Impact Injury Evaluation.* 807-819. Research Publication No. GMR-1910. Warren, MI: General Motors Corporation, 1975.

Knots

Ashley, Clifford W. *The Ashley Book of Knots.* Garden City: Doubleday & Co., Inc., 1944.

Hubacek, John. "Figure 8 Knot Holds Up in Rescue Service Application." *Fire Engineering* (October 1983): 52-53.

O'Campo, Leo. "Consider the Carabinier." *Fire Engineering* (April 1983): 29-30.

Peterson, Richard E. "Triple Sliding Hitch—Useful Knot for Use with Lifelines." *Construction Newsletter* (Jan-Feb. 1985): 5.

Rope Rescue Manual. Santa Barbara, CA: CMC, 1987.

Ladders

ANSI A14.1-1982 Safety Requirements for Portable Wood Ladders. Published by American Society of Safety Engineers, Des Plaines, IL.

ANSI A14.1a-1985 Supplement to ANSI A14.1-1982.
_____.

ANSI A14.2-1982 Safety Requirements for Metal Ladders.
_____.

ANSI A14.2a-1985 Supplement to ANSI A14.2-1982.

_____.

ANSI A14.3-1992 Safety Requirements for Fixed Ladders.
_____.

ANSI A14.4-1979 (R1984) Safety Requirements for Job-Made Ladders. _____.

ANSI A14.5-1982 Safety Requirements for Portable Reinforced Plastic Ladders. _____.

ANSI A14.5a-1985 Supplement to ANSI A14.5-1982. _____.

Armstrong, Malcolm C. *Pilot Ladder Safety.* Woolahra, NSW, Australia: International Maritime Press.

Bjornstig, Ulf, and Jeanette Johnsson. "Ladder Injuries: Mechanisms, Injuries and Consequences." *Journal of Safety Research,* Vol. 23. (1992): 9-18.

Bureau of Labor Statistics. *A Survey of Ladder Accidents Resulting in Injuries.* Washington, DC: GPO, 1978.

"Fixed Ladders and Climbing Devices," Data Sheet 1-606, Revised 1983. *National Safety News* (April 1983): 59-61.

"Job-made Ladders." Data Sheet 1-568, Revised 1987. Chicago: National Safety Council.

"OSHA Ladder Requirements." *Best's Safety Directory: 1991.* Oldwick, NJ: A.M. Best. Co.

Rescue

Department of Fire Programs Heavy and Tactical Rescue Training Unit, Fire Services Board, Commonwealth of Virginia. "Vertical Rescue Rope II." June 1990.

Ellis, J. Nigel. "Plan Confined-Space Fall Protection Before and Beyond Required Rescue." *Occupational Health and Safety* (February 1992): 17-19.

Peleaux, John R. "Post-fall Rescue of Workers Using Fall Protection." *Professional Safety* (March 1991): 22-24.

Rekus, John F. "Safety in the Trenches." *Occupational Health and Safety* (February 1992): 26-37.

Stephens, Hugh M. and Richard Tooth. "A New Tank Rescue Procedure." *Professional Safety* (May 1984): 15-18.

Ropes, Synthetic Fibers and Hardware

American National Standard Institute. *Requirements for Safety Belts, Harnesses, Lanyards, Lifelines and Droplines for Construction and Industrial Use.* ANSI Z10.14 (1975). New York: ANSI, 1975.

"Bend Tests Made on Natural and Synthetic Fibers Ropes." *Technical Communications* (January 1971).

"Dynamic Tests on Nylon Rope." *All American Engineering.* (February 1942): Wilmington, DE.

The Effect of Loading on the Extension and Recovery of Ropes of Nylon and Dacron. DuPont Technical Information Bulletin X-92. Wilmington, DE; DuPont Co., 1958.

Haas, Frank J. *Knowing the Ropes.* Auburn, NY: The Cordage Group.

Hauser, R.L. and V. Frieber. *Critique of Steels for Safety Hardware.* Report #5346-72-3. Boulder, CO: Hauser Labs, 1972.

Himmelfarb, David. *Technology of Cordage, Fibers and Rope.* New York: Textile Book Publishing (Interscience), 1957.

Impact Resistance or Energy Absorbing Properties of Ropes of Nylon and Dacron. DuPont Technical Information Bulletin X-99. Wilmington, DE; DuPont Co., February 1959.

Koon, A.W. *Environmental Degradation of Ropes.* Auburn, NY: The Cordage Group, 1973.

Kosmath, E. and P. Kaminger. *Aging of Ropes, Report of the Safety Committee of the Austrian Mountaineering Club.* Narrow Fabric and Braiding Industry (Germany), Vol. 3, September 1975, and Vol. 4, December 1975.

Light and Weather Resistance of Fibers. DuPont Technical Information Bulletin X-203. Wilmington, DE: DuPont Co., April 1966.

Madigan, Doris L. "Sunlight Degradation of Rope." *National Safety News* (March 1984): 54-56.

Newman, S.B. and H.G. Wheeler. *Impact Strength of Nylon and of Sisal Ropes.* Washington, DC; National Bureau of Standards, 1945.

Paul, Walter. "Review of Synthetic Fiber Ropes." U.S. Coast Guard Academy Research Project, August 1970.

Properties of Ropes of Dacron and DuPont Nylon. DuPont Technical Information Bulletin X-226. Wilmington, DE; DuPont Co., February 1969.

Rope Knowledge for Riggers. Auburn, NY: The Cordage Group, 1973.

Rope Technical Data. Auburn, NY: The Cordage Group, 1973.

Walker, C.R. "Comparison of Natural Fiber and Synthetic Fiber Ropes." *Transmission and Distribution* (September 1969): 48-53.

BIBLIOGRAPHY

Scaffolds

Bureau of Labor Statistics. *A Survey of Scaffold Accidents Resulting in Injuries.* NTIS Accession No. PB208009. BLS, 1978.

National Institute for Occupational Safety and Health. "Preventing Electrocutions During Work with Scaffolds Near Overhead Power Lines." NIOSH Publication No. 91-110. Cincinnati, OH: NIOSH, August 1991.

Scaffold Industry Association. *Suspended Scaffold Pocket Handbook.* Van Nuys, CA: SIA, August 1992.

Slips and Trips

Adler, S.C. and B.C. Perman. *A History of Walkway Slip Resistance at the National Bureau of Standards.* NBS Special Publication 565. Denver: National Bureau of Standards, 1979.

Allcott, G.A. *Slips, Trips and Falls—Working Surfaces and Industrial Stairs.* Morgantown: US Department of Health, Education and Welfare, 1979.

Amato, John. "How Sears Helps Minimize Slips and Falls." *National Safety News* (November 1978): 59.

American Society for Testing Materials. *Measuring Surface Frictional Properties Using the British Pendulum Tester.* ANSI/ASTM E.303-74. Philadelphia: ASTM, 1974.

_____. *Static Coefficient of Friction of Polish-coated Floor Surfaces as Measured by the James Machine.* ASTM D-2047-75. Philadelphia: ASTM, 1975.

_____. *Static Coefficient of Friction of Shoe Sole and Heel Materials as Measured by the James Machine.* ANSI/ASTM F 489-77. Philadelphia: ASTM, 1977.

Anderson, C. and J. Senne, eds. *Walkway Surfaces: Measurement of Slip Resistance.* ASTM Special Technical Publication 649. American Society for Testing Materials, 1978.

Andres, Robert O. and Don B. Chaffin. "Ergonomic Analysis of Slip-Resistance Measurement Devices." *Ergonomics* 28, No. 7 (1985): 1065-1079.

Archea, J., B. Collins and F. Stahl. *Guidelines for Stair Safety,* Building Science Series 120, Washington, DC: National Bureau of Standards, 1979.

Barrett, G.F.C. "Observations on the Coefficient of Friction of Shoe Soling Materials." *Rubber Journal* (December 1, 1956).

Brauer, Roger L. *Safety and Health for Engineers.* New York: Van Nostrand Reinhold, 1993.

Braun, R. and R.J. Brungraber. *A Comparison of Two Slip-Resistance Testers.* 58. Walkway Surfaces Symposium, American Society for Testing and Materials, Philadelphia, PA, 1978.

Brungraber, R.J. *A Portable Tester for the Evaluation of the Slip-resistance of Walkway Surfaces.* NBS Technical Note 953. Washington, DC: National Bureau of Standards, 1977.

_____. *An Overview of Floor Slip-resistance Research with Annotated Bibliography,* NBS Technical Note 895. Washington, DC: National Bureau of Standards, 1976.

Carlson, S. *How Man Moves, Kinesiological Methods and Studies.* London: Heinemann, 1972.

National Academy of Sciences. *Causes and Measurement of Walkway Slipperiness,* NAS Technical Report No. 43, Washington, DC: NAS, 1961.

Chaffin, D.G. and R.O. Andres. *Evaluation of Three Surface Friction Measurement Devices for Field Use.* Ann Arbor: University of Michigan, Center for Ergonomics and Safety, 1982.

Cohen, H. Harvey and D.M.J. Compton. "Fall Accident Patterns." *Professional Safety* (June 1982): 16-22.

Cramp, P.A. *Preliminary Study of the Slipperiness of Flooring.* Washington, DC: National Bureau of Standards, 1974.

Cunningham, D.M. *Components of Floor Reaction During Walking.* Berkeley: University of California, Institute of Engineering Research, 1950.

Davis, P.R. "Human Factors Contributing to Slips, Trips and Falls." *Ergonomics,* 26, No. 1 (1983): 51-59.

Day, S.S. and E. Shamburger. "Factors Controlling Skid Resistance of Hard Floor Surfaces." *Hospitals* 39 (April 16, 1965).

Day, S.S., H.D. Bowen and R.J. Hader. *Skid Resistance of Floor Surfaces and Finishes.* Technical Bulletin No. 200. Raleigh: University of North Carolina, 1980.

Doering, R.D. "A Systems Approach...Slips and Falls Accident Analysis." *National Safety News* (February 1981): 47-50.

_____. "Defining a Safe Walking Surface." *National Safety News* (August 1974): 54.

Draganich, L.F., T.P. Andriacchi, A.M. Strongwater and J.O. Galanti. "Electronic Measurement of Instantaneous

Foot-floor Contact Patterns During Gait." *Journal of Biomechanics* (1980): 13.

Edosomwan, Johnson A. and Tarek M. Khalil. "Accident Prevention in Slips and Falls." *Professional Safety* (June 1981): 30-35.

Ekkebus, C.E. and W. Kelley. "Measurement of Safe Walkway Surfaces." *Soap/Cosmetics/Chemical Specialties* (February 1973).

"Electronic Step-meter Reveals Mechanics of Walking." *Technical News Bulletin* (National Bureau of Standards) 35(4) (1951): 50.

English, William. *Slips, Trips & Falls.* Columbia, MD: Hanrow Press, 1989.

Falls on Floors. Data Sheet 495. Chicago: National Safety Council, April 1987.

Floor Mats and Runners. Data Sheet 595. Chicago: National Safety Council, 1967.

"Forces and Energy Changes in the Leg During Walking." *American Journal of Physiology* (1939): 125.

Fox, W.F. *Body Weight and Coefficient of Friction as Determiners of Pushing Capability.* Human Engineering Special Studies Memo No. 17. Cape Canaveral: Lockheed Aerospace, 1967.

Friction Measurements on Soles and Heels with Particular Reference to Women's Top-piece Materials. Publication TM 1355. SATRA, 1967.

Fundamental Studies of Human Locomotion and Other Information Relating to the Design of Artificial Limbs. Report to National Research Council, Berkeley, 1947.

Gavan, F.M. and J.G. Vanaman. "Significant Variables Affecting Results Obtained with the James Machine." *Materials Research and Standards* (November 1968).

Grieve, D.W. "Slipping Due to Manual Exertion." *Ergonomics* 26, No. 1 (1983): 61-72.

Harper, F.C., W.J. Warlow and B.L. Clark. *The Forces Applied to the Floor by the Foot in Walking.* National Building Studies research paper No. 32. London: Department of Scientific and Industrial Research, 1961.

Hodgin, Leslie, contributing editor. "Footwear Industry Makes Strides in Slip Resistance." *Occupational Health and Safety* (December 1992): 26-29.

Holden, T.S. and R.W. Muncey. "Pressures on the Human Foot During Walking." *Australian Journal of Applied Science* 4, No. 3 (1953): 405-417.

Irvine, C.H. "A New Slipmeter for Evaluating Walkway Slipperiness." *Materials Research & Standards* (MISTRA) 7, No. 12 (December 1967): 535-542.

_____. "Evaluation of Some Factors Affecting Measurements of Slip Resistance of Shoe Materials on Floor Surfaces." *Journal of Testing and Evaluation* 4(2) (1976).

_____. "Shoe Sole Slipperiness on Structured Steel." *Materials Research and Standards* (1970) 10(4)(b).

Jacobs, N.A., J. Skorecki and J. Charnley. "Analysis of the Vertical Component of Force in Normal and Pathological Gait." *Journal of Biomechanics* (1980): 13.

James, D.I. "A Broader Look at Pedestrian Friction." *Rubber Chemistry and Technology Review* (1980): 53.

James, D.I. and W.G. Newell. *A New Concept in Friction Testing (Report No. 20).* Shawbury, England: Rubber and Plastics Research Association (RAPRA), 1978.

Johnson, B.S. *A Discussion of Some Factors Influencing Slip Resistance Measurements.* Philadelphia: Franklin Research Company, 1958.

Manning, D.P. *Deaths and Injuries Caused by Slipping, Tripping and Falling Accidents.* Surrey, England: University of Surrey, 1982.

Miller, J.M. *A Bibliography of Coefficient of Friction Literature Relating to Slip Type Accidents.* Ann Arbor: University of Michigan, Department of Industrial Engineering, 1983.

_____. "Slippery Work Surfaces: Towards a Performance Definition and Quantitative Coefficient of Friction Criteria." *Journal of Safety Research* 14, No. 4 (Winter 1983): 145-158.

Outline of the Proposed Investigation for Determining the Slip Resistance of Floor Treatment Materials. Subject 410. New York: Underwriters Laboratory, 1974.

Palena, Maximillian. "Slip is a Sliding Motion." *National Safety News* (November 1978).

Perkins, P.J. *Measurement of Slip Between the Shoe and Ground During Walking.* Special Technical Publication No. 649. Philadelphia: American Society for Testing Materials, 1978.

"Prevention of Slips and Falls." *Safety Newsletter* (June 1972).

Redfern, M.S. and B. Bidanda. "Effects of Shoe Angle, Velocity, and Vertical Force on Shoe/floor/slip Resistance." *Advances in Industrial Ergonomics and Safety IV.* London: Taylor and Francis, 1992.

BIBLIOGRAPHY

Redfern, M.S. and D. Bioswick. "The Prevention of Slips and Falls in Industry." *Occupational Health & Safety* (July 1987).

Redfern, M.S. and D.B. Chaffin. "Slip Resistance Measurements in Industry." *Trends in Ergonomics/Human Factors IV*. Amsterdam: Elsevier, 1987.

Redfern, M.S., D.B. Chaffin and A. Marcotte. "A Dynamic Coefficient fo Friction Measurement Device for Shoe/floor Interface Testing." *Journal of Safety Research*, Volume 21 (1990): 61-65.

_____. "The Effects of Floor Types on Standing Tolerance in Industry." *Trends in Ergonomics/Human Factors IV*. Amsterdam: Elsevier, 1988.

Reed, M.E. *Standardization of Friction Testing of Industrial Working Surfaces*. Cambridge, MA: Comstock & Westcott Inc., 1975.

Riley, M.W. and R.C. Arnold. "Relating Human Static Work of Standing and the Coefficient of Friction between the Shoe and Floor Using a Link-system Model." *Proceedings of the Human Factors Society*, 22nd Annual Meeting, Santa Monica, CA, 1978.

Rosen, Stephan I. *The Slip and Fall Handbook*. 2 vols. and supplement. Columbia, MD: Hanrow Press, 1993.

Santos, F. "Factors in Detecting and Correcting Floor Slipperiness." *National Safety News* (October 1966).

Schuster, D.K. "Slip—An Investigation of Practical Accident Prevention." *Die Berufsgenossenschaft Betriebssicherheit* (September 1966).

Shawbury, James D.I. *Rubbers and Plastics on Shoes and Flooring: The Importance of Kinetic Friction*. London: Rubber and Plastics Research Association of Great Britain, 1982.

Sherman, Roger M. "Preventing Slips that Result in Falls." *Professional Safety* (March 1992): 23-25.

_____. "Slip and Fall Accident Prevention Simplified." *Professional Safety* (February 1986): 40-43.

Sigler, P.A., M.N. Geib and T.H. Boone. "Measurement of Slipperiness of Walkway Surface." *Journal of Research* 40 (1948): 339-346.

Sigler, P.A. *Relative Slipperiness of Floor and Deck Surfaces*. Report BMS 100. Washington, DC: National Bureau of Standards, 1943.

"Slip Study Suggestions and Solutions." *National Safety News* (September 1972).

"Slipping, Tripping & Falling Accidents." *Ergonomics* 26 (1983).

"Slips and Falls." *National Safety News* (September 1972).

"Solving the Problem of Unsafe Surfaces Begins with Selecting Correct Flooring." *National Safety News* (August 1980).

Strandberg, L. and H. Lanshammer. "Dynamics of Slipping Accidents." *Journal of Occupational Accidents* 3 (1981): 153-162.

Swensen, Eric E., Jerry L. Purswell, Robert E. Schlegel, University of Oklahoma - Norman, and Ronald L. Stanevich, National Institute of Occupational Safety and Health (NIOSH). "Coefficient of Friction and Subjective Assessment of Slippery Work Surfaces." *Human Factors* (February 1992): 67-77.

Szymusiak, Susan M. and Joseph P. Ryan. "Prevention of Slip and Fall Injuries, Part I." *Professional Safety* (June 1982): 11-15.

_____. "Prevention of Slip and Fall Injuries, Part II." *Professional Safety* (July 1982): 30-35.

Turnbow, Charles E. *Slip and Fall Practice*. Santa Ana, CA: James Publishing Group.

"Walking & Working Surfaces." *National Safety News* (April 1977): 82.

Wilson A. and P. Mahoney. "Measuring Functional Properties of Soles and Heels." *Rubber World* (March 1972).

Stair Falls

Archea, John, B.L. Collins, and Fred I. Shahl. *Guidelines for Stair Safety*. Building Science Series 120. Washington, DC: National Bureau of Standards, 1979.

Carson, D.H., J.C. Archea, S.T. Margulis, and F.E. Carson. *Safety on Stairs*. NBS Building Science Series 108. Washington, DC: National Bureau of Standards, 1978.

Esmay, M.L. and L.J. Segerlind. "Analysis of Frictional Characteristics of Stairway Tread Covering Materials." *Transactions of the American Society of Agricultural Engineers* 7, No. 2 (1964).

Illuminating Engineers Society of North America. *Lighting Handbook, 8th ed*. New York: IES, 1993.

Johnson, Daniel A. "Factors to Consider When Investigating Accidents on Stairs." *Safety News* (August 1991).

Kurtz, Edwin B. *Lineman's Handbook*. New York: McGraw-Hill, 1942.

Lovested, Gary. "First Steps to Safer Stairways Include Design Criteria." *Construction Newsletter* (National Safety Council), (November-December 1980).

Pauls, Jake L. "What Can We Do to Improve Stair Safety?" *Building Standards Magazine* (May, June, July and August 1984): 9-16.

Templer, John Arthur. "Stair Shape and Human Movement." Ph.D. diss., Columbia University, 1975.

U.S. Department of Labor, Bureau of Labor Statistics. *Injuries Resulting From Falls on Stairs.* Bulletin 2214. Washington, DC: GPO, 1984.

U.S. Department of Labor. "Walking and Working Surfaces and Personal Protective Equipment (Fall Protection Systems); Notices of Proposed Rulemaking." *Federal Register* (April 10, 1990).

Statistics

Accident Analysis and Prevention, Vol. 24, No. 5: (October 1992) 437-558.

Associated General Contractors Manual of Accident Prevention in Construction. Washington, DC: December 1971, December 1992.

Brett, Phillip. "Wave Goodbye to Work-site Falls." *Safety & Health* (National Safety Council) (September 1993): 54-56.

Ellis, J. Nigel. "Anchorage Planning: The Key to Fall Protection." *Safety & Health* (National Safety Council) (September 1991): 66-70.

"Guidelines for Roof Anchorages for Fall Arrest Systems," Regulation 527/88. Ontario Ministry of Labour, Ontario, Canada, September 1991.

Hadipriono, Fabian C. "Expert System for Construction Safety I: Fault-Tree Models," *Journal of Performance of Constructed Facilities* (American Society of Civil Engineers) Vol. 6, No.4 (November 1992).

_____. "Expert System for Construction Safety II: Knowledge Base." *Journal of Performance of Constructed Facilities.*

Pine, John C. "Firefighter Injuries and Illnesses in Louisiana." *Speaking of Fire* (Oklahoma State University) (Spring 1992).

Rinefort, Foster C. "The Economics of Safety." *Professional Safety* (May 1992): 42-45.

"Safety Guidelines for Window Cleaning." Chicago: International Window Cleaning Association, 1992.

Sulowski, Andrew C. *Principles of Fall Protection, 1st ed.* Ontario, Canada: International Society for Fall Protection (ISFP), 1992.

US Department of Labor, Occupational Safety and Health Administration. "Analysis of Construction Fatalities - OSHA Database 1985-1989." Washington, DC: November 1990.

Weber, J. Owen. "The Front-line Supervisor's Role in Safety." *Professional Safety* (May 1992): 34-39.

Training

National Institute for Occupational Safety and Health. *OSHA Instruction 3-1.1.* DHHS (NIOSH) Publication No. 90-100. Cincinnati, OH: NIOSH, 1989.

Work Methods at Heights

"Nobody Does It Better." *Continental Airlines Magazine* (August 1986): 38-52.

Videos on Fall Protection

LeBow, Dwight R. Rald Industries, Freeport, TX.
The Pin-Hole Safety Connection.

DSC Video, Dynamic Scientific Controls, 3101 N. Market, Wilmington DE 19802.
Scaffold Erection and Dismantling Fall Protection.

Ironworkers Local 711. Montreal, Quebec, Canada.
Various educational materials.

National Constructors Association, 1730 M Street N.W., Washington, DC 20036.
A Couple of Seconds to Die (Belts, Lanyards, Lifelines...).
Ladders and Stairways.
Planning to Prevent Falls.
Watch Your Step (Floor Openings, Covers, Rails and Nets).
West-1.

Whitman, Gerald. Whitman's Welding Service, Shenandoah Junction, WV 25442.
Safety Post System.

INDEX

-A-

ABC's of Fall Protection, 40-48
Access systems, 113-15
"Accident Facts," 2, 16
Aerial lift, 54
    fall protection, 152-53
    safety rules for, 166
Aerospace Medical Research Laboratory (Wright-Patterson AFB), 82
American National Standards Institute (ANSI), 9
    A10.8-1969, 160
    A10.8-1988, 160
    A10.14-1991 Standard, 10, 37, 92, 96
    A14.3-1992, 97-98
    A14.4, 155
    A92, 153
    Z10 Standard, 44
    Z117.1-1989, 156-57, 160
    Z359 Standards, 11, 163
    Z359.1, 11, 87-88, 158, 188
    Z359.2, 163
    Z535.3-1991, 36, 163
American Society of Safety Engineers, 11, 40
American Society for Testing and Materials
    A10.14 Subcommittee, 9-10
    Committee on Safety and Traction Footwear, 34
    Z117.1 Standard, 11
    Z133, 207
Anchorage(s), 40-42, 105
    criteria for testing, labeling and recertifying, 135
    points, 18-19, 80-82, 132-38, 146, 202
    portable, 102
    for rope grab system, 148
    roof, 136-37, 147
    strength requirements, 17-18
    structures, 53, 207
Andres, Robert O., 35
Angled descent, 118
Angles, recommended for stairs, ramps and ladders, 36
ANSI. *See:* American National Standards Institute (ANSI)
Architects, competency of, in writing safety specifications, 18

-B-

Backup protection, 52
Basketcage protection, 97
Beck, Don, 124
Belts, 12, 39-40, 91-93
    cleaning, 128
Body

supports, 42-46, 91-94
    Support Pentagon, 45
    weight as an element in fall hazards, 38
Boatswain's Chair Systems, 150, 160
Brinkley, Jim, 82
British Standards Institute, 82
Building(s)
    fall protection guidelines for managers/owners of, 18-19
    maintenance, procedures for elevated exterior, 145-51
    perimeters at roof level, 150
Bureau of Labor Statistics (BLS)
    1984 study of falls by, 5, 13, 52, 138
    Supplementary Data System, record of falls, 2
Business Roundtable Report A-3, "Improving Safety Performance" (1982), 7

-C-

Cable(s), 98
    lifeline, retracting, 106, 108–109
    shear, 202-203
    with shock absorbers, 194
Canada, fall protection regulations in, 12
Canadian Standard Association (CSA), 188
    fall arrest equipment component standards, 12
    Z259.11 Standard, 94
Carabiner locking snaphook, 123
Chaffing Report (1978), 38
Chapanis, Alphonse, 48
Cleaning synthetic ropes, belts and harnesses, 128
Climbing
    assists, 100, 101
    protection system, considerations in the selection of a, 104
    and/or traversing, 54
Cold hazards, 126
Competent persons
    defined by OSHA, 166
    employing, 138-39
Confined space(s), 46-48, 155-63
    access into, 160, 162-63
    NIOSH classification of, 111, 155
    considerations for fall protection when entering, 71-72
    entry and retrieval from, 111-15
    lifeline and rescue system, selecting, 114
    rescue, 206
    retrieval planning, 48, 54
    Standard, 1910.146, 12
    worker suspension issues, 160-62
Connecting means, 46-48
Construction. *See also:* Steel
    accidents, Workers' Compensation Data Base, 1985-1988, 4, 7
    cost of insurance for, 22
    falls in, 2, 4-7
    fall protection, 167

fatalities related to activities, 81
injuries due to falls, 2, 5-6
Consulting engineers, fall protection guidelines for, 19
Contractors guide for use of suspended scaffolds, 147-51
Control measures, prioritizing, 79-80
Controlled descent devices, 116
The Cordage Group, 100
Corporate counsel, fall protection guidelines for, 20
Corrosion and dirt hazards, 126
Crawford, Harry, 82
Cutting edges, 126

-D-

D-ring(s), 150
locations, 92
Debris nets, 90
Descent devices, 116-18, 147
DuPont Safety Management Services Newsletter, 72
Duty to warn,
responsibility of architect and general contractor regarding, 17

-E-

Electrical hazards, 126
Elevated
falls from one level to another, 37
platforms, standards addressing fall protection for scaffolds and, 148
work task, sample analysis of an, 78
Emergency escape, 101, 112-20
angled, 118
means of, 53-54
retrieval, 112
Emergency descent system, 119
Employers, fall protection guidelines for, 20
English, William, 35
Equipment. *See also:* Fall arrest equipment
and prefab manufacturers, fall protection guide lines for, 21-22
Error(s). *See also:* Fall hazards
common safety, and their probability of occurrence, 79
probabilities, 79
Escape, means of, 53-54
European Community (EC) standards for fall protection, 12

-F-

Fall(s)
arrest, 156
arrest forces, calculation of vertical, 188-92
classification of, 2
in construction, 2, 4-7

costs of, 6-7, 72
distribution of injuries resulting from, by industry, 5
elongation and deceleration distance considerations in, 210
free, 210
incidence of, in 1992, 2
occurrence of, 5
from one level to another, 37
signage, 36
Fall arrest equipment, 12, 71, 86-128. *See also:* ANSI Z359.1
cleaning, 128
components, 91, 148-51
inspection and maintenance of, 127-28, 208-209
installation and use of engineering guide, 200-203
interpretation of dynamic loads in tests of, 82-84
for light and heavy workers, suggested testing of, 89
mixing and matching, 125
residual hazards associated with the use of, 120-28
safety rules for, 166
Fall force testing results, 83
Fall hazard(s), 120-28
analysis, 67-69, 76
control of, 54, 68-69
due to heat, 126
elements of a, 37-39
electrical, 126
exposure to, 52, 76
in exterior building maintenance, 145-51
responsibility for, 16-18
risk of, 76-79
from roll-out, 122-25
swing fall, 122
Fall protection, 53, 101
ABC's of, 40-48
aerial lift, 152-53
confined space, 12, 48, 54, 71-72, 111-15, 155-63
connectors, 28-30, 70
connecting means, 46-48
construction, 167
escape and rescue standards, 184-87
equipment requirements, 9, 48
guidelines, 18-22, 208-210
on metal roof decks, 105
methods, outdated, 204-207
myths, 26-29
planning, 167-68
policies, 58
programs, 59-67, 71
providing, 58-72, 208
on scaffolds and elevated work platforms, 147-51
solutions, hierarchy of, 86
steel erection, 30
standards, USA and Canada, 10
systems, evaluating, 53
systems, two-dimensional, 110
by worker activity, 53-54
workers' needs for, 52-53
Federal Register, construction injury statistics listed in the, 5

INDEX

First-Worker-Up Devices, 100
First aid and medical assistance, 171
Fixed ladders, 97
Flexible cable carrier, 97
Floor surfaces, 34
Force test demonstration results, 83
Free-fall
    considerations, 210
    distance, 38, 46-47
Friction buckle, 92
Full body harnesses, 93-94

-G-

General contractors, fall protection guidelines for, 20
Grab, manually operated, 103
Grain Storage and Handling Industry Standard
    (Proposed), 1910.272, 11
Group evacuation, 118
Guardrails, safety rules for, 166

-H-

Handrails, stair, 35
Harnesses
    cleaning, 128
    full-body, 40, 42-44, 93-94
    required for confined-space entry, 111
Heat hazards, 126
Hitch knots, 204-205
Hoists. *See:* Winches
Horizontal
    rail system, 109
    travel, 54
Horizontal lifeline(s), 107-12, 147
    forces, calculation of, 193-96
    systems, permanent, 107-109
    systems, semi-permanent, 109-110

-I-

Illumination on stairs, 35
Industrial Equipment Association, 116
Insurance, cost of, 22
International Standards Organization (ISO)
    standard for fall arrest equipment, 12
    Technical Advisory Group, 9
Ironworker(s)
    fatalities, 1985-1989, 81
    study of accidents by, 78

-K-

Keylock, 110-111, 113

Knots, 96-97, 204-206

-L-

Ladder(s), 153-55
    falls, study by OSHA of, 37
    fixed, 97
    recommended angles for, 36
    step, 154-55
Lanyard(s), 94-95
    hitch knots, testing of, 205-206
    for a rope grab system, 149-50
    self-retracting, 99-100, 103, 106-107
Lifeline(s), 48, 107-11 *See also:* Lanyard(s); Self-retract-
   ing lanyards
    criteria for vertical and horizontal, 200-202
    for a rope grab system, 148-49
    termination requirements, 202
    vertical, 209
Lighting levels on stairs, 35
Lineman's belt and strap, 93
Load arresting systems, 120
Locking snaphook, 123-25
Lowering devices, manually operated 117-18

-M-

Material Safety Data Sheets, 17
Maximum Arresting Force (MAF), estimating, 188
MIL-S-87966 (1980), 97
Mine Safety and Health Administration (MSHA), 12
Mobile grab, 103-105
Mobile work positioning systems, 54
MSHA *Fatal Grams*, 12

-N-

National Bureau of Standards report on stairway falls,
   35, 188
National Engineering Labs (Scotland), 82
National Fire Protection Association (NFPA), *Life Safety
   Code*, 115
National Institute of Occupational Safety and Health
   (NIOSH)
    accidents relating to floor openings, reported by,
      37, 53
    Criteria Document 8-106, 111, 115
    definition of confined space by, 111, 155
    Hazard Alert #86-110 (January 1986), 112
    study of falls from derricks by, 5
National Safety Council, 2
New York State Code, recent owner's liability rulings
   under, 7
NFPA 101, 35
NIOSH. *See:* National Institute of Occupational Safety
   and Health (NIOSH)

224   INTRODUCTION TO FALL PROTECTION, SECOND EDITION

-O-

Obstructions, 210
Occupational Safety and Health Administration, 11
    1910.21-32 Subpart D (proposed), Walking and
      Working Surfaces, 11, 155
    1910.28, 160
    1910.30, 160
    1910.38, 115
    1910.66 (proposed), Powered Platform Industry, 11,
      66, 147, 150, 153
    1910.66, Appendix C, 124, 156-57, 163, 166, 188,
      193, 208-210
    1910.67, 153
    1910.119, process safety rules, 17
    1910.129-131, 11
    1910.146, Confined Space Standard, 12, 111, 156-59
    1910.270, Oil and Gas Well Drilling and Servicing
      Industry, 118
    1910.272, Grain Storage and Handling Industry, 11
    1926 (proposed) Subparts L and M, 11, 150
    1926 Subpart X, Stairs and Ladders, 11
    1926.21, 170
    1926.451, 145, 160
    1926.500, 142, 145
    1926.502 (proposed), 114, 142
    1926.850, 142
    1926.1053, 117, 155
    2:1 factor of safety, 138
    "Fatal Facts" newsletter, 2-3, 12
    General Industry Standards, Section Subpart I, 11
      guidance on fall planning, 208-210
    ladder requirements (1926.1050-1053; 1910.27),
      153
    measurement of free falls by, 38
    Oil and Gas Well Drilling and Servicing Industry
      Standard (Proposed), 1910.270, 11
    Program Directive 100-57, 97
    Training Institute, study of ladder falls by the, 37
Ontario Ministry of Labour, guidelines for roof anchor-
    ages for fall arrest systems, 136-37
OSHA. *See:* Occupational Safety and Health
    Administration

-P-

Pater, Robert, 36
Pauls, J.L., 35
Personal protective equipment, 39-49, 91-120. *See also:*
    Lifeline(s)
      for climbing, 97-107
      providing, 80
Personal rescue systems, 118-20
Personnel nets, 90
Planning
    anchorage points, 132-38
    fall protection, 167-68
    safe roof work, 145
Portable

    anchorages, 102
    tripods, 112-13
Powered Platform Industry Standard, 1910.66, 11
"Puppy-dog" system, 111

-Q-

Quantitative risk appraisal, 77-79

-R-

Rail(s), 98-99
    System, horizontal, 109
Ramps, recommended angles for, 36
Rescue, 209
    from above ground level, 119
Restraint/positioning suspension, 52
Retrieval
    means of, 52
    or rescue, 156
Rigid rail carrier, 97, 99
Risk, 54-55
    appraising, 80
Roll-out, 95-96, 122-25
Roof(s)
    anchorages, 136-37, 147
    flat, 143-45
    openings, falling through, 142
    work, guide for, 142-46
Rope(s)
    cleaning synthetic, 128
    grab system, 148-51
    synthetic, shear of, 202-203
    used in temporary systems, 110

-S-

Saddle belt, 93
Safety
    analysis, of an elevated work task, 78
    errors, common, 79
    monitoring system, 142
    policy,
    responsibility for setting, 17
Safety net(s), 90-91
    extensions, 91
    safety rules for, 166
Scaffolds, 151-52
    guide for contractors who use suspended, 147-51
    safety rules for, 166-67
    standards addressing fall protection on, and elevat
      ed platforms, 148
The Scaffold Act of Montana, 7
Self-retracting lanyards, 99-100, 103
    locking, 106-107
    lowering, 107-11
Semi-permanent lifeline systems, 109

INDEX

Shock absorption, 38-39
Signage, 36
The Slip and Fall Handbook, 36
Slip and Fall Practice, 36
Slips, 34, 36-37
Snaphook(s), 95-96, 147, 150
    carabiner, 123
    locking, 123-25
    safety, considerations for, 96, 210
Society of Illuminating Engineers, 36
Stair steps, 36
Stairway falls, 35-36
Steel
    erection, safety rules for, 167
    fabrication suppliers, fall protection guidelines for, 20
    ladder use during erection of, 154
Steinberg, Harold, 116, 188
Stepladders, 153-55
Stockpickers, safety rules for, 167
Storage of synthetic materials, 128
The Structural Work Act of Illinois, 7
Subcontractors, fall protection guidelines for, 20
Sulowski, Andrew, 188
Swing falls, 122

-T-

Templer, J.A., 35
Temporary systems, 110-11
Tie-off techniques, outdated, 204
Training
    considerations, 209
    emergency escape, 118
    to meet OSHA safety regulations, 170-71, 208
Trips, 34-37
Tongue buckle, 93
Tripods, portable, 112-13
Two-dimensional travel, 54
Tying off, problems with, 25-26

-U-

Underwriters Laboratory
    Standard 1323, 160
    Standard 1523, 116
United Auto Workers Union (UAW), 55
U.S. Coast Guard requirements for offshore rig egress, 117
USS Wire Rope Engineering Handbook, 193, 195

-V-

Vertical
    cable systems, 98
    descent, 116-18
    lifelines, 108, 209
    rail systems, 98-99
    Rope Grab Lifeline Systems, 101-105

-W-

Walking and working surfaces
    1910.21-32 Subpart D, 11
    guidelines for, 53
Wang, Chen, 82, 188
Winches, use for confined space access, 157-63
Window cleaner(s), 145
    belt system for, 93
Wire rope, 110
Work positioning equipment, 138
    maintenance and inspection guide for, 127
Work tasks, classifying, 79
Workers' activities at elevation, fundamental groups of, 54
Workers' Compensation
    Data Base, 1985-1988, 4, 7
    and general liability premium rates for various industries, 22-23
    laws, 7

ABOUT THE AUTHOR

J. Nigel Ellis, Ph.D., CSP, P.E., is a leading authority in the field of industrial fall protection. He is chief executive officer of Research and Trading Corporation (RTC) of Wilmington, Delaware, producers of an extensive line of fall protection, controlled descent, and confined space entry rescue systems. He also is president of Dynamic Scientific Controls (DSC), a consulting firm which specializes in fall hazard control planning and training, and which provides courses in Fall Protection – Principles and Applications of Fall Hazard Control – at the DSC Training Center in Wilmington. Dr. Ellis also instructs in the Fall Arrest Systems course for the OSHA Training Institute. A registered Professional Engineer in Safety Engineering, he resides in Wilmington.

A Board Certified Safety Professional (CSP) in two specialties, Dr. Ellis is a professional member of the American Society of Safety Engineers and the National Safety Council on the Construction Section Executive Committee. His company is a member of the American National Standards Institute, Scaffold Industry Association, and the National Safety Council.

In addition, Dr. Ellis has helped develop Occupational Safety and Health Administration (OSHA) standards on fall protection and emergency descent. He was the only fall protection professional to testify before an OSHA hearing on fall protection standards in the oil and gas well drilling and servicing industry. He also testified at the OSHA Power Platform hearing for window cleaner fall protection in 1986, and similarly for construction in 1988 and for confined space in 1989.

Dr. Ellis is a member of the following ANSI, ASTM, and SAE committees:
ANSI Z359 Fall Protection Equipment
ANSI A10.14 Fall Protection Equipment in Construction
ANSI A14.3 Fixed Ladders
ASTM Steel Stack Access
SAE J185 Off-The-Road Vehicles -Access and Egress
ANSI A120 Building Exterior Maintenance
ANSI Z117.1 Confined Spaces
ISO TC94/SC4 International Fall Protection/ANSI Tag

He is a past chairman of the Fall Protection Group of the Industrial Safety Equipment Association.

Dr. Ellis has lectured and participated in panel discussions at seminars and conferences across the USA, and has authored many articles on fall protection, including the fall protection chapter of *Best's Safety Directory*, since 1973.

He entered the fall protection field in 1970, after coming to the USA from northern England in 1966. He received a Ph.D. in chemistry, as well as B.Sc. and M.Sc. degrees, from the University of Manchester.